BASIC MICROBIOLOGY
An Illustrated Laboratory Manual

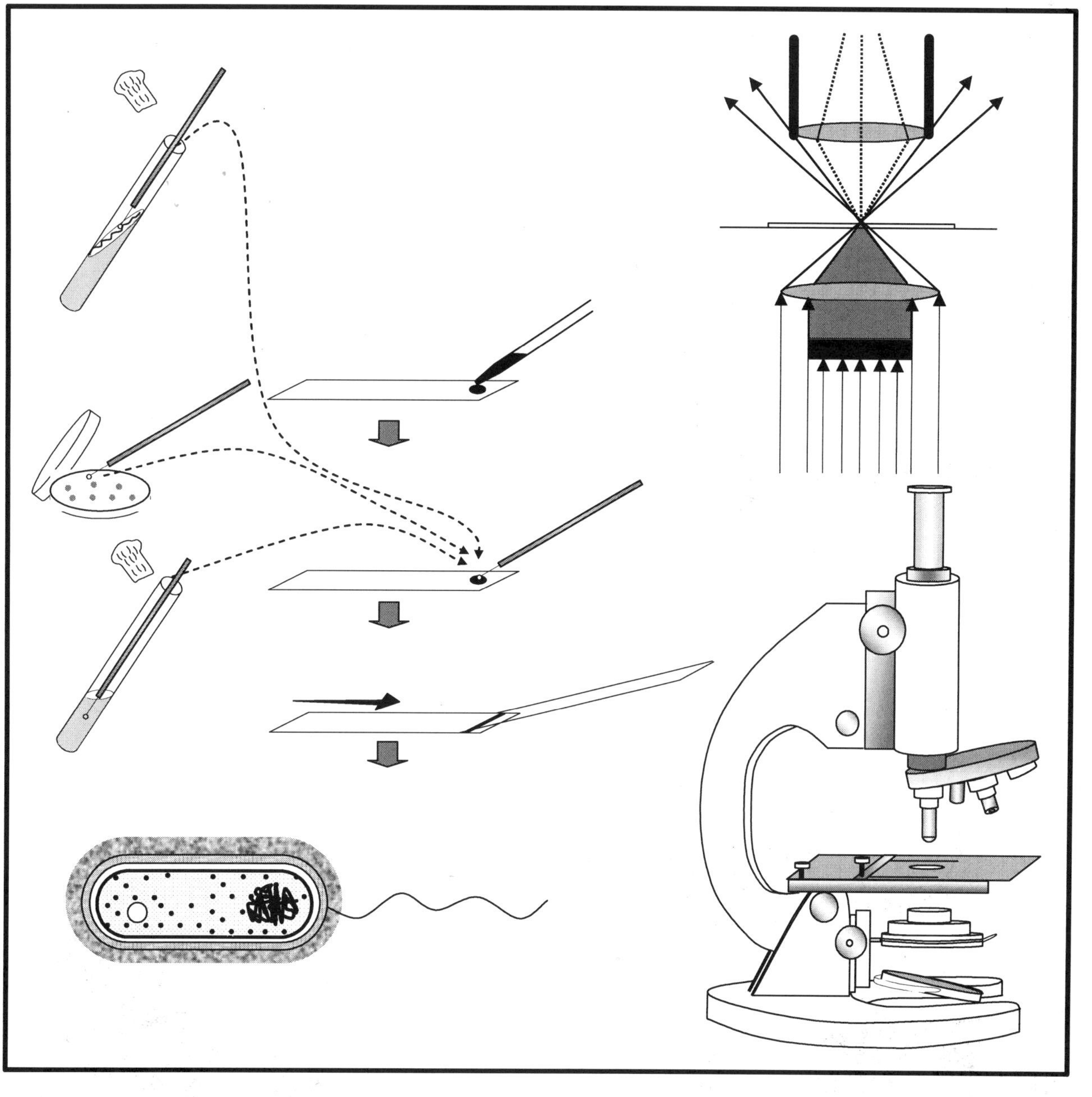

BASIC MICROBIOLOGY
An Illustrated Laboratory Manual

B. K. Khuntia
Associate Professor
College of Fisheries (OUAT)
Rangailunda, Berhampur - 760 007
Orissa

ASTRAL
Publishing Authors Across the Globe

2021

Daya Publishing House®

A Division of

Astral International Pvt. Ltd.

New Delhi - 110 002

First Published, 2011

ISBN 978-81-7035-682-0 (HB)

Published by : **Daya Publishing House®**
A Division of
Astral International Pvt. Ltd.
– ISO 9001:2015 Certified Company –
4736/23, Ansari Road, Darya Ganj
New Delhi-110 002
Ph. 011-43549197, 23278134
E-mail: info@astralint.com
Website: www.astralint.com

Digitally Printed at : **Replika Press Pvt. Ltd.**

To

My Father

SJ. JAYAKRISHNA KHUNTIA

&

Mother

SMT. TAAPOI KHUNTIA

Acknowledgement

I express my heartfelt thanks to Dr. (Mrs.) Indrani Karunasagar, Professor and Head, Department of Fishery Microbiology, College of Fisheries (KVAFSU), Mangalore, who taught me several courses and laid my foundation in the field of microbiology. I am grateful to Dr. S. K. Udgata, Associate Professor, Fishery Microbiology, College of Fisheries (OUAT), Rangailunda for thoroughly going through the whole manuscript and for his constant encouragement, valuable comments and constructive suggestions about the book. I am extremely thankful to my colleagues at College of Fisheries (OUAT), Rangailunda, who have extended their kind cooperation during writing of this book. Their critical suggestions have enabled me to upgrade the quality of the book.

I am indebted to my father Sj. Jayakrishna Khuntia and mother Smt. Taapoi Khuntia, whose generous blessings have enabled me to write the book. I owe a lot to my wife Sasmita, for her constant encouragement and deliberate support in bringing the book to the present form. I am thankful to my daughters Nilima and Banani for their patience and cooperation during writing of the book.

I am greatly obliged to Dr. S. Ayyappan, Director General, Indian Council of Agricultural Research, New Delhi for kindly writing a foreword to the book. I also extend my thanks to Daya Publishing House, New Delhi for publishing the book in such an excellent manner.

B. K. Khuntia

Foreword

Microorganisms are invisible living creatures, which have critical role in the maintenance of life on the earth. Some of them are extremely helpful and some others are deadly harmful. A thorough knowledge on these invisible living creatures will help in minimising their harmful effects and in harnessing their beneficial effects.

Microbiology, the science of microorganisms, had a subtle beginning in 1673 with the observation of small anilmalcules by Antoni van Leeuwenhoek under a crude microscope. Since then, a lot of advancement has been made in the techniques to study microorganisms. As they are invisible to naked eye, several techniques have been developed over the years to understand them and evaluate their importance. Moreover, many of the biological processes occurring in living systems could be understood through the study of microorganisms as simple models. Despite the fast advancement made in the field of microbiology, some of the basic techniques still remain vital in microbiological investigations. Though some of the techniques have been automated to reduce manpower requirement and to get faster results, the basic principles of the techniques have remained unchanged.

The book entitled, "Basic Microbiology : An Illustrated Laboratory Manual" authored by Dr. B. K. Khuntia, Associate Professor, College of Fisheries (Orissa University of Agriculture and Technology), Rangailunda, Berhampur, Orissa, contains most of the techniques required for the beginners, who enter into the field of microbiology and allied sciences. The step-wise description of the techniques along with the magnificent illustrations has brought the manual to a unique status. The concise description about the different microorganisms like bacteria, viruses, protozoa, microscopic fungi and microscopic algae will definitely give the users a background knowledge before starting their experiments in the respective fields.

The efforts made by Dr. Khuntia in preparing such an exhaustive and illustrated manual is praiseworthy. The manual will be of great use for students, teachers, researchers , laboratory personnel and all those involved in different branches of microbiology, pathology, food technology, biotechnology, molecular biology, environmental sciences, agriculture, diary science and fisheries.

S. Ayyappan
Director General
Indian Council of Agricultural Research
New Delhi

Preface

Microbiology is gaining much impetus in the present era, as the strides in science and technology are revealing the increasing importance of microbes on the quality of life on the earth. This book "Basic Microbiology: An Illustrated Laboratory Manual" is meant for the beginners who enter into the field of microbiology with some background knowledge in biology. All attempts have been made to make the text very clear and comprehensive through a number of illustrations. The manual covers most of the experiments that are required for the students entering into the field of microbiology. Looking at the abundant knowledge, which has been gathered in microbiology, it can be said that this manual is only an introductory aid in the field of microbiology.

The manual has 11 chapters with 55 experiments. The first chapter, 'Introduction' introduces the students into the world of microbes delineating their importance and branches of microbiology. A comprehensive account of bacteria, which is a prerequisite for most of the experiments has been given in the second chapter, 'Bacteria'. The third chapter, 'Microbiology laboratory' describes the infrastructures, equipments, glasswares, hardwares, chemicals and media required for a microbiology laboratory. The fourth chapter, 'Microscopes' completely covers the principles and operation of various types of microscopes. The various techniques used for the observation of microbes under microscopes have been described in the fifth chapter, 'Microscopic techniques'. The sixth chapter, 'Cultivation of bacteria' deals with the growing of bacteria in culture media, isolation of different species of bacteria and enumeration of bacteria in different samples. The seventh chapter, 'Biochemical tests of bacteria' describes the biochemical activities of different bacteria, which are helpful in their identification. The eighth chapter, 'Cultivation of viruses' deals with the growing of viruses in the laboratory and their enumeration. The procedure for the identification of free-living and parasitic protozoa has been delineated in the ninth chapter, 'Identification of protozoa'. The tenth chapter, 'Identification of microscopic fungi' describes the techniques of cultivating microscopic fungi and their identification. The eleventh chapter, 'Identification of microscopic algae' gives the identifying characteristics of few microscopic algae of general importance.

It is hoped that the manual will be of immense use for teachers, scientists, students and other laboratory personnel. For the beginners, who enter into the field of microbiology, the manual may serve as the door to the vast empire of microbiology. It will be instrumental for their diversification into several branches of microbiology like medical microbiology, industrial microbiology, food microbiology, agriculture microbiology, veterinary microbiology, fishery microbiology as well as other advanced branches of science like biotechnology and molecular biology.

B. K. Khuntia

E-mail: basantak@yahoo.com

Contents

List of Figures

List of Tables

1

Introduction

A. What are Microorganisms ?

Microorganisms (*Gk: micros:* small; *organismos*: organisms) or microbes are living forms, whose size is so small that they are usually not visible to naked human eye.

B. Types of Microorganisms

Microorganisms include bacteria, viruses, protozoa, microscopic fungi and algae. They are defined as follows.

1. **Bacteria**: They are prokaryotic, unicellular microorganisms, which lack chlorophyll[1] pigments.
2. **Viruses**: Viruses are ultra-microscopic, non-cellular living particles, composed solely of a nucleic acid (DNA or RNA) core, surrounded by a protein envelope called capsid.
3. **Protozoa**: They are eukaryotic, unicellular microorganisms, which lack cell wall.
4. **Microscopic fungi**: They are eukaryotic, heterotrophic microorganisms that fail to show any cellular differentiation into true tissues like root, stem or leaf and in which vascular system is absent.
5. **Microscopic algae**: They are eukaryotic, autotrophic microorganisms that fail to show any cellular differentiation into true tissues like root, stem or leaf and in which vascular system is absent.

C. Importance of Microorganisms

Microorganisms are present in almost all places on the earth. Despite their minute size, they have tremendous importance in the maintenance of life on the earth. Due to the difference in the activities of different microbes, they influence life in different ways. Some of them are very helpful, for example, those which fix atmospheric nitrogen into biologically useful forms, those which help in curd formation, those which recycle dead materials by degrading them into simpler substances and those which help in preparation of wine (Figure 1.1). Some other microbes are very harmful in that they cause diseases in plants and animals, spoil food or raw materials of food kept in normal conditions as well as they degrade rubber, paints, textiles, metals and even insulations on electric wires. Therefore, it is essential

1 The photosynthetic bacteria carry out photosynthesis by their bacteriochlorophyll pigments, which are different from true chlorophyll pigments in their chemical structure. Blue green algae, which belong to the Class Cyanophyceae are prokaryotic for which many consider them to be bacteria and group them as Cyanobacteria. However, they are actually not bacteria, as they contain true chlorophyll pigments.

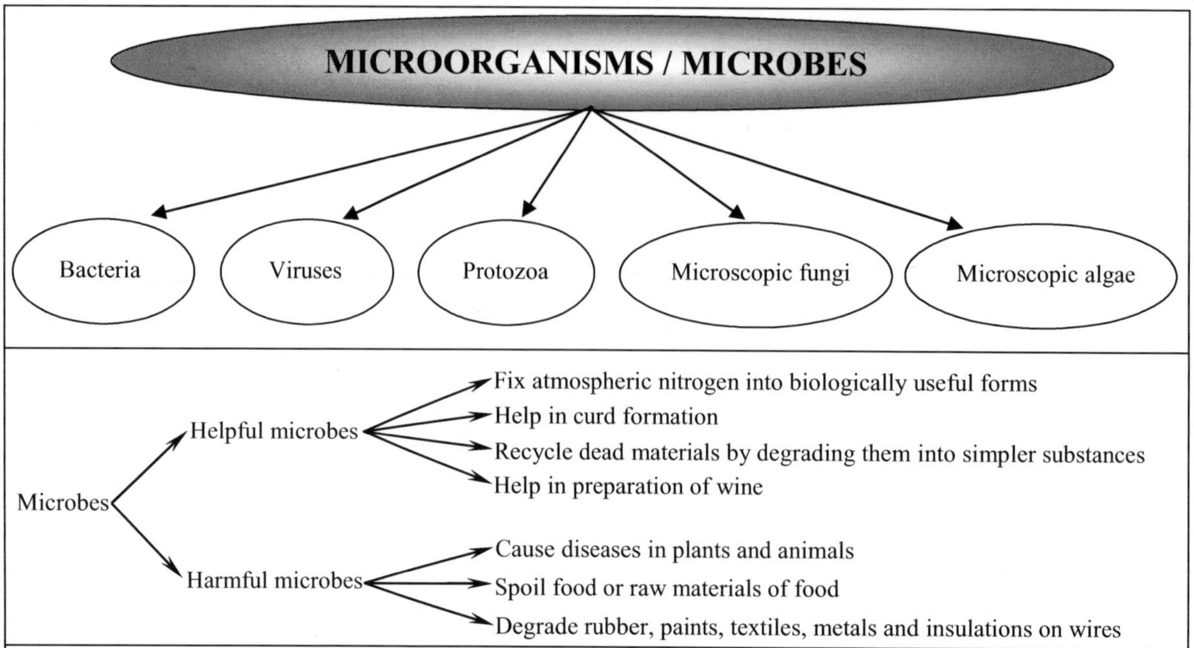

Figure 1.1: Microbes: Helpful and harmful

to study these microbes in details, so that by various techniques their harmful effects can be overcome and beneficial effects be utilised for enhancing quality of life on the earth.

D. What is Microbiology ?

The discipline of science, which deals with the study of microorganisms, is known as 'microbiology'. It has different branches as follows.

1. *Bacteriology* : Study of bacteria
2. *Virology* : Study of viruses
3. *Protozoology* : Study of protozoa
4. *Mycology* : Study of fungi
5. *Phycology* or *Algology* : Study of algae

2

Bacteria

A. Definition

Bacteria are prokaryotic, unicellular microorganisms, which lack chlorophyll pigments.

B. Size of Bacteria

The average diameter of spherical bacteria is 0.5-2.0μ (Figure 2.1). For rod-shaped or filamentous bacteria, length is 1-10μ and diameter is 0.25-1.0μ. One group of bacteria, called the Mycoplasmas, have individuals with size much smaller than these dimensions. They measure about 0.25 μ and are the smallest cells known so far. They were formerly known as pleuropneumonia-like organisms (PPLO). Viruses are still smaller, but as they are particles rather than cells, Mycoplasmas are considered to be the smallest cells known. Examples: *Mycoplasma laidlawii* and *M. gallisepticum.*

C. Shape and Arrangement of Bacteria

1. Spherical Bacteria

Bacteria, which are spherical or ovoid in shape, are called 'coccus' (plural: cocci) (Figure 2.2). Based on the arrangement of the cells they are of the following types.

(*a*) *Coccus*: The spherical bacteria cells, called cocci, are present as single individuals.

(*b*) *Diplococcus*: The cocci are arranged in pairs.

(*c*) *Streptococcus*: The cocci are arranged in chains, as the cells divide in one plane.

(*d*) *Tetrads*: The cocci are arranged in packets of four cells, as the cells divide in two plains.

(*e*) *Staphylococcus*: The cocci are arranged in grape-like clusters formed by irregular cell divisions in three plains.

(*f*) *Sarcinae (Octet):* The cocci are arranged in a cuboidal manner, as the cells are formed by regular cell divisions in three planes.

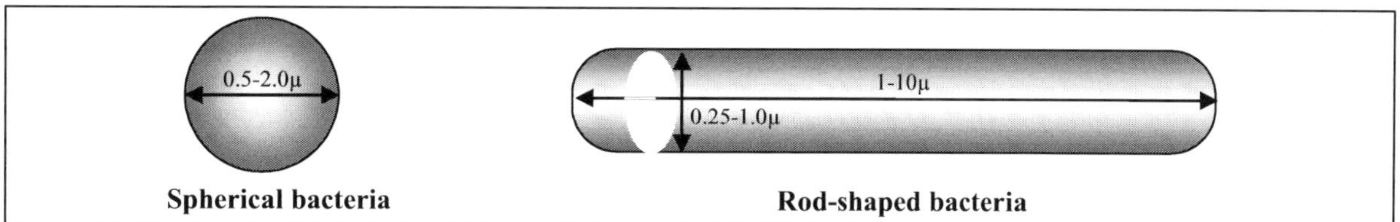

Figure 2.1: Size of bacteria

2. Rod-shaped Bacteria

The cylindrical or rod-shaped bacteria are called 'bacillus' (plural: bacilli). They are of three shapes as follows.

(*a*) *Bacillus:* They are rod-shaped bacteria. Based on arrangement they are of the following types.

(*i*) *Bacillus:* The rod-shaped bacteria cells, called bacilli, are present as single individuals.

(*ii*) *Diplobacillus:* The bacilli are arranged in pairs.

(*iii*) *Streptobacillus:* The bacilli are arranged in chains, as the cells divide in one plane.

(*iv*) *Trichomes:* The bacilli are arranged in chains with larger area of end-to-end contact between the cells.

(*v*) *Palisades:* The bacilli bend at the points of division following the cell divisions, resulting in a palisade arrangement resembling a picket fence and angular patterns that look like Chinese letters.

(*b*) *Coccobacillus:* These are so short and stumpy that they appear ovoid. They look like coccus and bacillus.

(*c*) *Vibrios:* They are comma-shaped bacteria with less than one complete turn or twist in the cell.

3. Spiral Bacteria

Unlike the vibrios, which have less than one complete turn or twist in the cell, the spiral bacteria are rod-shaped bacteria, which have more than one twist in the cell. They usually occur singly. They are of two types as follows:

(*a*) *Spirillum:* They have rigid spiral structure. Spirillum with many turns can superficially resemble spirochetes. They do not have outer sheath and endoflagella, but have typical bacterial flagella.

(*b*) *Spirochetes:* They are flexible and can twist and contort their shape. They have outer sheath and endoflagella, but lack typical bacterial flagella.

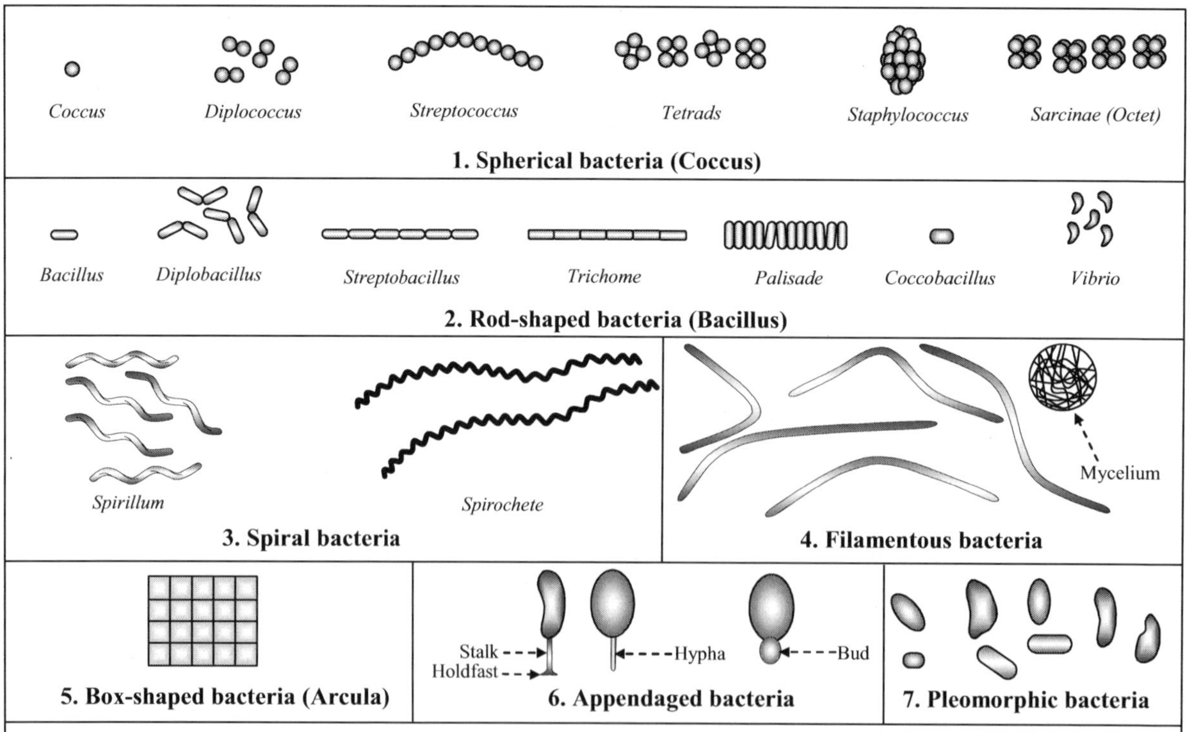

Figure 2.2: Shape and arrangement of bacteria

4. Filamentous Bacteria

They are very long thin filament-shaped bacteria. Some of them form branching filaments resulting in a network of filaments called 'mycelium'.

5. Box-shaped or Square-shaped Bacteria (Arcula)

They are flat, box-shaped bacteria with perfectly straight edges and sharp 90° angles at the corners. Smaller cells are usually perfectly squares (2X2µ), while larger cells are rectangular; about twice as long as they are wide (4X2µ). Each bacterium is a thin flexible sheet with smooth surface. After cell divisions, the cells remain attached to each other, producing large sheets of squares. It was first discovered in 1980 in natural salt ponds.

6. Appendaged Bacteria

They possess extension of their cells, as long tubes in the form of stalk or hypha, or as buds.

7. Pleomorphic Bacteria

These bacteria do not have any characteristic shape unlike all others described above. They can change their shape. In pure cultures, they can be observed to have different shapes.

D. Structure of Bacteria

The different parts of a generalised bacteria cell have been shown in Figure 2.3 and have been described as follows.

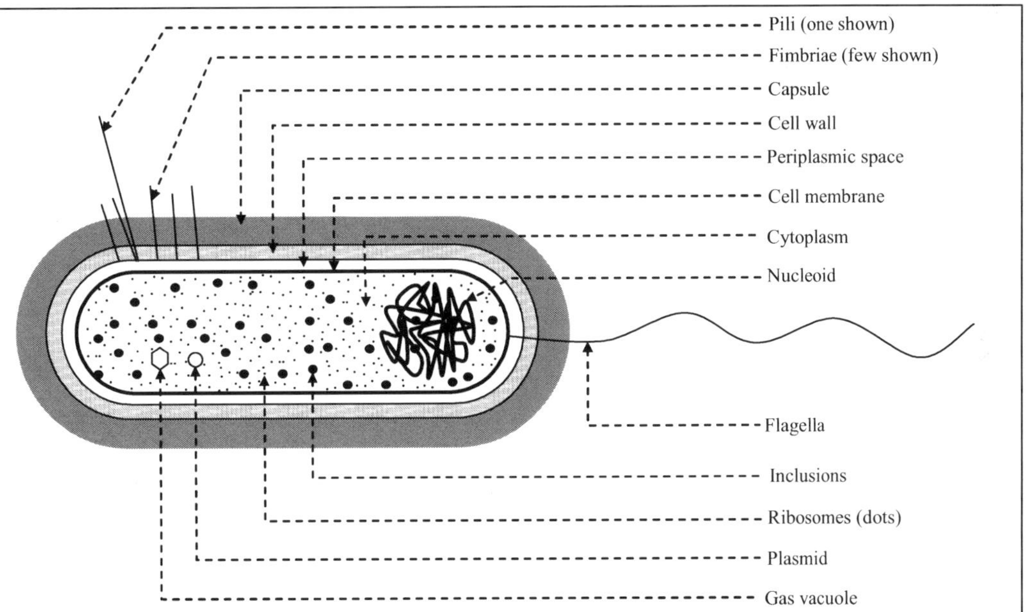

Figure 2.3: Structure of a generalised bacteria cell

1. Flagella

Bacterial flagella are thin filamentous hair-like helical appendages that protrude through the cell wall and are responsible for the motility of bacteria. Most of the motile bacteria possess flagella. Its length is about 10-15µ. Bacterial flagella are totally different from eukaryotic flagella in structure and mechanism of action. They are much thinner than the flagella or cilia of eukaryotic cells. No cell membrane is present over the bacterial flagella unlike in eukaryotic flagella. Moreover, bacterial flagella, unlike eukaryotic flagella, are somewhat rigid and do not whip back and forth, rather they spin much like the propeller of a boat for the movement of the cell. The bacterial flagella have three parts namely; (a) Basal Body, (b) Hook and (c) Filament (Figure 2.4).

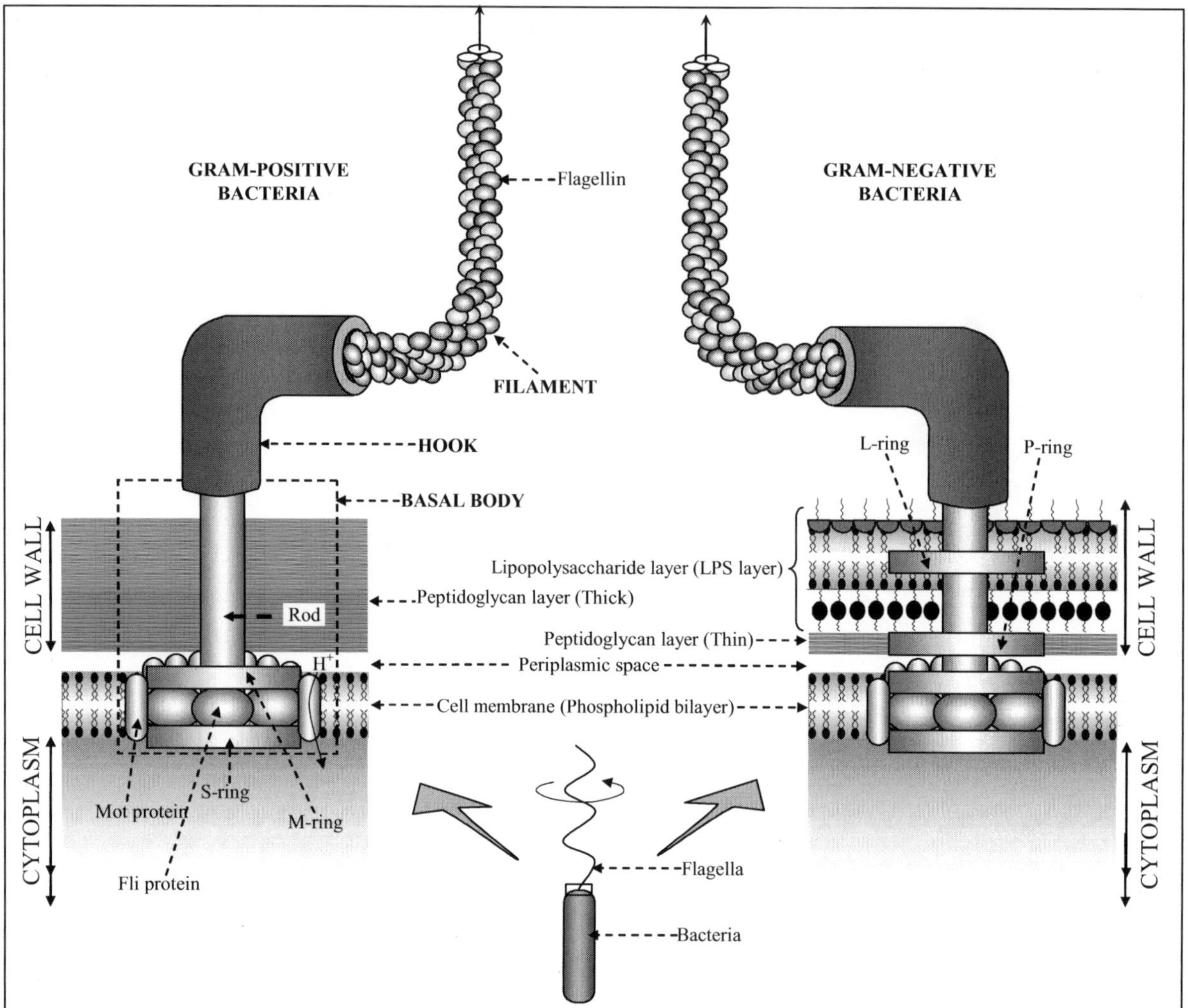

Figure 2.4: Structure of flagella of gram-positive and gram-negative bacteria

(*a*) Basal Body

It forms the base part of the flagellum and is anchored in the cytoplasmic membrane and cell wall. It provides anchorage to the flagella as well as functions as a motor, thereby imparting the rotary motion of the flagellum. It consists of a small central rod that passes through a system of rings. In case of gram-positive bacteria, in which the cell wall consists of a peptidoglycan layer alone, the basal body has only one pair of rings; the M-ring and the S-ring, both embedded in the cell membrane. Surrounding these rings are a group proteins called mot proteins. Proton movement across the cell membrane through these mot proteins produces the proton motive force (energy) required for the rotation of these two rings, which ultimately act as the motor for the propeller-like rotation of the flagellum. Another group of proteins, called fli proteins, is present sandwiched between these two rings. They function as motor switch, reversing the rotation of the flagellum in response to intracellular signals. In case of gram-negative bacteria, in which the cell wall consists of an outer lipopolysaccharide (LPS) layer in addition to the thinner inner peptidoglycan layer, the basal body has one more pair of rings; the L-ring embedded in the LPS layer and the P-ring in the thin peptidoglycan layer.

(*b*) Hook

A short hook connects the basal body to the filament of the flagellum. It is slightly thicker than the filament. The motor action of the basal body is transmitted to the filament through the hook.

(*c*) Filament

It is the long hair-like filamentous portion of the flagellum, which emerges from the hook. It is several times longer than the bacteria cell. It is made of a single type of protein, 'flagellin' whose molecular weight is about 40,000. Flagellin molecules form chains; three such chains inter-twine to form the flagellum. Unlike a hair, which grows at its base, the filament of a flagellum grows at its tip. Amino acids pass along the hollow center of the filament and add to its distal end. This process is called self-assembly, as all the information for the final structure of the filament resides in the protein subunits themselves. The filament is somewhat rigid and do not whip back and forth, rather it spins much like the propeller of a boat for the movement of the cell.

The spirochetes lack external flagella. However, they move with the help of a flagella-like structure located within their cells just beneath the outer envelope. These are called periplasmic flagella, axial flagella, axial fibrils or endoflagella.

Flagella are arranged in different ways in different bacteria. The arrangement of flagella on bacteria cells is called flagellation. Flagellation is of the following four types (Figure 2.5).

(*a*) *Monotrichous flagellation* (*Mono*: single; *trichous*: hair): A single flagellum is present at one end of the cell.

(*b*) *Lophotrichous flagellation* (*Lopho*: tuft; *trichous*: hair): A tuft or cluster of flagella is present at one end of the cell.

(*c*) *Amphitrichous flagellation* (*Amphi*: both; *trichous*: hair): Flagella are present at both the ends of the cell either singly or in tuft.

(*d*) *Peritrichous flagellation* (*Peri*: around; *trichous*: hair): Flagella are present throughout the surface of the cell.

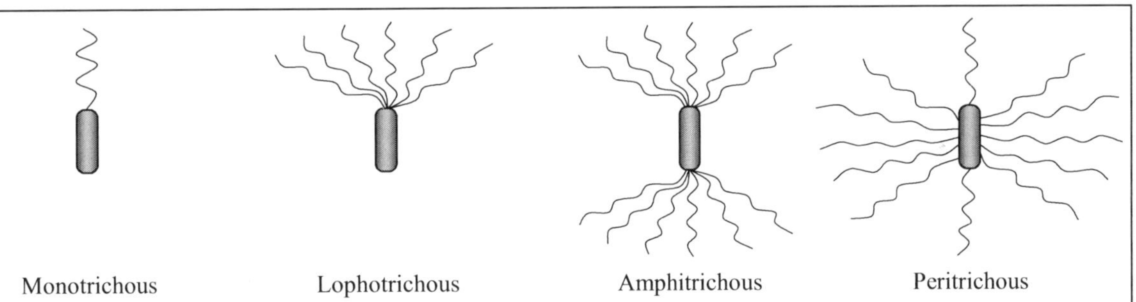

Figure 2.5: Types of flagellation

2. Fimbriae

Fimbriae are thin filamentous hair-like appendages, which are structurally similar to flagella, but are not involved in the motility of bacteria (Figure 2.3). Unlike flagella, they are considerably shorter and more numerous, but like flagella, they are made of protein molecules. Fimbriae are present in few species of bacteria, which help them to attach to the cells of other organisms and prevent them from being washed away by the flow of mucous or body fluid. Thus, it particularly helps the pathogenic bacteria to establish infection in the host body. They also help to form pellicles or biofilms on surfaces.

3. Pili

Pili are thin filamentous hair-like appendages, which are structurally similar to flagella, but are not involved in the motility of bacteria (Figure 2.6). They are also structurally similar to fimbriae, but are generally longer and only one or a few pili are present on the surface of a bacteria cell. It is made of a single type of protein, 'pilin', whose molecular weight is about 17,000. Pilin molecules are arranged helically to form a single rigid filament with a central hollow core. In some bacteria, genetic material is

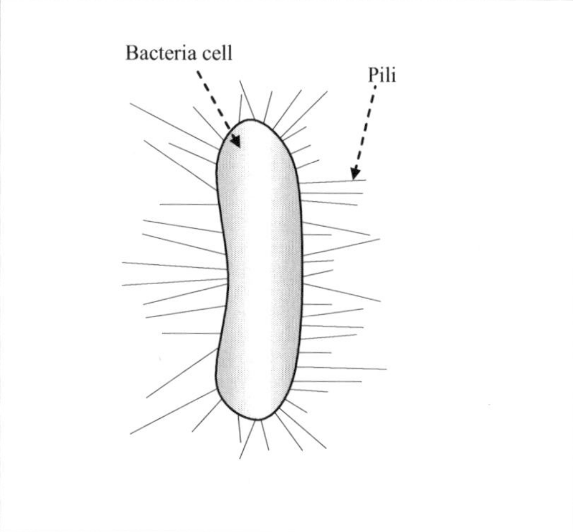

Figure 2.6: Electron microscopic view of pili

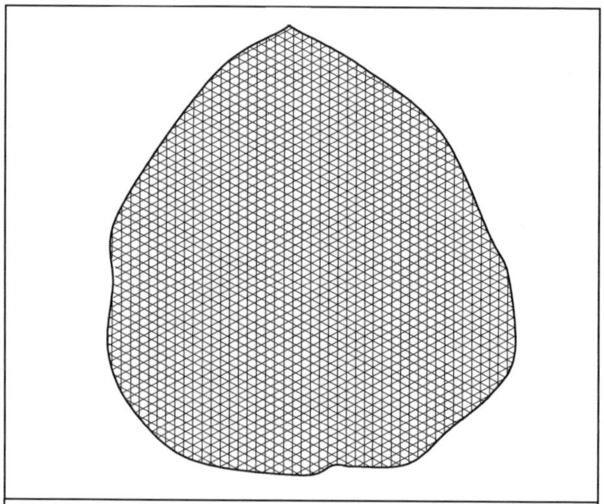

Figure 2.7: Electron microscopic view of S-layer

transferred through the hollow core of pili during conjugation (mating with another bacteria). Such pili are called fertility pili (F pili) or sex pili. In some pathogenic bacteria, pili act similar to fimbriae in attachment to the host cells and establishment of infection. The agglutinating action of pili results in the formation of films of bacteria that are visible on the surface of broth cultures.

4. S-Layer

S-layer (surface layer) is a layer found on the surface of most of the pathogenic bacteria, which is composed of a two-dimensional array of proteins with crystalline appearance in various symmetries, such as hexagonal, tetragonal or trimeric (Figure 2.7). The crystalline symmetry depends upon the composition of the proteins of the S-layer. It is associated with the cell wall structure (with the peptidoglycan layer in gram-positive bacteria and with the LPS layer in gram-negative bacteria). It functions as an external permeability barrier, allowing the passage of low molecular weight substances and excluding high molecular weight substances. It also provides protection to the pathogenic bacteria, against the host defense mechanism.

5. Capsule (slime layer or glycocalyx)

Many bacteria have a viscous slimy or gummy material outside the cell, surrounding the cell wall (Figure 2.8). It is made of macromolecules, which are not covalently attached to the bacteria. These surface macromolecules are mainly charged polysaccharides (glycoproteins or glycolipids) and are therefore called 'glycocalyx' (*glyco*: carbohydrates; *calyx*: part of flower below the petals extending outward from the stalk). Glycocalyx is defined as the polysaccharide-containing material lying outside the cell as a loose network of polymer fibers extending outward from the cell. They are synthesised and secreted by the bacteria, which bind to the receptors on the surface of the host tissues. Glycocalyx is not only found surrounding some bacteria cells; it is also found surrounding some plant and animal cells. Glycocalyx can be of three types as follows.

(*a*) Capsule

It is a polymer coat consisting of a dense, well-defined viscous layer closely surrounding the bacteria cells in many species. The viscous layer can be visualised by light microscopy using a special staining technique. The glycocalyx polymer fibers are organised in a tight matrix that excludes particles such as indian ink. Bacteria, which have capsule, are called capsulated bacteria, while those, which do not have capsule, are called non-capsulated bacteria.

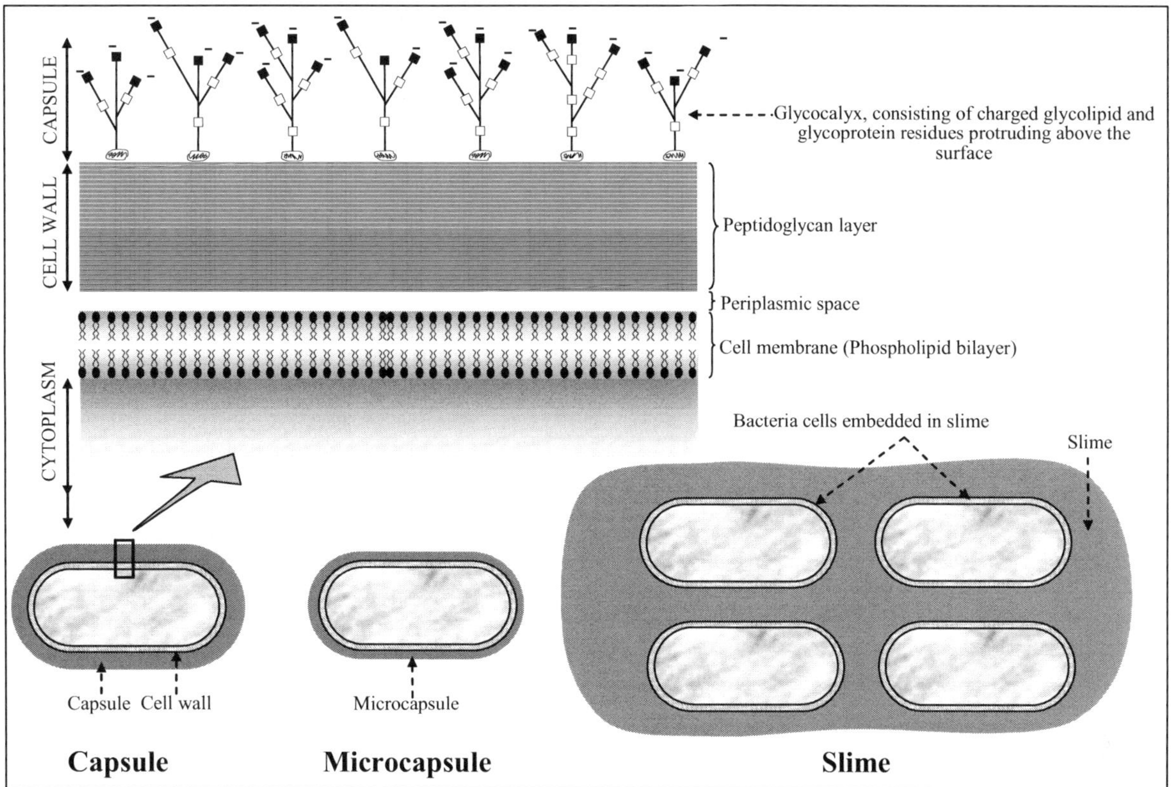

Figure 2.8: Capsule of bacteria

(*b*) Microcapsule

It is a viscous layer surrounding the bacteria cells, which is so thin that, it cannot be visualised by light microscopy.

(*c*) Slime

It is a diffuse mass of polymer fibers seemingly unattached to any single cell. The viscous layer is so thick that many cells are embedded in the slime matrix. The layer is easily deformed and do not exclude particles. It is difficult to be visualised by light microscopy.

The functions of capsule and slime are given below.

1. It prevents drying of cells, by binding water molecules.
2. It prevents attachment of bacteriophages (the viruses, which attack bacteria) onto the bacteria cells.
3. It provides virulence (the disease-producing ability) by inhibiting their recognition and subsequent destruction by phagocytes (white blood corpuscles or WBC).
4. It helps the pathogenic bacteria for its attachment to receptors on the surface of the host tissues to be infected.
5. It provides adherence between different bacteria cells.

6. Sheaths

Sheaths are long hollow tubular structures, which enclose chains of bacteria cells forming 'trichomes' (Figure 2.9). Sheathed bacteria are common in freshwater habitats that are rich in organic matter, such as polluted streams, trickling filters and activated sludge digestors in sewage

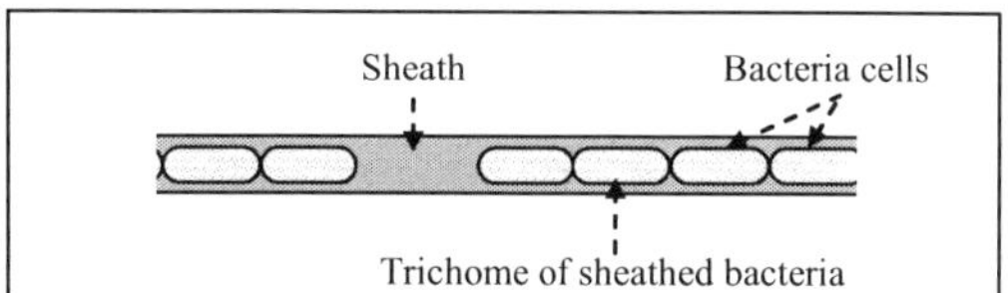

Figure 2.9: Sheath of bacteria

treatment plants. Sheaths can be easily visualised, when some of the cells, called 'the flagellated swarmer cells' of the trichome move out of the sheath leaving behind the empty sheath.

7. Prosthecae

Prosthecae are cytoplasmic extensions from bacteria cells, which form appendages like hypha, stalk or bud (Figure 2.2). They are smaller in diameter than the mature cells, contain cytoplasm and are bounded by cell wall. Bacteria having prosthecae are called prosthecate bacteria. Unlike the cell division in other bacteria, which takes place through binary fission producing two equivalent daughter bacteria cells, that in the prosthecates involves formation of a new daughter cell with the mother cell retaining its identity after the cell division is completed.

'Hyphae' are cellular appendages formed by direct cellular extension of the mother cell containing cell wall, cell membrane, ribosomes and occasionally DNA. It is formed by the lengthening of a small outgrowth of the bacteria cell at a single point. Such growth at a single point is called 'polar growth' in contrast to the 'intercalary growth' taking place in all other bacteria, in which growth of bacteria takes place throughout the surface. At the end of hypha, a bud is formed, which enlarges and produces a flagellum. The DNA in the mother cell replicates and a copy of the circular DNA is moved down the length of the hypha into the bud. A cross septum then forms separating the still developing bud from the hypha and mother cell. Now, the bud breaks from the mother cell and swims away as a daughter cell. Later the daughter cell loses its flagellum and gradually grows to become a mother cell ready for formation of hyphae and bud.

'Stalks' are cellular appendages used by certain aquatic bacteria for attachment to solid substratum. At the end of the stalk there is a structure called 'holdfast', by which the stalk is attached to the substratum. Besides providing attachment, stalk also increases the surface area of bacteria cell, which helps it in nutrient absorption and removal of wastes. In some bacteria, the stalks of several individuals remain attached to form 'rosettes'. Cell division in stalked bacteria occurs by the elongation of cell in the direction opposite to the direction of the stalk followed by fission. A single flagellum is formed at the pole opposite the stalk. The flagellated daughter cell so formed is called a 'swarmer'. It separates from the non-flagellated mother cell, swims around and attaches to a new surface forming a new stalk at the flagellated pole. The flagellum is then lost.

'Buds' are cellular appendages, which directly develop as daughter cells from the mother cells without the intervening formation of hyphae.

8. Cell Wall

Cell wall is the rigid structure that immediately surrounds the cell membrane of bacteria cells. The cell membrane of bacteria cells is a phospholipid bilayer similar to that of all other animal and plant cells (Figure 2.11). While animal cells lack cell wall, plant cells and bacteria cells have cell wall surrounding the cell membrane. However, unlike the cell wall of plant cells, which is composed mainly of cellulose, the cell wall of bacteria cells is composed mainly of peptidoglycan layers (Figure 2.10). Earlier, peptidoglycan was also called murein or mucopeptide. Peptidoglycan consists mainly of amino acids and sugars (*peptido*: chain of amino acids; *glycan*: sugar). Two sugars namely N-acetylglucosamine (NAGA) and N-acetylmuramic acid (NAMA) are bonded to each other alternately through glycosidic bonds (β-1-4 linkage) to form long parallel sugar chains. Attached to the NAMA molecules are short side chains of four or five amino acids bonded to each other through peptide bonds. Usually the amino acids are alanine, glutamic acid and either lysine or diaminopimelic acid (DAP). These short peptides form cross-linkages between adjacent sugar chains to form a network or layer. Though the glycosidic bonds in the sugar chains are very strong, these alone cannot provide rigidity in all directions. High rigidity is obtained, only when these chains are cross-linked by the peptide bonds in the cross-linking short peptides.

The composition of cell wall is not same for all the bacteria; rather there exist remarkable differences in its composition, based on which bacteria have been grouped as given below.

A. Based on Gram Staining

Based on the differences in the composition of cell wall, a special staining technique called 'gram staining', named after Dr. Christian Gram who developed it (*See* page 93-97), differentiates bacteria into two groups as follows.

(1) *Gram-positive Bacteria*

After staining a bacteria with crystal violet, if its cell wall resists decolourisation by washing with a decolourising agent (ethanol or acetone), it is a gram-positive bacteria. Examples: *Bacillus, Staphylococcus.*

(2) *Gram-negative Bacteria*

After staining a bacteria with crystal violet, if its cell wall allows to undergo decolourisation by washing with a decolourising agent (ethanol or acetone), it is a gram-negative bacteria. Examples: *Escherichia, Salmonella, Vibrio.*

Differentiation of bacteria into gram-positive and gram-negative groups provides the most important clue for proceeding further in proper direction for the identification of unknown bacteria.

Gram-Positive Cell Wall

The gram-positive cell wall is very simple. It is mainly made of a thick layer of peptidoglycan, which constitutes about 90% of the cell wall. This thick layer makes the gram-positive bacteria resistant to osmotic lysis. The wall may also contain teichoic acid, lipoteichoic acid and M protein, which are the major surface antigens of gram-positive cell wall. The teichoic acid is negatively charged and is partially responsible for the negative charge of the cell surface of bacteria. It also helps in the passage of ions through the cell wall. The lipoteichoic acid is teichoic acid, which is bound to the membrane lipids. The M protein helps some bacteria in causing diseases by preventing their engulfment by WBC. The antibiotics, penicillin (produced by the fungus, *Penicillium notatum*) and cephalosporin kill gram-positive bacteria by preventing peptidoglycan synthesis. Lysozyme (an enzyme found in tear, saliva, egg albumin and slime of fish) kills gram-positive bacteria by breaking the glycosidic bond (β-1-4 linkage) between NAGA and NAMA.

Gram-Negative Cell Wall

The gram-negative cell wall is very complex and more fragile than gram-positive cell wall. It has a thin layer of peptidoglycan, which constitutes only about 10% of the cell wall. It is surrounded by a thick protective coating called lipopolysaccharide (LPS) layer, which resists penetration of some potentially toxic chemicals into the bacteria cell. The LPS layer consists of 1) a lipoprotein layer and 2) an outer membrane. One surface of the lipoprotein layer is directly attached to the peptidoglycan layer and the other surface extends into the outer membrane. It functions as an anchor between the peptidoglycan layer and the outer membrane. The outer membrane is a protein-embedded phospholipid bilayer with 'unit membrane' structure similar to the cell membrane. The inner leaf of the outer membrane is a layer of phospholipid molecules alone. However, unlike the unit membrane, some of the phospholipid molecules in the outer leaf are replaced by LPS molecules. Each LPS molecule is made of a lipid portion called 'lipid A' covalently linked to a hair-like polysaccharide. When gram-negative pathogenic bacteria is killed inside the host's body, the lipid A, which is an internal component of gram-negative bacteria, is released, eliciting toxic reactions and disease symptoms. That is why, lipid A is also called 'endotoxin' (*endo*: internal). In contrast, 'exotoxin' is the toxic substance synthesised inside the bacteria cells and released to outside, which causes disease, if present in or enters into the host's body. Unlike other normal lipids like triglycerides, which are made of three fatty acids bonded to a glycerol, lipid A is made of fatty acids bonded to a disaccharide composed of two NAGA phosphates. The fatty acids in lipid A are commonly caproic, lauric, myristic, palmitic and stearic acids. The polysaccharide, which is bonded to lipid A at the other end of the disaccharide, is made of two portions; 1) the inner core polysaccharide and 2) the outer O-polysaccharide. The outer membrane also contains proteins called 'porins', which contain three identical subunits. Each subunit is cylindrical with a central pore, through which materials can pass. Thus, the porins make the outer membrane relatively permeable. Porins are of two types; 1) non-specific porins, which form water-filled channels for small substances of any type to pass through and 2) specific porins, which have specific binding sites for specific substances to pass through. Several materials (solutions, syringes, needles etc.), though are made free from pathogenic microbes by heat sterilisation, still retain the residual debris of the cell wall of gram-negative bacteria produced by killing them. If introduced into host body, this cell wall debris can induce disease symptoms. This broken cell wall debris, which can induce disease symptoms is called 'pyrogen'.

B. Based on Acid-fast Staining

Based on the differences in the composition of the cell wall, another special staining technique called 'acid-fast staining' (*See* page 97-100) differentiates bacteria into two groups as follows.

(1) *Acid-fast Bacteria*

A bacteria, which is extremely difficult to be stained, but once stained, it is equally difficult to remove the stain out of its cells, even with vigorous use of acid-alcohol as decolourising agent, is an acid-fast bacteria (acid-loving bacteria). Examples: *Mycobacterium* spp. [*M. tuberculosis* (TB bacteria), *M. leprae* (leprosy bacteria), *M. smegmatis* (natural bacteria of smegma), *M. marinum* (TB bacteria of marine fishes)]. They possess a thick waxy cell wall made of lipid materials.

(2) *Non-acid-fast Bacteria*

A bacteria, which is easy to be stained and is also easy to be decolourised by acid-alcohol as decolourising agent, is a non-acid-fast bacteria (non-acid-loving bacteria). Examples: All other bacteria except *Mycobacterium* spp. In these bacteria, the cell wall is not thick waxy.

Differentiation of bacteria into acid-fast and non-acid-fast groups provides the most important clue for the identification of *Mycobacterium* spp.

Wall-deficient Variants

Some bacteria naturally exist without cell wall. *Mycoplasma*, which is the smallest bacteria has no cell wall. It is protected from osmotic lysis by the presence of sterols in the cell membrane and by adopting a parasitic existence in osmotically favourable environment of eukaryotic hosts. Similarly, some marine bacteria lack cell wall, in which the osmotic lysis is prevented by the high salt concentration of seawater. Most of the gram-positive bacteria lose their cell wall (peptidoglycan) in presence of lysozyme. However, their cells survive if they are present in an isotonic environment such as pus-filled wounds. These wall-deficient bacteria consisting of only protoplasm enclosed by cell membrane are called 'protoplast' or 'L-forms' (L for Lister Institute in London). Once lysozyme is removed, they may resume growth by synthesising their cell wall. If the protoplast retains pieces of cell wall, such that the cell takes amoeboid shape, protruding out where there is no cell wall, it is called 'spheroplast'. Spheroplast is also formed, when peptidoglycan of gram-negative cell wall is removed by treatment with lysozyme. Here, the protoplasm is enclosed by two layers, the cell membrane and the LPS layer.

Functions of Cell Wall

(a) Protection form Lysis

It protects the bacteria cells from osmotic lysis, as most of them remain in hypotonic environments. This is because, the concentration of dissolved solutes inside the bacteria cells is considerably higher than that in the environment. This develops a considerable turgor pressure inside the cells, which may be comparable to the pressure inside an automobile tire. The cell wall helps to withstand this pressure.

(b) Shape and Rigidity

It provides shape and rigidity to the bacteria cells.

9. Periplasmic Space

It is the thin space between the cell wall and the cell membrane (Figures 2.10 and 2.11). It is filled with plasma called periplasm. The periplasm contains several proteins, of which three are important. They are, 1) hydrolytic enzymes, which help in the initial degradation of food molecules of bacteria, 2) binding proteins, which begin the process of transporting substrates and 3) chemoreceptors, which are involved in the chemotaxis response of bacteria. Chemotaxis means movement towards or away from a chemical.

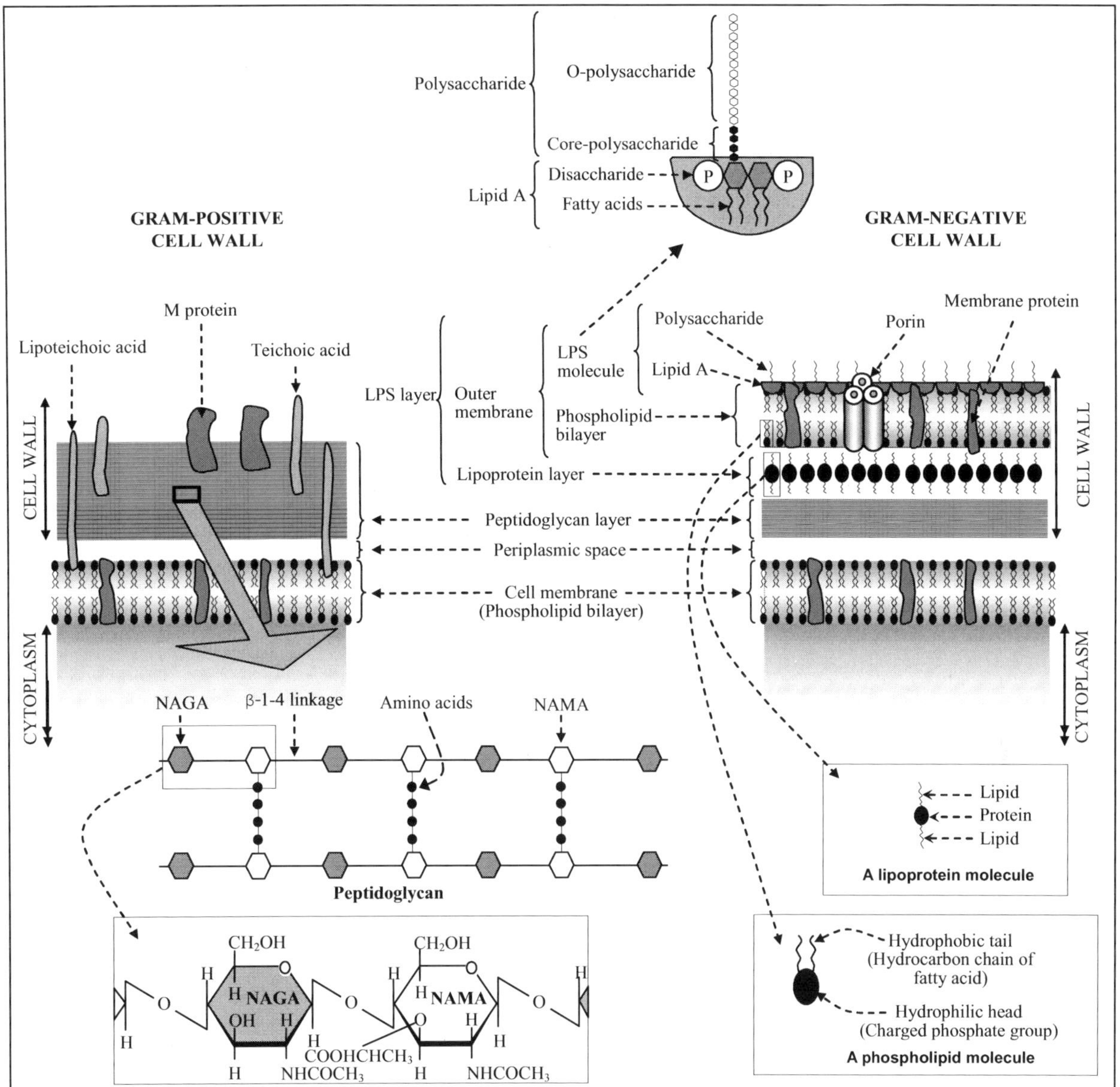

Figure 2.10: Structure of gram-positive and gram-negative cell wall

10. Cell Membrane

It is a thin membrane beneath the cell wall that completely encloses the protoplasm. It is also called 'cytoplasmic membrane' or 'plasma membrane'. It is a protein-embedded phospholipid bilayer (Figure 2.11). Two types of proteins are embedded in the bilayer. One type of proteins are tenaciously held in the bilayer and are called 'integral proteins'. The other type of proteins are loosely anchored on the surface of the bilayer and are called 'peripheral proteins'. The components of the membrane are not static; rather they are dynamic and are always in the state of motion like a 'fluid'. The proteins provide

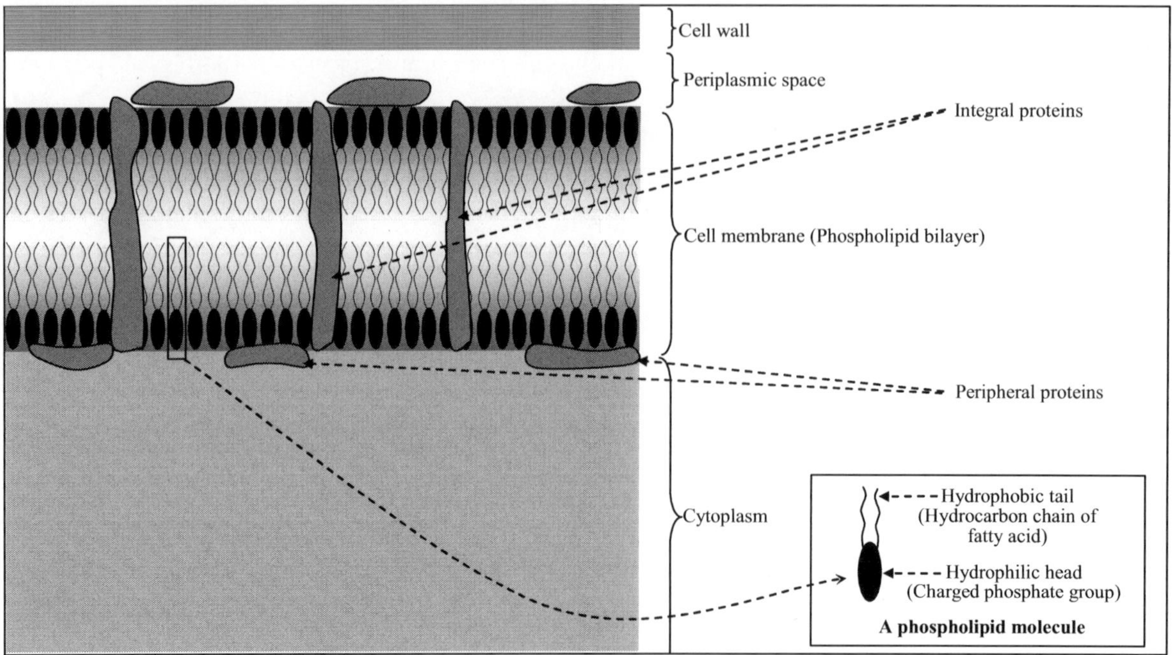

Figure 2.11: Structure of bacterial cell membrane

the membrane with a 'mosaic' appearance. That is why, the unit membrane is usually expressed through a 'fluid-mosaic model'. The phospholipid bilayer consists of two opposite facing layers each consisting of a layer of phospholipid molecules. Each phospholipid molecule has a head and a pair of tails emerging from it. The head is charged and hydrophilic (water-loving), for which it remains towards the aqueous environment. The tails are uncharged and hydrophobic (water-hating), for which they remain hidden inside the membrane away from the aqueous environment. Such a membrane is called 'unit membrane'. Sterols, which are present in the unit membrane of all the eukaryotes as the strengthening agent, are absent in the unit membranes of virtually all bacteria. However, molecules similar to sterols, called 'hopanoids' are present in several bacteria, which play a role similar to that of sterols in eukaryotes. One of the important hopanoids is 'diploptene', which has 30 carbon atoms.

Functions of Cell Membrane

(a) Permeability Barrier

The interior of the cell (the cytoplasm) consists of an aqueous solution of salts, sugars, amino acids, vitamins, coenzymes and a wide variety of other soluble materials. The hydrophobic nature of the cell membrane makes it a tight barrier. Although some small hydrophobic molecules may pass through the membrane by diffusion, hydrophilic and charged molecules (most of the water-soluble molecules) do not readily pass through it. These molecules are transported across it by specific transporting systems. Even a substance as small as a hydrogen ion (H^+) does not diffuse across the cell membrane. The only molecule that penetrates the membrane is water, which is sufficiently small and uncharged to pass between phospholipid molecules. Thus, the cell membrane is a critical barrier separating the inside of the cell from its environment and preventing the passive leakage of cytoplasmic constituents into or out of the cell. If the membrane is broken, the integrity of the cell is destroyed, the internal contents leak into the environment and the cell dies.

(b) Selective Barrier

The cell membrane is also a highly selective barrier. Specific proteins, called 'membrane-transporting systems' present on and in the cell membrane allow and facilitate transport of specific substances across it by active and passive transport. Structurally, the membrane transporting systems are proteins made of 12 alpha helices that wind back and forth through the membrane to form a channel, through which the substance to be transported is carried into or out of the cell. These proteins can bind to specific substances to be transported and move them into or out of the cell across the membrane as required. This enables a bacteria cell to concentrate specific substances inside the cell and remove specific substances from the cell to the outside. There are three types of membrane transport proteins, such as 1) Uniporters, which transport one type of molecule only in one direction across the membrane, 2) Symporters, which transport one type of molecule and always transport another type of molecule along with it in the same direction and 3) Antiporters, which transport one type of molecule and always transport another type of molecule in the opposite direction. Transportation of substances can take place in three ways, such as 1) Simple transportation, in which the transportation is done across the membrane by the energy from the proton motive force, 2) Group translocation, in which the transported substance is chemically altered during passage across the membrane and 3) ABC transportation (*A*TP-*b*inding *c*assette), in which a periplasmic-binding protein in the periplasm specifically binds to the substance, a membrane-spanning protein, which spans across the membrane transports it across the membrane and a cytoplasmic ATP–hydrolysing protein present in the cytoplasm supplies the energy for the transport event.

(c) Extracellular Hydrolysis

The cell membrane secrets many enzymes to outside for extracellular breakdown of large food particles into molecules, which can pass into the cell through the membrane.

(d) Respiration

Bacteria do not have mitochondria. Therefore, cellular respiration, to get energy from food materials, is performed in the cell membrane, which contains the enzymes of the respiratory chain. It is a device for energy conservation in the cell. The membrane can exist in an energetically 'charged' form, in which a separation of protons (H^+) from hydroxyl ions (OH^-) occurs across its surface. This charge separation is a form of metabolic energy, analogous to the potential energy present in a charged battery. The energised state of the membrane, referred to as a 'proton motive force' (PMF), is responsible for driving many energy-requiring functions in the cell, including some forms of transport, motility and the biosynthesis of the cell's energy currency, ATP.

(e) Photosynthesis

Phototrophic bacteria carry out photosynthesis by special organelles called 'chromatophores' which are formed by the invagination of the cell membrane. These organelles contain enzymes and pigments for photosynthesis.

(f) Absorption of Nutrients

Nutrients in the surrounding are directly absorbed into the bacteria cells through the cell membrane. 'Mesosomes' are membranous invaginations of the cell membrane into the cytoplasm, which increase the surface area for efficient absorption.

(g) Reproduction

Bacteria reproduce by binary fission. Each cell divides into two daughter cells. In the process, the cell membrane forms the new cell wall between dividing daughter cells.

11. Cytoplasm

The viscous fluid-like substance, which fills the compartment within the cell membrane, is called cytoplasm (Figures 2.10 and 2.11). It is a fluid made of water, enzymes and small molecules. Suspended in the fluid are a relatively transparent region of chromosomal material called 'nucleoid', ribosome granules and cytoplasmic inclusions, which store energy.

12. Nucleoid

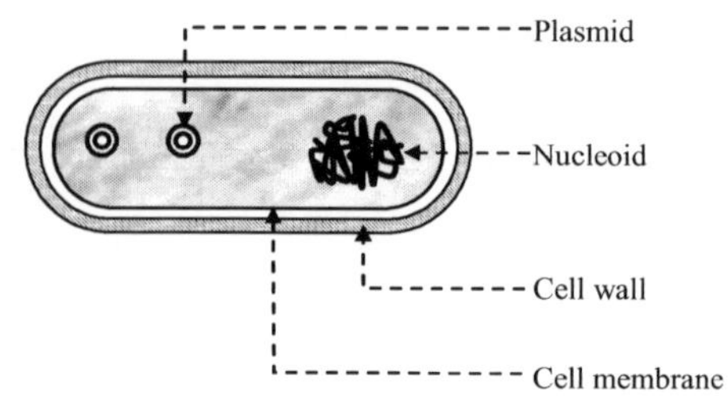

Figure 2.12: Nucleoid and plasmid

It is the aggregated mass of DNA that makes up the chromosome of bacteria (Figure 2.12). As bacteria are prokaryotes, their DNA is not confined within a membrane-bound nucleus, as it is in eukaryotes. However, it is not scattered throughout the cell, rather it tends to aggregate as a distinct structure within the bacteria cell and is called 'nucleoid' (Figure 2.12). Ribosomes are absent in the region of the nucleoid, because nucleoid DNA exists in a gel-like form that excludes particulate matter. Most bacteria contain only a single chromosome, which consists of a single circular double-stranded DNA, though some bacteria have linear chromosomal DNA. Usually the chromosomal DNA is extensively twisted and folded to 'supercoiled DNA', so as to accommodate it in the small space of the nucleoid. Supercoiled DNA is more compact than the free circularised DNA. Bacteria contain only a single copy of each gene on their chromosome and are therefore genetically 'haploid'. In contrast, eukaryotes contain two copies of each gene in their chromosomes and are thus genetically diploid. Gene can be defined as any segment of a DNA, which is responsible for a particular character of the host organism. Each character of an organism is specified by a particular gene, which consists of a particular segment of the DNA. The chromosomal DNA of bacteria contains the essential 'house-keeping genes', which are needed for basic survival of bacteria. This DNA is distributed between the two daughter cells during cell division. Besides the chromosomal genes, there are also non-chromosomal genes present outside the chromosome. For example, the plasmids contain specific genes, which confer special properties to bacteria. The sum total of all the genes present in a cell is called its 'genome'.

13. Plasmids

These are few non-chromosomal DNA found in the cytoplasm of some bacteria (Figure 2.12). Each plasmid consists of a small circular piece of double stranded DNA, which can replicate independently of the chromosome. Many plasmids are rather small, but some are quite large. However, no plasmid is as large as the chromosome. Plasmids do not have genes essential for bacterial growth or survival. They may have genes responsible for the resistance to antibiotics, for production of toxins or for production of surface appendages essential for attachment and establishment of infection. Thus, the plasmids contain the genes that confer special properties to bacteria, unlike the chromosomal DNA, which contains the essential house-keeping genes needed for basic survival of the bacteria. Some plasmids, which can integrate into the host chromosomal DNA are called 'episomes'. Plasmids can also be eliminated from the host bacteria cell by the process called 'curing'. Some plasmids are widely used in gene manipulation and genetic engineering.

14. Ribosomes

These are granular bodies present in the cytoplasm, in which protein synthesis takes place (Figure 2.3). They are so numerous that, their presence gives the cytoplasm a dark appearance. The size of each bacterial ribosome is 70 S (70 Svedberg), which consists of two subunits of 50S and 30S size. In contrast, the size of each eukaryotic ribosome is 80 S consisting of two subunits of 60S and 40S size.

15. Gas Vacuoles

Gas vacuoles are spindle-shaped gas-filled structures found in the cytoplasm (Figures 2.3 and 2.13). They are hollow cylindrical tubes, closed by a hollow conical cap at each end. Their number in a cell may vary from a few to hundreds. Their length and width vary in different bacteria, but the vacuoles of any given bacteria are more or less of constant size. They are hollow, but rigid. They are impermeable

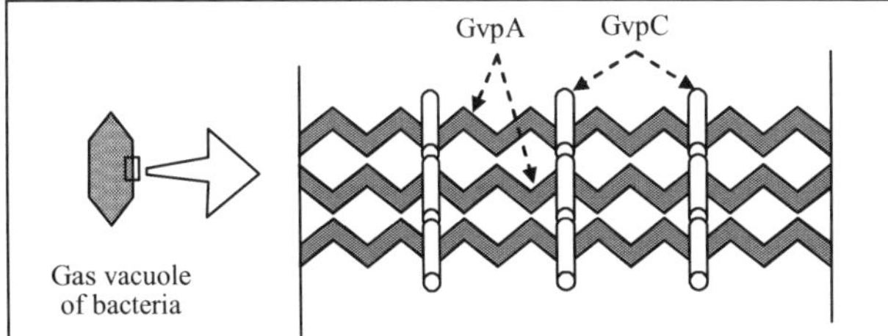

Figure 2.13: Structure of gas vacuole in bacteria

to water and solutes, but are permeable to most gases. Therefore, the composition of the gas inside them is the same as that of the gas, in which the organism is suspended. Gas is present in the vacuoles at about 1 atm. pressure. Therefore, rigidity of gas vacuole membrane is essential for the vacuole to resist the pressure exerted on it from outside. Due to this, it is composed of proteins able to form a rigid membrane rather than of lipids, which would form a fluid, highly mobile membrane. There are two types of proteins, which make the membrane. They are 1) GvpA and 2) GvpC (*G*as *v*acuole *p*rotein A and C). GvpA is the major gas vacuoles protein, which is small and highly hydrophobic (Figure 2.13). It is the shell protein and makes up 97% of the total protein of the gas vacuoles. Gas vacuoles are made of several GvpA protein molecules aligned as parallel 'ribs' forming a watertight surface. GvpA proteins fold as a β-sheet and thus, give considerable rigidity to the overall vacuole structure. GvpC is a larger protein, but is present in much smaller amount. It strengthens the shell of the gas vacuoles by acting as cross-linker, binding several GvpA ribs together like a clamp. The final shape of the gas vacuoles, which can vary in different organisms from long and thin to short and fat, is a function of how the GvpA and GvpC proteins are arranged to form the intact vacuoles. As the gas vacuoles are filled with gases, their density is about 5-20% of that of the cell proper. Thus, the intact gas vacuoles decrease the density of the bacteria cells, thereby conferring buoyancy to them. Most of the floating aquatic bacteria have gas vacuoles, which confer buoyancy and help them to float on the surface of water or anywhere in the water column. Gas vacuoles also act as a means of motility, allowing cells to float up and down in the water column in response to environmental factors. For example, aquatic phototrophic organisms benefit from gas vacuoles, which help them to adjust their position rapidly in the water column to regions where light intensity for photosynthesis is optimal. The gas vacuole membrane cannot resist high hydrostatic pressure and can collapse, leading to a loss of buoyancy. Once collapsed, gas vacuoles cannot be reinflated.

16. Inclusions

The non-living reserve materials suspended in the cytoplasm are called 'inclusions' (Figure 2.3). Most of the inclusions are bounded by a thin non-unit membrane consisting of lipids separating them from the surrounding cytoplasm. Their function is the storage of energy or structural building blocks. Different bacteria contain different types of inclusions. Some of the common inclusions found in bacteria cells are described below.

(*a*) Poly-β-hydroxybutyric Acid (PHB) Granules

These are granules consisting of poly-β-hydroxybutyric acid (PHB), which is a lipid-like substance. Monomers of β-hydroxybutyric acid are bonded to each other in a chain by ester linkages to form the polymer of poly-β-hydroxybutyric acid. The polymers aggregate into granules.

(*b*) Poly-β-hydroxyalkanoate (PHA) Granules

It is a collective term used to describe all classes of carbon/energy storage polymers found in bacterial cytoplasm. The most common PHA granules are the PHB granules. The length of the monomers in a polymer can vary, from as short as C_4 (in PHB granules) to as long as C_{18} (in other granules) in many bacteria.

(*c*) Volutin Granules

These are granules composed of polyphosphates. The basic dye, toluidine blue becomes reddish violet, when it combines with the polyphosphate granules. This phenomenon of colour change is called 'metachromasy'. Therefore, volutin granules are also called 'metachromatic granules'.

(*d*) Glycogen Granules

These are starch–like polymers made of glucose subunits. Glycogen granules are usually smaller than PHB granules. These are storage depots of carbon and energy in bacteria cells.

(*e*) Sulphur Granules

These are granules of elemental sulphur produced by its accumulation in the cytoplasm. Elemental sulphur comes from the oxidation of reduced sulphur compounds like hydrogen sulphide and thiosulphate. The granules remain as long as the source of reduced sulphur is present. As the source disappears, being utilised by the bacteria cells, the granules also disappear slowly.

(*f*) Magnetosomes

Magnetosomes are granules of the iron mineral magnetite, Fe_3O_4. They impart a permanent magnetic dipole to a bacteria cell, allowing it to respond to magnetic fields. A membrane containing phospholipids, proteins and glycoproteins surround each magnetosome. The membrane proteins play a role in precipitating Fe^{3+} (brought into the cell in soluble form by chelating agents) as Fe_3O_4 in the developing magnetosomes. The morphology of magnetosomes appears to be species-specific, varying in shape from square to rectangular to spike-shaped in certain bacteria. Magnetosomes are primarily found in aquatic bacteria. Bacteria that produce magnetosomes orient and migrate along geomagnetic field. This phenomenon is called 'magnetotaxis'. Bacteria, which show magnetotaxis, are called 'magnetotactic bacteria'. There is no evidence that magnetotactic bacteria employ the sensory systems of chemotactic or phototactic bacteria. Instead, the alignment of magnetosomes in a bacteria cell simply imparts magnetic properties to it, which then orients the cell in a particular direction in its environment. Thus, a better term to describe these organisms is ' magnetic bacteria'.

17. Endospore

It is a differentiated cell formed within the cell of certain gram-positive rod-shaped bacteria, which can withstand severe adverse conditions like heat, cold, radiation, ageing, toxic chemicals and lack of nutrients. Mostly, the following three genera of rod-shaped bacteria can produce endospores[1] in adverse conditions.

I. Aerobic rod-shaped bacteria
   1. *Bacillus* spp.

II. Anaerobic rod-shaped bacteria
   2. *Clostridium* spp.
   3. *Desulfotomaculum* spp.

---

1 There are two forms, in which bacteria can remain. They are a) vegetative forms and b) spores. All bacteria remain in their 'vegetative forms' if the environmental conditions are favourable for their normal metabolic activities. In this form, they take up nutrients, grow and reproduce. On the other hand, when the environmental conditions become severely adverse beyond their tolerance, they die. However, some bacteria, survive under such adverse conditions by changing themselves to highly resistant metabolically inactive forms called 'spores'. These bacteria are called the 'spore-forming bacteria' or 'spore-formers'. Of course, they can be killed by special techniques like autoclaving. Most other bacteria, which cannot form spores and die in their vegetative forms under adverse conditions are called 'non-spore-forming bacteria' or 'non-spore-formers'. Depending on the location where it is formed with respect to bacterial cell, spores are of two types. They are:

(*i*) *Endospore*: It is formed within the bacteria cell and released to outside as 'spore' to survive the adverse conditions. These are the most commonly found spores. Therefore, very often spore and endospore are used synonymously.

(*ii*) *Exospore*: It is produced external to the vegetative cell by budding at one end of the bacterial cell and released to outside as 'spore' to survive the adverse conditions. Unlike endospore, it lacks dipicholinic acid (DPA). Example: Methane oxidising bacteria of the genus *Methylosinus* and *Methylocystis*.

Cyst is a desiccation-resistant form of certain bacteria produced under adverse conditions, in which the whole cell is surrounded by a thick protective layer called 'coat'. Upon return of favourable conditions, the coat ruptures and the cell becomes active again. Thus, cyst is completely different from spore, which are released from the bacteria cell. Example of cyst forming bacteria is *Azotobacter*.

Structure of Endospore

The structure of the endospore is much more complex than that of the vegetative cell in that it has many layers. The layers from outside towards inside are given below (Figure 2.14).

(*a*) *Exosporium*: It is the outermost layer, which is a thin, delicate covering, made of proteins.

(*b*) *Spore coat*: It is made of layers of spore-specific proteins. It acts like a sieve that excludes large toxic molecules like lysozyme, is resistant to many toxic molecules and may also contain enzymes that are involved in the germination of the spore.

(*c*) *Cortex*: It is made of loosely cross-linked peptidoglycan.

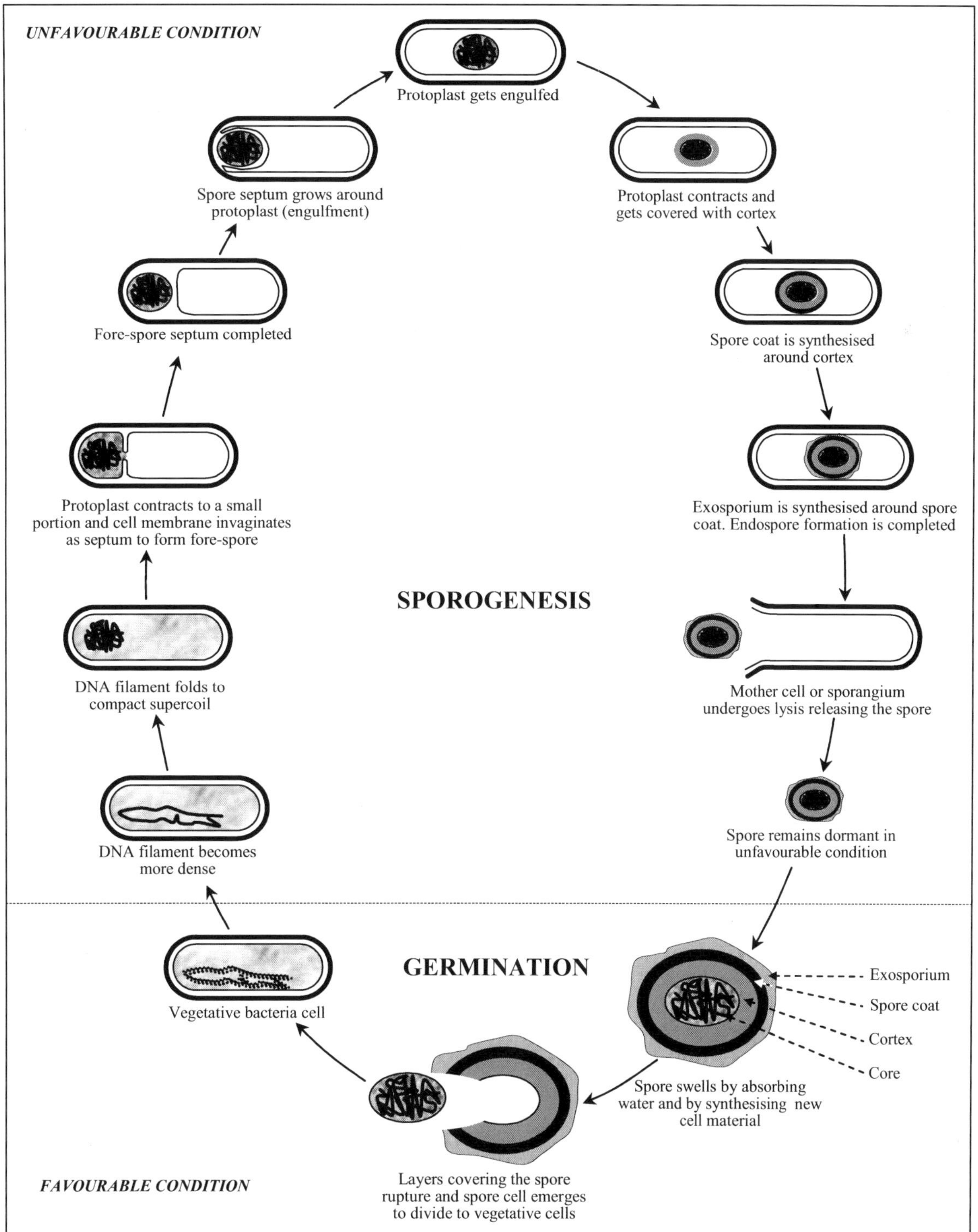

Figure 2.14: Spore cycle in bacteria

(*d*) *Core*: It contains the usual structures of bacteria cell, which includes the cell wall (core wall), enclosing the spore protoplast. The spore protoplast consists of the cell membrane, cytoplasm, nucleoid, ribosomes, inclusions and so on.

Thus, the spore differs structurally from the vegetative cell primarily in the kinds of structures found outside the core wall.

Properties of the Endospore Core

The core of a mature endospore differs greatly from the vegetative cell, from which it is formed. The properties of the endospore core are as follows.

(*a*) One chemical substance that is characteristic of endospores, but not present in vegetative cells is dipicolinic acid (DPA). It is located in the core.

(*b*) Spores are also high in calcium ions, most of which are combined with dipicolinic acid. The calcium-dipicolinic acid complex of the core represents about 10% of the dry weight of the endospore.

(*c*) Besides having an abundant calcium-dipicolinic acid (Ca-DPA) content, the core is in a partially dehydrated state. The core of a mature endospore contains only 10-30% of the water content of the vegetative cell and thus, the consistency of the core cytoplasm is that of a gel. Dehydration of the core greatly increases the heat resistance of the endospore as well as confers resistance to chemicals, such as hydrogen peroxide (H_2O_2) and causes the enzymes present in the core to remain inactive.

(*d*) In addition to the low water content of the spore, the pH of the core cytoplasm is about one unit lower than that of the vegetative cell.

(*e*) The core contains high levels of core-specific proteins called 'small acid-soluble spore proteins' (SASPs). These are synthesised during the sporulation process and have two functions. First, they bind tightly to the DNA in the core and protect it from potential damage from UV radiation, desiccation and dry heat. Second, they function as the source of carbon and energy for the outgrowth of new vegetative cell by the process of germination.

Spore Cycle

In adverse conditions, a spore is produced within a vegetative cell by dehydration and contraction of the cell contents (Figure 2.14). This spore, formed inside the bacteria cell, is called 'endospore'. If adverse conditions worsen, the cell ruptures releasing the endospore, which now becomes an independent dormant cell called 'spore'. The process, by which a vegetative cell produces a spore, is called 'sporogenesis' or 'sporulation'. The spore remains in the inactive dormant form till the adverse conditions persist. Upon return of favourable conditions, the spore comes back to the vegetative form and becomes active again. The layers covering the spore rupture and the spore gives rise to a metabolically active vegetative cell. The process, by which a spore changes to a vegetative cell, is called ' germination'. The cyclic process of change from vegetative form to spore under adverse conditions and back to vegetative form under favourable conditions is called 'spore cycle'. The two halves of the spore cycle are given below.

A. Sporulation

Sporulation involves a very complex series of events in cellular differentiation (Figure 2.14). Many genetically directed changes in the cell underlie the conversion from a moist, metabolically active cell to a dry, metabolically inactive but extremely resistant spore. The structural changes occurring in sporulating cells can be divided into several stages. The entire sporulation process takes about few hours. Genetic studies have shown that as many as 200 genes are involved in a typical sporulation process. During sporulation, the synthesis of some proteins involved in the functioning of vegetative cells ceases and synthesis of specific spore proteins starts. These proteins are called 'small acid-soluble spore proteins'

(SASPs). This is accomplished by activation of a variety of spore-specific genes including *spo, ssp* (which encodes SASPs) and many other genes in response to the adverse environmental condition. The proteins encoded by these genes catalyse the series of events changing a vegetative cell to a spore. The spore gains its heat resistance by several mechanisms, which have not yet been clearly explained. However, it is clear that the impervious layers, such as spore cortex and spore coat protect the spore from any physical damage. A major factor influencing the heat resistance of a spore is the amount and state of water within it. During sporulation, the protoplasm is reduced to a minimum volume, as a result of the accumulation of Ca^{2+}, small acid-soluble spore proteins (SASPs) and synthesis of dipicolinic acid, which leads to the formation of a gel-like structure. At this stage, a thick cortex forms around the protoplast core. Contraction of the cortex results in a shrunken, dehydrated protoplast with a water content of only 10-30% of that of a vegetative cell. The water content of the protoplast and the concentration of SASPs determine the heat resistance of the spore. If the spore has low concentration of SASPs and high water content, it shows low heat resistance. If it has high concentration of SASPs and low water content, it shows high heat resistance. Water moves freely in and out of the spore. Thus, it is not the impermeability of the spore coat, rather the gel-like material in the spore protoplast, that excludes water.

B. Germination

An endospore may remain dormant for many years, but can convert back to a vegetative cell relatively rapidly. This process involves three steps; activation, germination and outgrowth. 'Activation' involves activating the spore and making it ready for germination. 'Germination' involves loss of microscopic refractility of the spore and loss of resistance to heat and chemicals. The spore loses calcium-dipicolinic acid and cortex components. Moreover, the SASPs are degraded. 'Outgrowth' involves visible swelling due to water uptake as well as synthesis of new DNA, RNA and proteins. The cell emerges from the broken spore coat and eventually begins to divide. The cell then remains in vegetative growth until environmental conditions are favourable.

While sterilising a material to make it bacteria-free, the bacteria present in it are killed by some method. However, if the material contains spore-formers, it becomes difficult to sterilise it. The more is the number of spores in the material, the higher is the stress required to sterilise it. For colonies of spore-forming bacteria grown on agar plates or slants, as the age of bacteria increases, they form spores due to ageing, nutrient deficiency and accumulation of metabolites.

E. Growth of Bacteria

Cellular Growth and Reproduction

An individual bacteria cell grows in size, when environmental conditions are favourable for its growth. Each cell grows to approximately double its size (Figure 2.15). In case of spherical bacteria, the diameter of the cell doubles, while in others, the cell elongates to double its original length. Such growth is called 'cellular growth'. After a bacteria cell attains almost double its size, it divides into two cells by a process called 'binary fission'. Thus, reproduction of bacteria takes place through binary fission. The term binary implies that each mother bacteria cell divides (*fission*: division) to two (*bi*: two) daughter bacteria cells. During division, the cell membrane and cell wall at the middle of the mother cell grow inward from opposite sides till they meet each other and form a partition wall called 'septum'. The septum divides the cell into two equal halves, which later on pinch off to form two new daughter bacteria cells. During growth of the mother cell, its DNA molecule replicates to two similar DNA molecules, so that each daughter cell receives one DNA molecule. Other cellular substances are also divided equally between the two daughter cells.

Growth of Bacteria

In case of higher plants and animals, growth implies an increase in the size of an individual. Although each bacteria cell also grows by increase in its size, such cellular growth is difficult to be

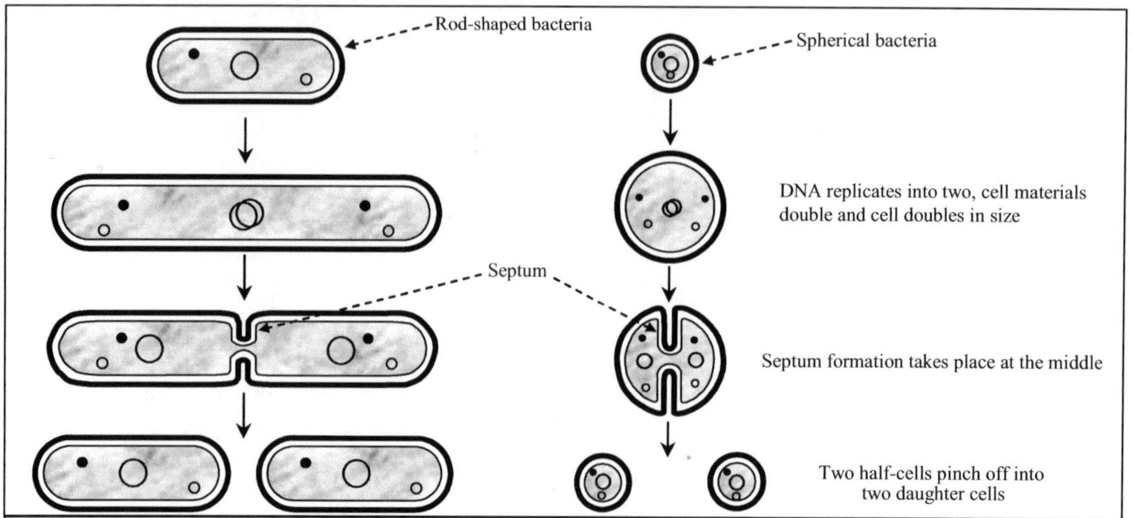

Figure 2.15: Cellular growth and reproduction in rod-shaped and spherical bacteria

perceived ordinarily and is of little importance; rather it is the number of cells produced at the end of a certain time interval, which can be perceived and has definite importance. That is why, 'growth of bacteria' is defined as an increase in the number of bacteria cells. 'Growth rate' of bacteria is defined as the increase in the number of bacteria cells per unit time. The time required for a given population of bacteria to double is called 'generation time' or 'doubling time'. It varies among bacteria from few minutes to few hours.

Exponential or Logarithmic Growth

As growth of bacteria takes place through binary fission, a single bacterium (1) grows as 1,2,4,8,16 and so on, which can also be expressed as 1×2^0, 1×2^1, 1×2^2, 1×2^3, 1×2^4,......1×2^n respectively. This type of growth, in which the number of cells doubles during each unit time (generation time), is called 'exponential growth' or 'logarithmic growth'. Logarithmic growth is much faster than arithmetic growth (1, 2, 3, 4, 5, 6, 7,......) or geometric growth (1, 2, 4, 8, 16, 32,......). Though, apparently it follows geometric growth, after few generations it grows as 1, 10, 100, 1000, 10000,...... (10^0, 10^1, 10^2, 10^3, 10^4,......) whose logarithmic values are 0, 1, 2, 3, 4,...... respectively. If the initial number of bacteria is N_0 instead of 1, then after 'n' number of generations, the final number of bacteria (N) will be $N_0 \times 2^n$. Thus, the final number of bacteria can be obtained using the following equation.

$$\boxed{N = N_0 \times 2^n}$$

where,

N: Final number of bacteria,

N_0: Initial number of bacteria and

n: Number of generations.

The equation to find out the number of generations (n), is derived from the above equation as follows.

$$N = N_0 \times 2^n$$

$$\Rightarrow \log N = \log (N_0 \times 2^n) \quad \text{(taking log of both the sides)}$$

$$\Rightarrow \log N = \log N_0 + \log 2^n \quad (\because \log a \times b = \log a + \log b)$$

$$\Rightarrow \log N = \log N_0 + n \log 2 \quad (\because \log a^x = x \log a)$$

$$\Rightarrow \quad \log N - \log N_0 = n \log 2$$

$$\Rightarrow \quad n \log 2 = \log N - \log N_0$$

$$\Rightarrow \quad n = \frac{\log N - \log N_0}{\log 2}$$

$$\boxed{n = 3.3 (\log N - \log N_0)}$$

Growth Curve

Growth of bacteria takes place in four phases as given below. A plot of log of bacteria number versus time gives a typical curve called 'growth curve' (Figure 2.16).

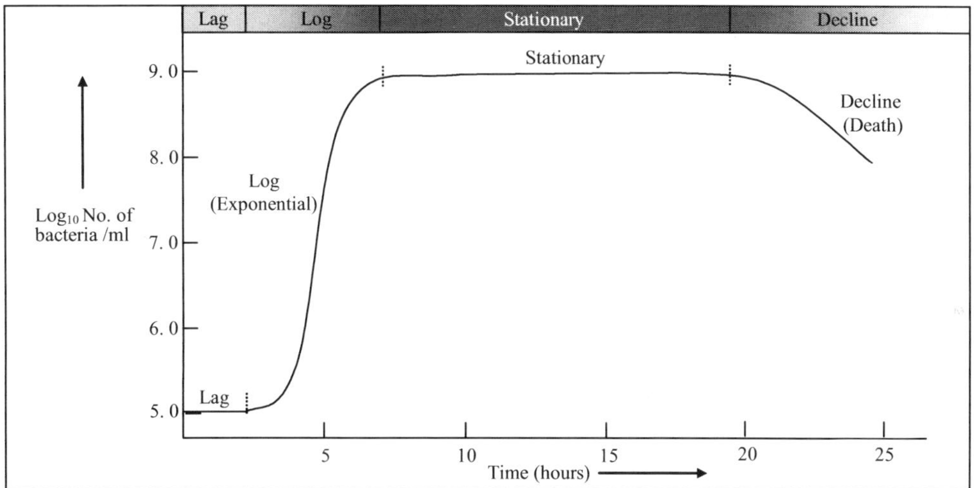

Figure 2.16: Growth curve of bacteria

1. Lag Phase

When an inoculum of bacteria is inoculated into a suitable fresh culture medium, normal logarithmic growth usually does not begin immediately; rather it starts after a certain lapse of time. This lapse of time between the inoculation and beginning of the normal logarithmic growth of bacteria is called 'lag phase'. During this period, the bacteria acclimatises to the new environment of the fresh culture medium, which is not the same as the environment, from which it has been taken. In this phase, the bacteria grows very slowly through division by binary fission. Therefore, in the growth curve, the lag phase slopes upward only slightly. A lag phase usually does not occur, if the inoculum is taken from an exponentially growing culture and is inoculated into a fresh culture medium similar to that, from which it has been taken and maintained under similar conditions of growth.

2. Log Phase (Exponential Phase)

During this period, the bacteria grows at the fastest rate in a logarithmic (exponential) manner. Maximum growth takes place during this phase. Generation time and growth rate remain almost constant. Therefore, in the growth curve, the log phase shows a steep rise from the end of the lag phase.

3. Stationary Phase

In the stationary phase, the number of cells in the culture remains almost constant. An indefinite exponential growth is impossible and can be compared with the story of a poor beggar making fool of a king by asking for a simple alms; double the match sticks every day for a year starting with one. (1,2,4,8,16,32,64,128,256,512,1024,2048,4096,8192,16384,32768,65536,131072,262144,524288, 1048576, 2097152, 4194304, 8388608,16777216, 3354432, 6708864, 13417728, 26835456, 53670912,......only in one month). It has also been calculated that a bacterium weighing only 10^{-12} gram and having a generation time of 20 minutes, if grows exponentially for 48 hours, would produce a population weighing about 4000 time the weight of the earth. Exponential growth does not continue indefinitely and ceases after some time because of two reasons: a) The culture medium becomes so over-populated that, essential nutrients present in it are used up and become unavailable after sometime and b) Due to over-population, toxic waste metabolites produced by the bacteria accumulate to inhibitory levels. These lead to the beginning of death of the bacteria cells in the culture. Although cells reproduce by binary fission and growth continues unabated, the number of cells produced almost equals the number of cells dying. This leads to the stationary phase.

4. Decline Phase (Death Phase)

In this phase, the number of bacteria cells in the culture decreases. As more and more toxic metabolites accumulate in the medium, more and more cells start dying. This leads to more cells dying than produced. As a result, the number of cells decreases. The death phase also occurs exponentially (logarithmically), but at a much slower rate than that of the exponential growth phase.

F. Environmental Factors Influencing Growth of Bacteria

Environmental factors have tremendous influence on the growth of bacteria. Each species of bacteria has an optimum set of environmental conditions for its growth. Based on their requirements of environmental conditions, bacteria can be categorised as follows (Table 2.1 and Figure 2.17).

1. Depending on the Requirement of Oxygen/Air for Growth

(*a*) Aerobic Bacteria (Aerobes)

Bacteria requiring the presence of free oxygen (or air) for their growth are called aerobic bacteria or aerobes. Examples: *Bacillus, Micrococcus.*

(*b*) Anaerobic Bacteria (Anaerobes)

Bacteria, which can grow only in the absence of free oxygen, are called anaerobic bacteria or anaerobes. They are killed by oxygen, for which they are also called obligate anaerobes (*obligate*: strict). Example: *Clostridium.*

(*c*) Facultatively Anaerobic Bacteria (Facultatives)

Bacteria growing in the presence or absence of free oxygen are called facultatively anaerobic bacteria or facultatives. Examples: *Salmonella, Vibrio, Listeria.*

(*d*) Microaerophilic Bacteria (Microaerophiles)

These bacteria can grow better in the presence of very little free oxygen. Examples: *Streptococcus, Lactobacillus, Campylobacter.*

2. Depending on the Optimum Temperatures for Growth

(*a*) Thermophilic Bacteria (Thermophiles)

They are high-temperature-loving bacteria (*thermo*: high temperature; *philic*: loving), which have high optimum temperatures for growth, of 45-80°C. Bacteria belonging to this group are quite rare. Such bacteria are found in natural hot springs. Certain bacteria causing spoilage of canned foods belong to this group. Examples: *Bacillus stearothermophilus, Clostridium thermosaccharolyticum, Desulphotomaculum (Clostridium) nigrificans.*

(*b*) Mesophilic bacteria (Mesophiles)

They are moderate-temperature-loving bacteria (*meso*: moderate temperature; *philic*: loving), which have moderate optimum temperatures for growth, of 20-45°C. Majority of the bacteria naturally encountered belong to this group. Most of the pathogens belong to this group. Examples: *Salmonella, Escherichia, Staphylococcus, Clostridium botulinum.*

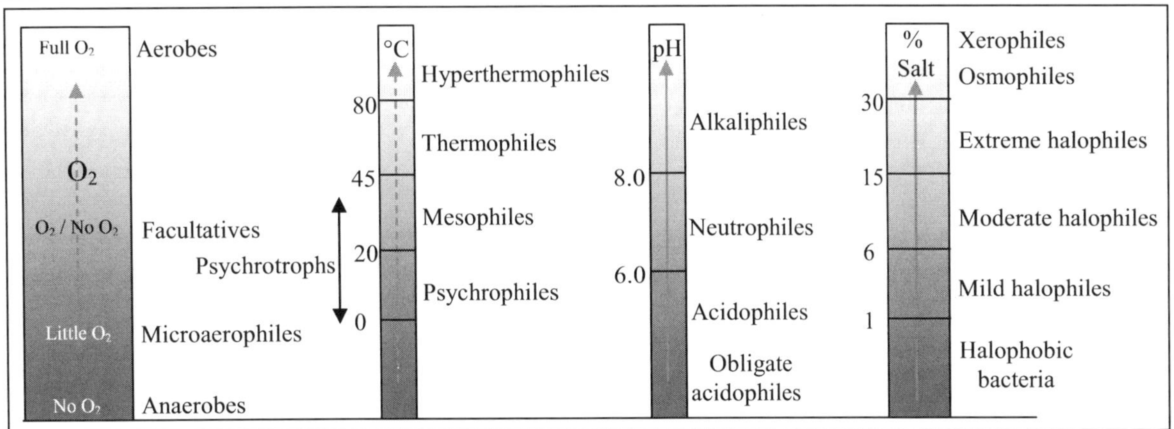

Figure 2.17: Types of bacteria based on optimum requirements for growth

Table 2.1: Types of bacteria based on optimum requirements for growth

Based on Oxygen Requirement		***Based on pH Requirement***	
Aerobes	(Need O_2)	Acidophiles	pH< 6.0
Anaerobes	(Need absence of O_2)	Neutrophiles	pH 6.0–8.0
Facultatives	(O_2/No O_2)	Alkaliphiles	pH > 8.0
Microaerophiles	(Need very little O_2)	Obligate acidophiles	Only low pH
Based on Optimum Temperature for Growth		***Based on Salt and Water Requirement***	
Thermophiles	45-80°C	Halophobic bacteria	< 1% salt
Mesophiles	20-45°C	Mild halophiles	1-6% salt
Psychrophiles	0-20°C	Moderate halophiles	6-15% salt
Hyperthermophiles	80°C or above	Extreme halophiles	15-30% salt
Psychrotrophs/ Psychrotolerants	20-40°C (Tolerate 0-20°C)	Halotolerants	Tolerate and grow at some concentrations of salt
		Osmophiles	Grow in high osmotic environments
		Xerophiles	Grow in very dry environments

(*c*) Psychrophilic Bacteria (Psychrophiles)

They are low-temperature-loving bacteria (*psychro*: low temperature; *philic*: loving), which have low optimum temperatures for growth, of 0-20°C. They are found in environments that are constantly cold and may be rapidly killed even by brief warming to room temperature. Therefore, truly psychrophilic bacteria are not usually encountered. Example: *Polaromonas vacuolata.*

(*d*) Hyperthermophilic Bacteria (Hyperthermophiles)

They are very-high-temperature-loving bacteria (*hyperthermo*: very high temperature; *philic*: loving), which have very high optimum temperatures for growth, of 80°C or above. Examples: *Thermococcus celer, Pyrolobus fumarii.*

(*e*) Psychrotrophic or Psychrotolerant Bacteria (Psychrotrophs/Psychrotolerants)

They can grow at 0-20°C, but have moderate optimum temperatures for growth, of 20-40°C. Thus, unlike psychrophilic bacteria, which are cold-loving, psychrotrophic bacteria are not cold-loving, rather they can tolerate cold. Although they can grow even at 0°C, they do not grow very well in such cold conditions. They grow optimally at moderate temperatures. They are found in soil and water of temperate climates and in chilled foods like refrigerated milk, iced fish and chilled meat. Examples: *Pseudomonas, Alteromonas, Acinetobacter.*

3. Depending on the Optimum pH for Growth

(*a*) Alkaliphilic Bacteria (Alkaliphiles)

They grow best at pH higher than 8.0.

(*b*) Neutrophilic Bacteria (Neutrophiles)

They have optimum pH for growth between 6.0 and 8.0

(*c*) Acidophilic Bacteria (Acidophiles)

They grow best at pH lower than 6.0.

(*d*) Obligate Acidophilic Bacteria (Obligate Acidophiles)

They can grow only at low pH and cannot grow at high pH or even at neutral pH. Example: *Thiobacillus ferrooxidans, Picrophilus oshimae.*

4. Depending on the Requirement of Water and Salt for Growth

(*a*) Halophobic Bacteria

They die at salt concentrations above 1%. They are the salt-hating bacteria.

(*b*) Halophilic Bacteria (Halophiles)

They require at least some salt (NaCl) for their growth. They are of three types as follows.

(*i*) *Mild halophiles:* These halophiles require NaCl at low concentrations of 1-6% for their growth. Example: *Vibrio fischeri*

(*ii*) *Moderate halophiles:* They require NaCl at moderate concentrations of 6-15% for their growth.

(*iii*) *Extreme halophiles:* These bacteria require NaCl at high concentrations of 15-30% for their growth. Example: *Halobacterium salinarum*

(*c*) Halotolerant Bacteria (Halotolerants)

They can tolerate and grow at some concentrations of salt, but growth is best in absence of salt. Example: *Staphylococcus aureus*

(*d*) Osmophilic Bacteria (Osmophiles)

These bacteria are able to grow in high osmotic environments, which contain high concentration of solutes (salt or sugar).

(*e*) Xerophilic Bacteria (Xerophiles)

They can grow in very dry environments.

G. Control of Bacterial Growth

It is often desirable to inhibit growth of bacteria or to destroy them in different materials. For example, in food preservation methods, a number of steps are taken to destroy bacteria or to inhibit their growth in the food, as they are the main causative agents of food spoilage. Moreover, uncontrolled growth of bacteria in the tissues of plants and animals causes cell destruction by a process called 'infectious disease'. In general, growth of bacteria can be controlled in four ways as given below (Figure 2.18).

(a) Decontamination
(b) Inhibition
(c) Destruction
(d) Sterilisation

(*a*) Decontamination

It is a method that reduces, to a greater or less extent, the initial number of bacteria in a given material by their removal. For example, the washing of floor or top of fish processing table with water

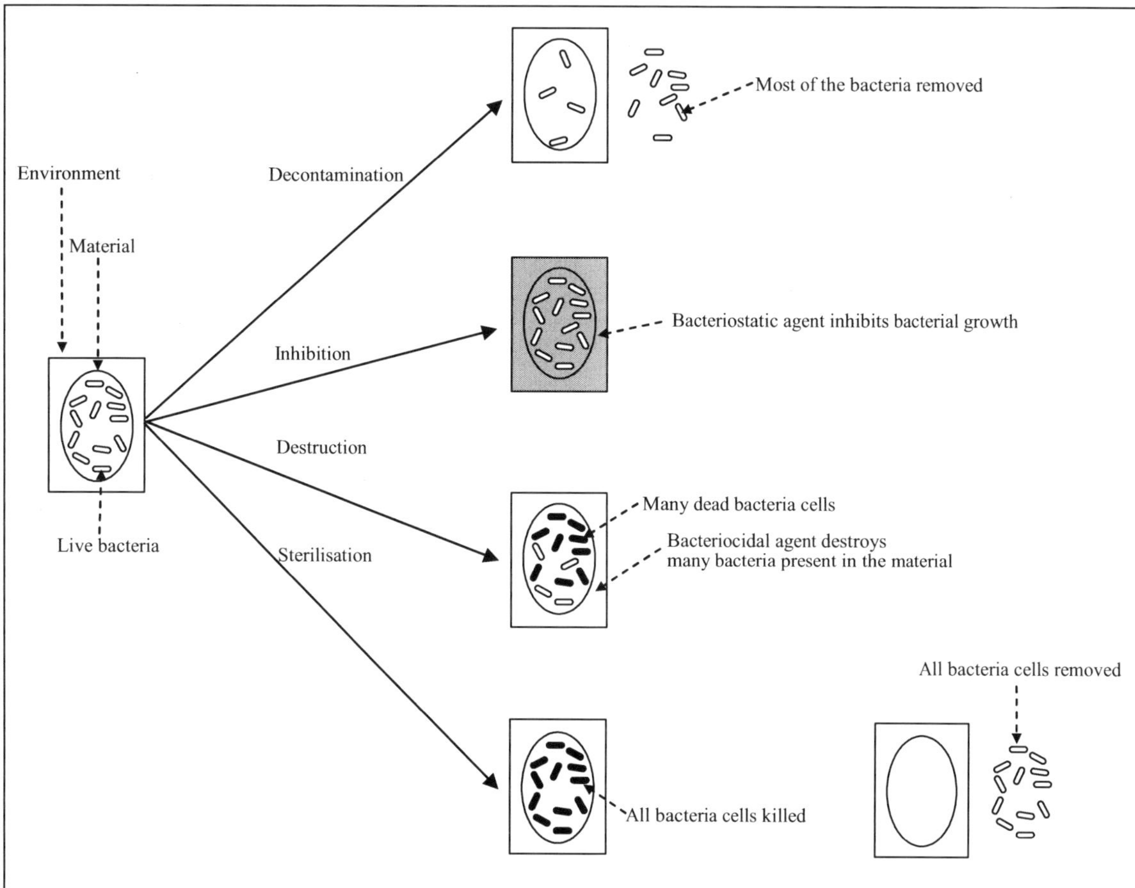

Figure 2.18: Different ways of controlling bacterial growth

removes most of the contaminating bacteria. Washing of fish with water removes most of the bacteria from its body surface. Similarly, gills and gut of fish, which harbour large number of bacteria, are removed during processing to reduce the bacterial load. Washing and deskinning of fruits and vegetables also reduce the bacterial load. Purification of water by filtration is also a decontamination method.

(*b*) Inhibition

Here, the growth of bacteria in a given material is inhibited. As a result, they cannot grow and their number remains almost unchanged. Agents that inhibit bacterial growth are called 'bacteriostatic agents' (*bacterio*: of bacteria; *static*: unchanged). If the agent is removed, growth of bacteria starts again. In freezing preservation of foods, the very low temperature of storage and in drying preservation of foods the reduced moisture content do not allow bacteria to grow; rather few of them die. If these agents are removed, bacteria again start growing and spoil the foods. Thus, freezing and drying are bacteriostatic in nature.

(*c*) Destruction

In this method, bacteria present in a given material are destroyed to a greater or less extent, thereby reducing the initial number. Agents that destroy or kill bacteria are called 'bacteriocidal agents' (*bacterio*: of bacteria; *cidal*: killing). Examples are heating and exposing to chemical agents that can kill bacteria.

(*d*) Sterilisation

It is the process of rendering a given material completely free of microbes either by killing them (bacteriocidal) or removing them from the material (decontamination). For example, in the sterilisation of bacterial culture media, they are given such a high heat treatment that, all the bacteria present in them die. In filter sterilisation, the bacteria cells are removed by filtering them out.

Microbial Control Measures

The different measures taken to control microbial growth are as follows:

1. Cleaning
2. Low temperature
3. High temperature
4. Filter sterilisation
5. Radiation sterilisation
6. Removal of moisture
7. Modified atmosphere packaging
8. Lowering of pH
9. Use of chemicals

1. Cleaning

Cleaning involves sweeping, wiping, washing and brushing of a material, which removes most of the microbes present on it. For examples, sweeping the floor, wiping the table after a meal, washing of floor or cloths, brushing of teeth are steps aiming at decontaminating the material, thereby controlling microbial growth.

2. Low Temperature

Low temperature retards the growth of a large group of microbes and thereby controls microbial growth. Exposure to low temperature can be done in two ways as follows.

(i) Chilling

It is a process of lowering the temperature of a material to about 0°C, but not below it. The low temperature retards the growth of a large group of microbes and thereby controls microbial growth in the material. For example, fish is chilled, usually by icing, which retards the growth of the spoilage microbes and thereby preserves it over few days.

(ii) Freezing

It is a process of lowering the temperature of a material below 0°C. The low temperature retards the growth of a large group of microbes and thereby controls microbial growth in the material. Microbial growth is completely arrested below –10°C. For example, fish and meat are frozen usually below –20°C, which completely arrests the growth of the spoilage microbes and thereby preserves it over months together.

3. High Temperature

As temperature rises beyond the maximum temperature for growth of microbes, lethal effects occur. Thus, very high temperature destroys microbes and thereby controls microbial growth. Exposure to high temperatures can be done in the following ways.

(i) Sunlight

The high temperature of sunlight kills many microbes. The water of ponds and tanks usually get severe microbial contamination, but sunlight kills a large number of microbes and thereby reduces the contamination considerably. The UV radiation of sunlight also kills many microbes.

(ii) Dry Heat

Dry heat kills microbes by oxidation of cell components, whereas moist heat kills by coagulation or denaturation of cellular proteins of the microbial cells. Dry heat is applied in the following ways.

(*a*) *Hot air oven*: All glasswares and materials like powders, wax and oil, which should not come in contact with moisture are sterilised in hot air oven at 180°C for 3 hours. Indicator organism for sterility test of an oven is *Clostridium tetani*, which grows in Robertson cooked meat or thioglycolate agar medium.

(*b*) *Incineration*: It is a process of sterilisation by burning a material to ashes. Loops and needles are burnt to red hot on bunsen burner. Infected materials and carcasses of laboratory animals are incinerated before disposing.

(*c*) *Flaming*: It is a process of sterilisation of materials like scalpel, scissors and glass spreader, which are first dipped in spirit and then just run over the flame allowing the spirit to catch fire and burn off. They are not allowed to become red hot.

(iii) Moist Heat

Moist heat kills microbes by coagulation of their proteins. Moist heat is more effective than dry heat in that, it takes less time, particularly under high pressure, when temperature is above 100°C. It is applied in the following ways.

(*a*) *Pasteurisation*: Pasteurisation is a process of heat treatment upto 100°C using moist heat, which kills certain types of microbes in a given material, but does not kill all the microbes present in it. Milk, juices, cream and certain alcoholic beverages are preserved by pasteurisation. It kills certain pathogenic microbes as well as some spoilage microbes, thereby increasing the storage life of perishable liquids considerably. Pasteurisation of milk is done in two ways, *viz.* flash pasteurisation (71°C for 15 seconds) and bulk pasteurisation (63-66°C for 30 minutes).

(*b*) *Boiling*: It is a process of heating materials in boiling water at 100°C for about 30 minutes. Syringes and needles for hospital uses are boiled in water before use. Cooking of food is also a boiling process.

(*c*) *Tyndalisation*: It is a process of fractional heat sterilisation using moist heat, performed over three days, so as to sterilise a material completely. Some microbiological media containing heat-labile sugars, which get destroyed by autoclaving, are sterilised by tyndalisation. The material to be sterilised is heated by steam at 100°C for 20 minutes every day for three consecutive days. The heat treatment on the first day kills the vegetative forms of bacteria. During the first day incubation, the spores, which survive the heat treatment, germinate. The second day heat treatment kills these germinated bacteria. The second day incubation allows any residual spores to germinate. The third day heat treatment kills these germinated bacteria, thereby sterilising the material completely.

(*d*) *Autoclaving*: It is a process of heat sterilisation, in which the material to be sterilised is heated at 121°C for 15 minutes by super-saturated steam (steam with temperature above 100°C) in an autoclave. An autoclave is a sealed device that generates and maintains steam under pressure. Under normal atmospheric pressure, the maximum temperature that can be attained in an open water bath is 100°C. When water is heated in a closed chamber like autoclave, steam is produced and the steam pressure inside the chamber increases, as steam is not allowed to escape from the chamber. The high pressure raises the boiling point of water in the chamber and temperature much above the boiling point of water (>100°C) is attainable in the chamber. Autoclaving is done for complete sterilisation of materials like microbiological media and diluents, by moist heat. Sometimes, glasswares are also sterilised by autoclaving after covering them with craft paper. Autoclaving completely kills the spores as well as the vegetative forms, thereby ensuring complete sterility in the material. Autoclaves are of two types, vertical and horizontal. The indicator of heat sterilisation in autoclave is *Bacillus stearothermophilus*, the most heat resistant bacteria. Sterility can also be ensured by using a colour solution called Brownis tube (changes from red to green, when heated at 121°C for 15 minutes) or Johnson tape (changes from half light green + half white to half black + half white, when heated at 121°C for 15 minutes).

4. Filter Sterilisation

Filter sterilisation is a process of passing a liquid or gas through a filter having very small pores, which do not allow microbes to pass through, but allow the liquid or gas. The liquid or gas that comes out from the filter is free of microbes and is therefore sterile. Here, the sterilisation is achieved by decontamination. Filter sterilisation is done for sterilising heat-sensitive liquids or gases. The four major types of filters used are as follows.

(i) Mechanical Microfilters (Depth Filters)

These filters do not have uniform pore size. Examples are asbestos pad in Seitz filter, diatomaceous earth in Brokefield filter, porcelain in Chamberland-Pasteur filter and sintered glass discs in other filters. They are also called depth filters, because they trap particles in the tortuous paths created throughout the depth of the structure. As they are rather porous, depth filters are often used as pre-filters to remove larger particles from a solution, so that clogging does not occur in the final filter sterilisation process. They are also used for the filter sterilisation of air in industrial processes.

(ii) Membrane Filters

The most common type of filters for sterilisation in the field of microbiology are the membrane filters. They have uniform pore size. They are composed of polymers with high tensile strength, such as cellulose acetate, cellulose nitrate or polysulphone, manufactured in such a way that they contain a large number of micropores. The size of the pores can be precisely controlled during manufacture of the filters by controlling the polymerisation process. About 80-85% of the filter area is occupied by the pores, which provides for a relatively high fluid flow rate. To further enhance the flow rate, vacuum pump is used. Generally, the membrane filtration assembly is heat-sterilised separately from the membrane filter and the assembly is assembled aseptically at the time of filtration. (Figure 2.19). The indicator organism of filtration sterilisation is *Cerratia marcescens* (0.75μ).

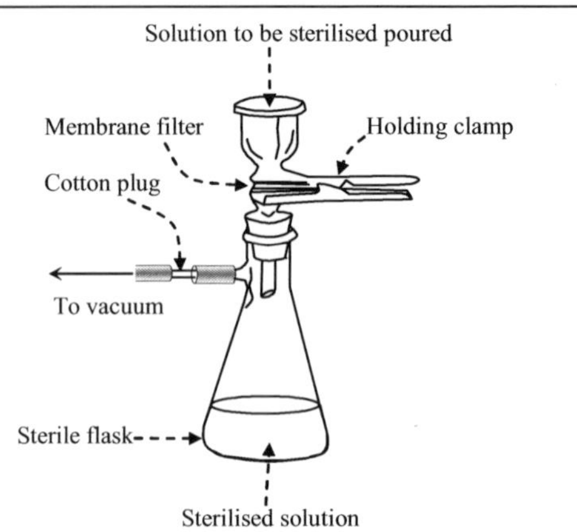

Figure 2.19: Membrane filtration assembly

(iii) Nucleation Track Filters (Nucleopore Filters)

These filters are manufactured by treating very thin polycarbonate films (10μ thick) with nuclear radiation and then etching the films with a chemical. The radiation causes localised damage in the film and the etching chemical enlarges these damaged locations into pores. The size of the pores can be precisely controlled by the strength of the etching solution and the etching time. These filters are commonly used in scanning electron microscopy of microorganisms.

(iv) High Efficiency Particulate Air (HEPA) Filters

The HEPA filters with laminar flow of air are used to deliver clean air into an enclosure, such as a cubicle or room, so as to produce a dust-free sterilised chamber. Aseptic transfer of microbes and sterilised materials is done in the microbiology laboratory inside such laminar flow chambers, which is pre-sterilised by a UV lamp.

5. Radiation Sterilisation

Energy transmitted through space in a variety of forms is generally called radiation. Most important among them is the 'electromagnetic radiation', which includes microwaves, ultraviolet (UV) radiation, light rays, gamma rays, X-rays and electrons. Though all forms of electromagnetic radiations have the potential to control microbial growth, each type of radiation acts through a specific mechanism as given below.

(i) Microwave Radiation

Its antimicrobial effect is due, at least, to its thermal (heating) effects.

(ii) UV Radiation

Radiation with wavelength between 220 and 300 nm is called UV radiation. It has sufficient energy to cause breaks in DNA, leading to the death of the exposed microorganisms. It also causes mutation by formation of pyrimidine (particularly thymine) dimers in nucleic acids. This mutation is lethal, when the gene (fragment of DNA responsible for a particular character) for a vital function stops to work. This near-visible light is useful for disinfecting surfaces, air and other materials like water that do not absorb the UV light. It is used to disinfect the laminar flow chamber. As it has low penetration power, it cannot penetrate solid, opaque, light-absorbing surfaces. Its usefulness is therefore limited to the disinfection of exposed surfaces.

(iii) Ionising Radiations

Among the electromagnetic radiations, those which have energy sufficiently high (more than 10eV) to ionise cell components, so that the cells can no longer perform critical functions and consequently, damage the cells are called 'ionising radiations'. The different types of ionising radiations include the following.

(*a*) *α-rays, β-rays and γ-rays*: They are produced by disintegration of nuclei of radioactive elements like ^{60}Co, ^{90}Sr and ^{127}Cs.

(*b*) *X-rays and high speed electron beams*: They are produced by powerful electrical accelerators.

Ionising radiations are produced by the formation of charged subatomic particles (electrons, protons, neutrons) from atoms or molecules. These radiations ionise the exposed material to electrons (e^-), hydroxyl radicals (OH*) and hydride radicals (H*). Each of these particles is capable of degrading and altering biopolymers like DNA and proteins. The ionisation and subsequent degradation of DNA and proteins lead to the death of the irradiated cells. As γ-ray has high penetration power, it can penetrate solid, opaque, light-absorbing surfaces and sterilise most of the materials. Currently, it is used for sterilisation in food industries (to sterilise ground meat and fresh meat products like hamburger and chicken) as well as for sterilisation of spices, disposable labware and medical supplies like surgical items, drugs and tissue grafts. The high penetration capacity of γ-rays makes it useful in sterilising bulk quantities of materials. As it is detrimental to human cells too, high precautions are needed in its use. On the other hand, high-speed electron beams have less penetration capacity and consequently are less hazardous. They are used to sterilise smaller individually wrapped articles.

6. Removal of Moisture

All microbes need moisture for their growth and activity. Therefore, removal of moisture present in a material retards the growth of the microbes present in it. It can be done in the following ways.

(i) Drying

It includes sun drying and artificial drying in mechanical driers.

(ii) Dehydration

It implies drying under controlled conditions.

(iii) Salting

In salting, salt removes moisture by osmosis.

(iv) Freeze-drying or Lyophilisation

It implies drying under low temperature.

(v) Accelerated Freeze-drying

It is freeze-drying at a very fast rate.

All these methods are adopted in the preservation of fish and many other materials. Lyophilised bacteria are sent to different laboratories in sealed ampoules.

7. Modified Atmosphere Packaging

Modified atmosphere packaging (MAP) is used to extend the shelf life of fresh fish, meat, fruits and vegetables during chilled storage. They are packed in airtight containers, within which the atmosphere is modified desirably by flushing-in of required gases in required proportion. The three major gases used commercially are CO_2, N_2 and O_2.The extension of shelf life in MAP is the result of the antimicrobial activity of these gases. CO_2 has bacteriostatic effect, N_2 inhibits the growth of aerobic microorganisms and O_2 inhibits the growth of strictly anaerobic microorganisms.

8. Lowering of pH

Low pH retards the growth of a large group of microbes and thereby controls microbial growth in the material, which harbours them. For example, the low pH of curd, marinades and pickles retards the growth of spoilage microbes and thereby preserves them over months together.

9. Use of Chemicals

The chemicals that kill or inhibit the growth of microorganisms are called 'antimicrobial chemicals'. Such substances may be synthetic chemicals or natural products. Those chemicals, which kill bacteria, fungi or viruses are called bacteriocidal, fungicidal or viricidal chemicals, while those, which do not kill, but only inhibit their growth are called bacteriostatic, fungistatic or viristatic chemicals respectively. The effectiveness of a chemical in inhibiting the growth of a species of bacteria is determined by a factor called minimum inhibitory concentration (MIC). MIC is defined as the minimum amount of an antimicrobial chemical needed to inhibit the growth of a test microorganism. The effectiveness of a chemical against a given organism is also determined by measuring the zone of inhibition in the agar diffusion technique. Antimicrobial chemicals are of the following categories.

(i) Disinfectants (Germicides)

These are antimicrobial chemicals used to kill the microbes present only on inanimate objects (Table 2.2).

(ii) Antiseptics

These are antimicrobial chemicals used to kill the microbes present only on the body surface of living organism, which are exposed to external infection. They are sufficiently non-toxic to be applied to living tissues (Table 2.2).

(iii) Sterilants

These are antimicrobial chemicals, which, under appropriate circumstances, can kill all microbial life and can actually be used to sterilise inanimate objects and surfaces (Table 2.2).

(iv) Preservatives

These are antimicrobial chemicals used in processing of foods including fish, meat and vegetable products to retard or prevent microbial spoilage (Table 2.3).

(v) Chemotherapeutic Agents

These are antimicrobial chemicals, which can be used internally to control infectious diseases in man and animals and are not toxic to them. These are commonly used as medicines. These are of three types namely synthetic agents, antibiotics and bacteriocins.

(*a*) *Synthetic agents*: Most of the synthetic agents are prepared synthetically and include 'growth factor analogs' like sulpha drugs (sulphanilamide), isoniazide, flurouracil, bromouracil and 'quinolones' like norfloxacin, nalidixic acid and ciprofloxacin.

Table 2.2: Commonly used antiseptics, disinfectants and sterilants*

Antiseptics	***Uses***
Alcohol (60-85% ethanol or isopropanol in water) [a]	Skin
Phenol-containing compounds (hexachlorophene, triclosan, chloroxylenol, chlorhexidine)	Soaps, lotions, cosmetics, body deodorants
Cationic detergents, especially quaternary ammonium compounds (benzalkonium chloride)	Soaps, lotion
Hydrogen peroxide [a] (3% solution)	Skin
Iodine-containing iodophor compounds in solution [a] (Betadine®)	Skin
Organic mercury compounds (mercurochrome)	Skin
Silver nitrate	Eyes of newborn to prevent blindness due to infection by *Neisseria gonorrhoeae*
Disinfectants and Sterilants	
Alcohol (60-85% ethanol or isopropanol in water)[a]	Disinfectant and sterilant for medical instruments, laboratory surfaces
Cationic detergents (quaternary ammonium compounds)	Disinfectant for medical instruments, food and dairy equipment
Chlorine gas	Disinfectant for purification of water supplies
Chlorine compound (chloramines, sodium hypochlorite, chlorine dioxide)	Disinfectant for dairy and food industry equipment, and water supplies
Copper sulphate	Algicide in swimming pools, water supplies (disinfectant)
Ethylene oxide (gas)	Sterilant for temperature–sensitive laboratory materials such as plastics
Formaldehyde	3%-8% solution used as surface disinfectant, 37% (formalin) or vapor used as sterilant
Gluteraldehyde	2% solution used as high-level disinfectant or sterilant
Hydrogen peroxide	Vapor used as sterilant
Iodine-containing iodophor compounds in solution[a] (Wescodyne®)	Disinfectant for medical instruments, laboratory surfaces
Mercuric dichloride[b]	Disinfectant for laboratory surfaces
Ozone	Disinfectant for drinking water
Peracetic acid	0.2% solution used as high-level disinfectant or sterilant
Phenolic compounds[b]	Disinfectant for laboratory surfaces

a: These can act as antiseptics, disinfectants, or even sterilants depending on concentration, length of exposure and form of delivery.

b: These produce environmentally hazardous waste products, especially when used at high concentration and in high volumes.

* *Source*: Madigan, M.T., Martinko, J.M. and Parker, J. (2000) Brock Biology of Microorganisms, 9th edition, Prantice Hall International, Inc., New Jersey, USA, 991pp.

(*b*) *Antibiotics*: These are antimicrobial chemicals produced by certain microorganisms that inhibit or kill other microorganisms. These are natural products, not prepared synthetically. An antibiotic that acts on both gram-positive and gram-negative bacteria is called a 'broad-spectrum antibiotic'. In contrast, an antibiotic, which acts only on a single group of bacteria, is called a 'narrow–spectrum antibiotic'. Antibiotics are of the following types.

1. *β-Lactam Antibiotics*: These antibiotics possess β-lactam ring. All of them are potent inhibitors of cell wall synthesis. They include the following.

(*i*) *Penicillins*: Penicillin G (Benzylpenicillin produce by the fungus *Penicillium notatum*), Methicillin, Oxacillin, Ampicillin, Carbenicillin

(*ii*) Cephalosporins: Ceftriaxone

(*iii*) Cephamycins

2. *Aminoglycoside Antibiotics*: They contain amino sugars bonded by glycosidic bonds to other amino sugars. They include the following.

(*i*) Streptomycin

(*ii*) Kanamycin

(*iii*) Neomycin

3. *Microlid Antibiotics*: They contain large lactone rings connected to sugar moieties. They include the following.

(*i*) Erythromycin

(*ii*) Oleandomycin

(*iii*) Spiramycin

(*iv*) Tylosin

4. *Tetracyclines*: They contain a naphthacene ring structure. They include the following.

(*i*) Tetracycline

(*ii*) 7-Chlortetracycline (Aureomycin) (CTC)

(*iii*) 5-Oxytetracycline (Terramycin) (OTC)

5. *Aromatic compounds*: They contain aromatic ring structure. They include the following.

(*i*) Chloramphenicol

(*ii*) Novobiocin

(c) *Bacteriocins*: They are antimicrobial chemicals produced by some bacteria that kill closely related species of bacteria or even different strains of the same species. They include the following.

1. *Colicin*: It is produced by the bacteria, *Escherichia coli.*
2. *Subtilisin*: It is produced by the bacteria, *Bacillus subtilis.*
3. *Nisin A*: It is produced by the lactic acid bacteria (LAB), *Lactobacillus acidophilus.*

Table 2.3: Preservatives used in food processing

(*a*)	Ammonia
(*b*)	Chlorine
(*c*)	Sulphur dioxide
(*d*)	Acids: Formic acid, acetic acid, propionic acid,benzoic acid and sorbic acid
(*e*)	Salts of acids: Sodium formate, potassium formate,calcium formate, sodium acetate, potassium acetate, calcium acetate, sodium diacetate, sodium propionate, sodium benzoate, potassium sorbate,sodium sorbate
(*f*)	Sulphites: Sodium sulphite, potassium sulphite, sodium bisulphite, potassium bisulphite, sodium metabisulphite, potassium metabisulphite
(*g*)	Nitrates: Sodium nitrate, potassium nitrate
(*h*)	Nitrites: Sodium nitrite, potassium nitrite
(*i*)	Hexamethylene tetramine
(*j*)	Esters of parahydroxy benzoic acid
(*k*)	Hydrogen peroxide
(*l*)	Phosphate peroxide: Sodium pyrophosphate peroxide,potassium pyrophosphate peroxide, disodium hydrogen phosphate peroxide, dipotassium hydrogen phosphate peroxide
(*m*)	5-aminohexahydropyrimidines
(*n*)	Tert-butyl hydroperoxide

3

Microbiology Laboratory

A. Infrastructures

Experiment 1

***Aim*: To study the infrastructure components of a microbiology laboratory.**

An ideal sophisticated laboratory should have the following infrastructures, which should preferably be designed as shown in Figure 3.1.

1. Main laboratory
2. Instrument room
3. Stock culture room
4. Electron microscopy chamber
5. Inoculation chamber
6. Store room
7. Laboratory animal house
8. Store for animal feeds, medicines etc.
9. Chamber of the laboratory head
10. Staff room
11. Office room
12. Library
13. Seminar hall
14. Toilets
15. Garage

1. Main Laboratory

Most of the laboratory activities are performed in the main laboratory. It should have sufficient space inside. A concrete shelf with glazed tile or marble top should project from the wall for keeping the equipments and for performing routine works. Few sunmica-top laboratory tables with shelves, sinks and gas connections should be kept in the lab. Prepared chemicals and reagents should be kept on the shelves of the tables. Disinfectant solution should be kept on each table in a bottle along with a sponge pad. Before and after each experiment, the table-top must be cleaned with the disinfectant solution using the sponge pad. A dispose jar containing germicide solution such as lysol with a thick

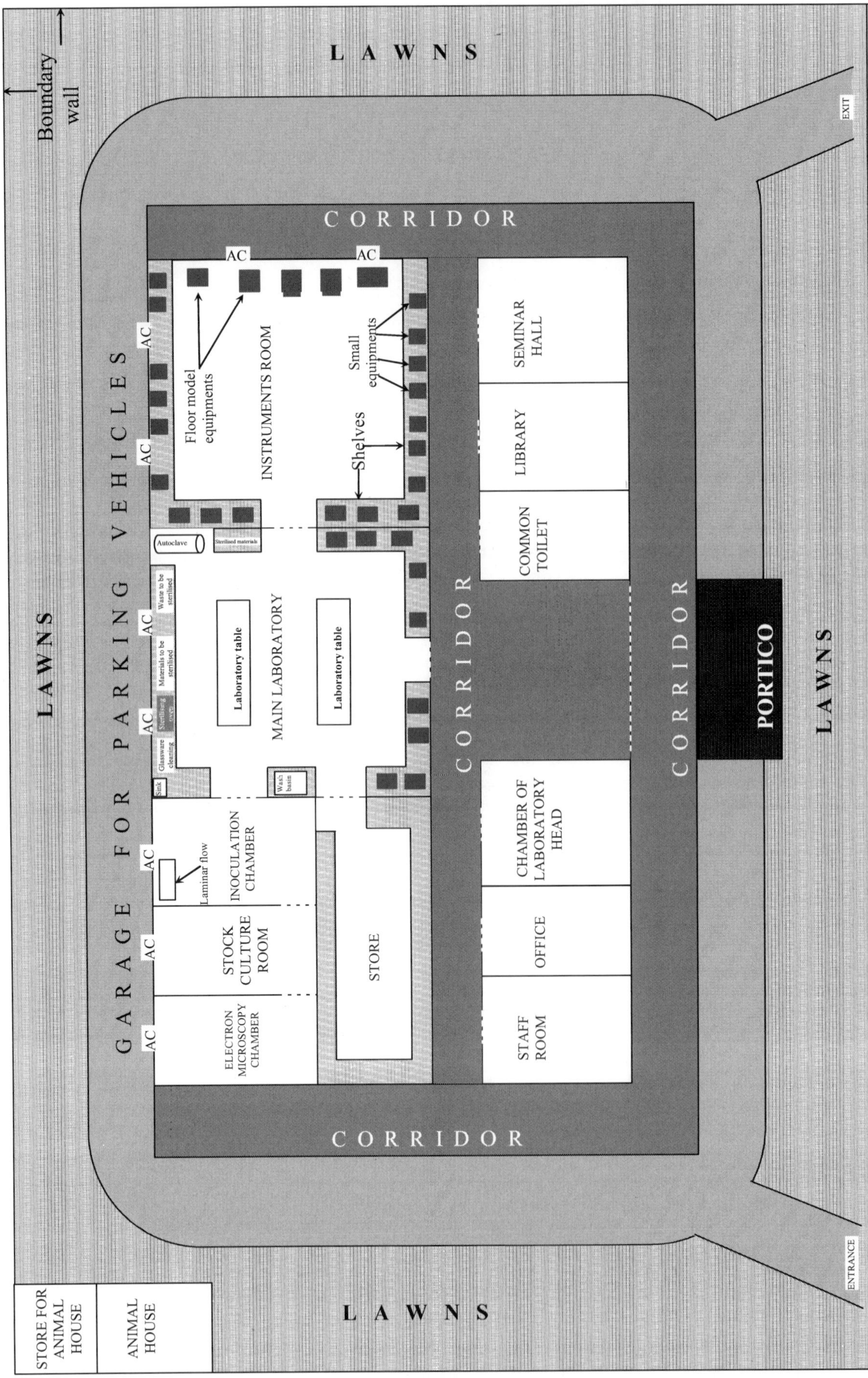

Figure 3.1: Plan of a microbiology laboratory (not to scale)

layer of cotton at its bottom should be kept on or near each table for the pipettes to be disposed into it after use. At one corner of the lab, an autoclave, preferably a double-jacketed horizontal autoclave, should be kept. Space should be left out on the concrete shelf for different purposes labeled accordingly such as, 'waste to be sterilised', 'sterilised materials', 'materials to be sterilised', 'light microscopy', 'glassware cleaning' etc. Equipments, such as oven, microbiological incubator, BOD incubator, single-pan balance, double-pan electrical balance, ultrapure water purification system, distilled water plant, shaking water bath, TLC apparatus, UV lamp, magnetic stirrer, homogeniser etc. should be kept on the shelf as shown in Figure 3.1.

2. Instrument Room

This room should be kept neat and clean, as most of the sophisticated instruments are kept in it. It should be air-conditioned to make it dust-free and to reduce humidity as well as to avoid high ambient temperatures. Otherwise, accumulation of dust particles on and inside the instruments as well as exposure to high room temperatures decreases the longevity of the instruments. At the same time, high humid conditions lead to the rusting of their metallic components and fungal growth on optical parts, such as microscope lenses and phototubes of spectrophotometers. The instruments to be kept on the floor of the room include fridge, refrigerated centrifuge and ultracentrifuge. Other equipments, such as single-pan precision balance, Quebec colony counter, electronic colony counter, particle counter, electrophoresis apparatus, UV-cum-visible double beam spectrophotometer, computer, gas chromatography (GC), high performance liquid chromatography (HPLC), pH meter, trinocular research microscope with photomicrographic attachment, projection microscope, fluorescence microscope, dark-field microscope, phase-contrast microscope and PCR thermocycler should be arranged on a continuous concrete shelf projecting from the wall as shown in Figure 3.1.

3. Stock Culture Room

In routine microbiological analysis, very often it is required to isolate different types of bacteria in samples, to maintain the isolated bacteria as pure cultures and to identify them in subsequent days by performing several tests. After identification, it is required to compare them with standard pure cultures of the same species obtained from international standard microbiology laboratories such as, American Type Culture Collection (ATCC) of the USA; National Collection of Type Cultures (NCTC) of England and Pasteur Culture Collection (PCC) of France. These laboratories maintain and supply the standard pure cultures of known bacteria. If a pure culture of unknown bacteria is found to differ from similar standard pure cultures of known bacteria in morphology, staining reactions, biochemical reactions and serological tests, then it is sent to the international standard laboratories. After thorough testing in these laboratories, if it is found to differ from the known bacteria, then it is declared 'new' and is published in the International Journal of Systematic Bacteriology of the American Society of Microbiologists. It is given a new name (a new genera, or new species or new strain) based on its closeness to the known bacteria.

The standard pure cultures of known bacteria obtained from the international laboratories are maintained in the stock culture room. Isolated pure cultures of unknown bacteria (stock cultures) are also maintained in this room for further identification. Great care is taken in this room, so that the pure cultures do not get contaminated with other bacteria, which, otherwise, would lead to erroneous results.

4. Electron Microscopy Chamber

The electron microscope is installed in this room and the room is air-conditioned.

5. Inoculation Chamber

This room is meant for inoculation of bacteria *i.e.* transfer of bacteria from one container to another. Sometimes, unwanted microbes, usually floating in air on dust particles, may enter into the containers and contaminate the pure stock culture as well as the inoculated ones. To overcome this, the room is kept extremely hygienic. The walls should be plastic-painted and the room should be air-conditioned.

There should be a laminar flow chamber with gas connection, for inoculation of bacteria. A bottle of disinfectant solution, a sponge pad and a dispose jar should be kept beside the laminar flow chamber as in case of tables in the main lab.

6. Store Room

The store room should be closed from all sides with entrance into the main lab. There should be no window; otherwise the chemicals may get spoiled. There should be a number of concrete shelves for storage of chemicals, reagents, glasswares and other such items. The room should not be opened unless needed. The chemicals should be arranged alphabetically on the shelves for easy location.

7. Laboratory Animal House

Laboratory animals, such as guinea pig and rabbit are required for *in-vivo*[1] (in natural condition) studies as well as to get blood. These animals are reared in the animal house located slightly away from the main building. The house is designed in such a way that it is well-ventilated and can be easily cleaned daily. This keeps the room hygienic and the animals remain disease-free.

8. Store for Animal Feeds, Medicines etc.

It is a small room adjacent to the animal house where animal feeds, medicines and other such items required for rearing the animals are stored.

9. Chamber of the Laboratory Head

This room is meant for the head of the unit. It should have excellent official interior decoration, which should be maintained properly.

10. Staff Room

This room is meant for the scientists and other research personnel.

11. Office Room

This room is meant for the administrative staff of the laboratory.

12. Library-cum-Reading Room

In this room the books should be kept on shelves or inside glass-fitted cupboards (almirahs). There should be a catalogue in wooden box for easy reference. Computer-assisted cataloguing should also be done. Recent journals should be displayed on slanting display boards. Tables and chairs should be arranged for reading inside the library.

13. Seminar Hall-cum-Display Room

The seminar hall should be furnished with required furniture. Besides, there should be a black board, a projection screen, an LCD projector, an overhead projector, a slide projector, an epidiascope, video equipments and audio systems. Important charts, diagrams, photos, particularly those highlighting the achievements of the laboratory and ongoing research works should be displayed on the walls. The windows should have deep colour curtain to make the room dark, when required for visual presentations.

14. Toilets

The chamber of the head of the laboratory, office room, staff room and seminar hall should have separate toilets in addition to a common toilet.

15. Garage

There should be a garage behind the building for parking of the vehicles, so as to avoid erratic parking. The space surrounding the building should have lawns with tall plants like deodar or pine near the boundary walls.

---

1 *in-vivo*: In natural condition *e.g.* in animals, in pond water etc.

in-vitro: In controlled conditions in laboratory *e.g.* on agar plates, in tissue cultures etc.

B. Equipments

Experiment 2

***Aim*: To study the working principle and operation of equipments used in microbiology laboratory.**

A modern microbiology laboratory should be furnished with the following equipments. An asterisk,*, indicates that the equipment is not essential in an ordinary laboratory for undergraduate courses.

1. Hot Air Oven for Sterilisation

It is used for sterilisation of glasswares, such as test tubes, pipettes and petri dishes. Such dry sterilisation is done only for glasswares. Liquid substances, such as prepared media and saline solutions cannot be sterilised in oven, as they lose water due to evaporation. The glasswares are sterilised at 180°C for 3 hours. An oven (Figure 3.2) has a thermostat-control, using which the required constant temperature can be obtained by trial and error. The thermostat dial reading is approximate and the exact temperature is read by introducing a thermometer into the oven or on a built-in L-shaped thermometer. In a modern oven (Figure 3.3), there is a digital temperature display and automatic temperature controller to set the desired temperature easily. Time is set by a digital timer. After loading the glasswares, the door is closed and oven switched on. The required temperature is set. After the oven attains the set temperature, the required time of sterilisation is set on the timer. The oven switches off automatically after the set time. The oven is opened, only after its temperature comes down near to room temperature. Otherwise, if the door is opened, while the inside of the oven is still very hot, cold air may rush in and crack the glasswares.

*2. Drying Oven

For preparation of certain reagents, the glasswares, after proper cleaning and rinsing with distilled water, are required to be dried. They are dried inside the drying oven at 100°C till the glasswares dry up completely.

3. Autoclave

Autoclave is the nucleus of a microbiology laboratory. It is used not only to sterilise liquid substances such as prepared media and saline (diluent) solutions, but also to sterilise glasswares, when required. It has the same working principle as a domestic pressure cooker. The maximum temperature that can be obtained by boiling water in an open container is 100°C (boiling point of water). This temperature is sufficient to kill only the non-spore formers, but it is difficult to kill the spore-forming bacteria at this temperature, as they escape by forming heat resistant spores. It takes very long time to kill the spores at this temperature. On the other hand, when water is boiled in a closed container, due to increased pressure inside it, the boiling point elevates and steam temperature much beyond 100°C can be obtained. This high temperature is required to kill all the bacteria including the heat resistant spore-formers. Steam temperature increases with increase in steam pressure (Table 3.1).

Table 3.1: Temperatures attainable at different steam pressures

Steam Pressure (Pounds/inch^2 or psi)	*Temperature (°C)*
0 (free-flowing steam)	100
10	115
15	**121**
20	126
25	130

In operating a standard vertical autoclave, (Figure 3.4) sufficient water is poured into it. If water is too less, the bottom of the autoclave gets dried during heating and further heating damages it. If it has an in-built water heating element, (Figure 3.5) water level should be maintained above the element. On the other hand, if there is too much water, it takes long time to reach the required temperature. The

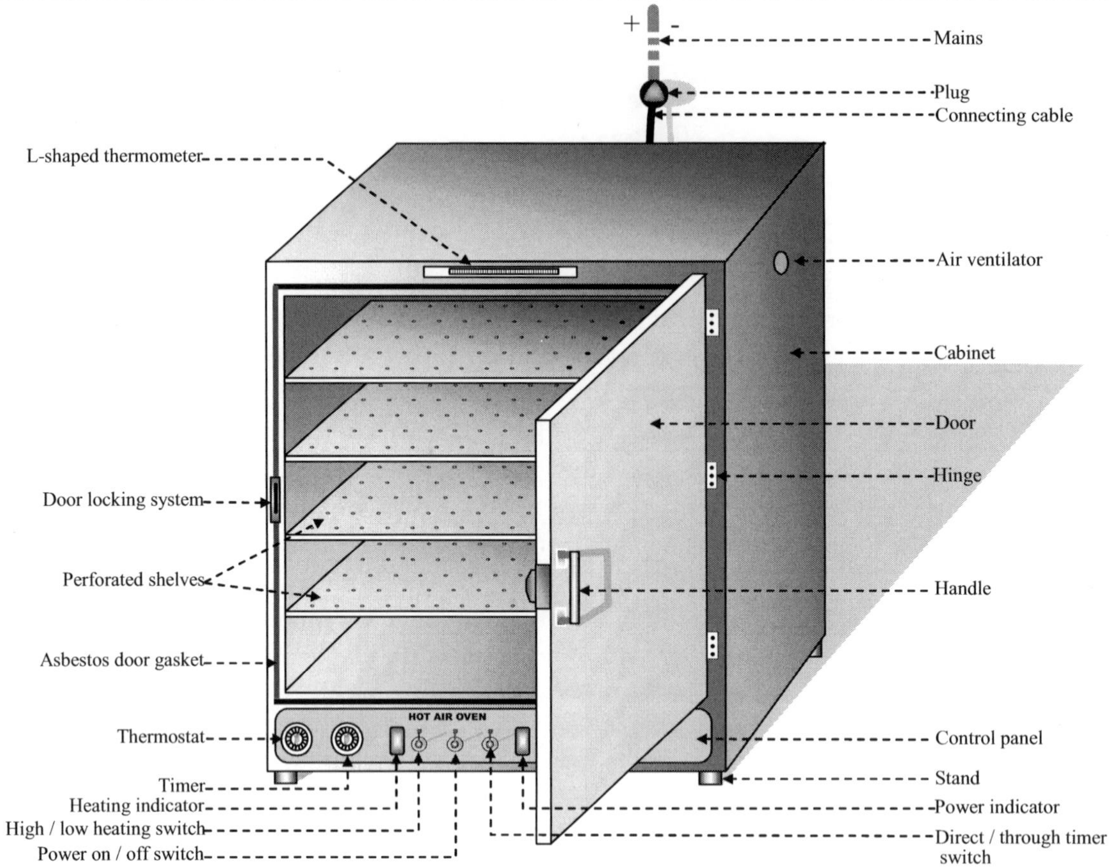

1. **Mains:** It is the source of electric current for the equipment. The oven runs using alternating current (AC) supplied through a three-ply cable. The three wires are phase (+), neutral (-) and earthing (E). The earthing helps in the safe operation of the oven against electric shock due to any short-circuit in the oven.
2. **Plug:** A three-pin plug (15 ampere capacity) provides non-sparking interface between the oven and the mains.
3. **Connecting cable:** A three-ply cable connects the mains with the oven.
4. **Air ventilator:** Air ventilator is a port (hole), through which the moisture-laden air escapes out from the oven.
5. **Cabinet:** It is the main body of the oven consisting of a double-walled cuboidal enclosure. The outer wall is made of mild steel sheets while the inner wall is made of anodised aluminium or stainless steel. From the inner wall, there are inward projections (battens) to support the sliding shelves. The space between the two walls is filled with glass wool to provide thermal insulation. The insulation minimises heat loss from the oven and reduces consumption of electric current, thereby working the oven efficiently.
6. **Door:** It is the insulated wall, which closes the insulated cabinet of the oven.
7. **Hinge:** It holds the door to the cabinet.
8. **Handle:** It is used to open the door by pulling.
9. **Control panel:** It is the panel or switchboard containing all the switches and indicators, with which the functions of the oven can be controlled.
10. **Stand:** It supports the total weight of the oven along with its contents.
11. **Power indicator:** It indicates supply of electric current to the oven by glowing.
12. **Direct / through timer switch:** This switch gives option to operate the oven directly or through the timer. In case of direct operation, the oven has to be switched off after the required time. Through timer option operates the oven through the timer, which starts functioning and switches off the oven after the set time.
13. **Power on / off switch**: It controls the entry of electric current into the oven.
14. **High/low heating switch**: High heating is done initially to quickly heat the oven near to the desired temperature, after which the low heating is done throughout the operation period to maintain the high temperature.
15. **Heating indicator:** It glows when the heating cycle goes on and the heating elements heat the oven.
16. **Timer:** It is used to set the required time, after which the oven switches off automatically.
17. **Thermostat:** It is used to set the temperature required. After the set temperature is reached, it automatically maintains the oven at that temperature constantly by alternate heating and no-heating cycles. During the heating phase, the heating elements heat the oven. During the no-heating phase, heating by these elements is discontinued and the oven is allowed to cool by radiating heat to the surrounding.
18. **Asbestos door gasket:** It provides an almost airtight seal between the cabinet and the door, thereby preventing the outside air from entering into the cabinet. This ensures an isolated hot environment inside the oven, without being influenced by the outer environment.
19. **Perforated shelves:** The materials to be sterilised are kept on the shelves. The perforations ensure proper circulation of the hot air inside the oven. The shelves are removable.
20. **Door locking system:** It locks the door tightly to the cabinet.
21. **L-shaped thermometer:** It is fitted at the top panel of the oven. One of its arms having graduations for temperature reading, remains along the top panel, so that the temperature can be easily read and the other arm, which has the mercury bulb at its end, remains protruded slightly into the oven.

Figure 3.2: A conventional hot air oven

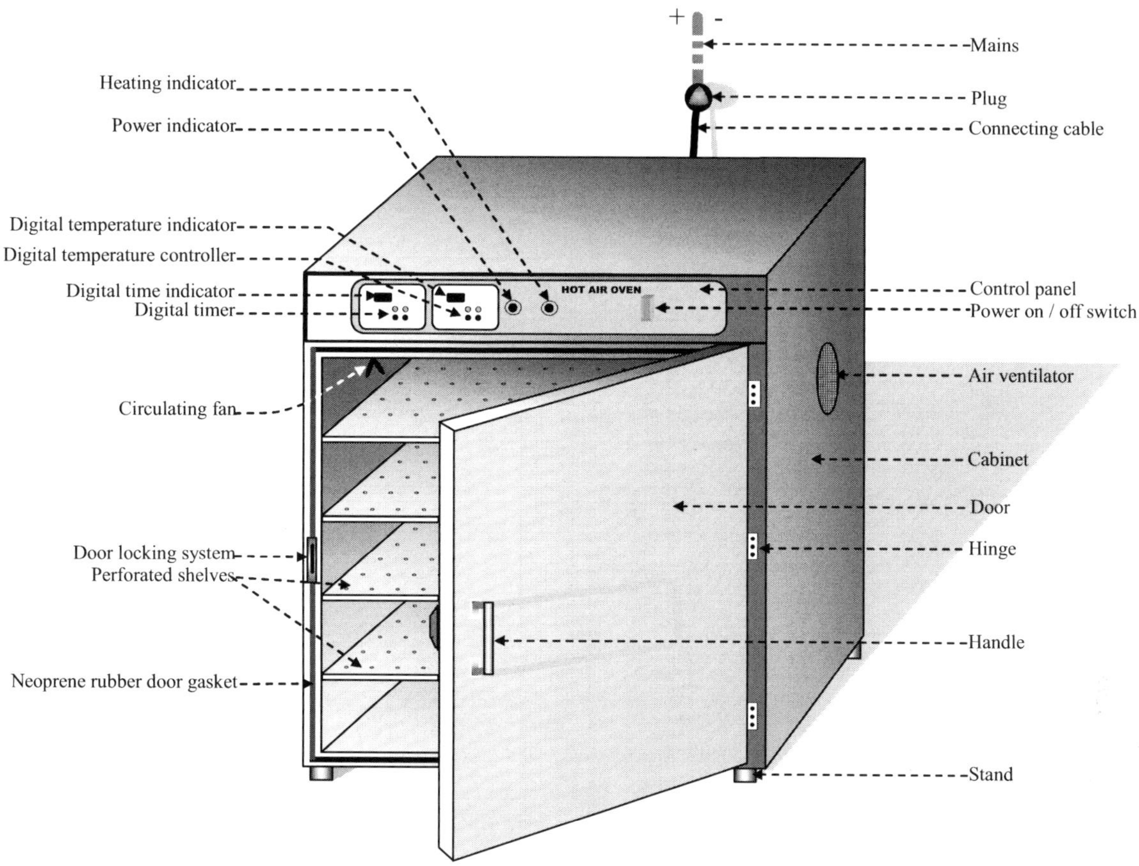

1. **Mains:** It is the source of electric current for the equipment. The oven runs using alternating current (AC) supplied through a three-ply cable. The three wires are phase (+), neutral (-) and earthing (E). The earthing helps in the safe operation of the oven against electric shock due to any short-circuit in the oven.
2. **Plug:** A three-pin plug (15 ampere capacity) provides non-sparking interface between the oven and the mains.
3. **Connecting cable:** A three-ply cable connects the mains with the oven.
4. **Control panel:** It is the panel or switchboard containing all the switches and indicators, with which the functions of the oven can be controlled.
5. **Power on / off switch**: It controls the entry of electric current into the oven.
6. **Air ventilator :** Air ventilator is a port (hole), through which the moisture-laden air escapes out from the oven.
7. **Cabinet:** It is the main body of the oven consisting of a double-walled cuboidal enclosure. The outer wall is made of mild steel sheets while the inner wall is made of stainless steel. From the inner wall, there are inward projections (battens) to support the sliding shelves. The space between the two walls is filled with glass wool to provide thermal insulation. The insulation minimises heat loss from the oven and reduces consumption of electric current, thereby working the oven efficiently.
8. **Door:** It is the insulated wall, which closes the insulated cabinet of the oven.
9. **Hinge:** It holds the door to the cabinet.
10. **Handle:** It is used to open the door by pulling.
11. **Stand:** It supports the total weight of the oven along with its contents.
12. **Neoprene rubber door gasket:** It provides an almost airtight seal between the cabinet and the door, thereby preventing the outside air from entering into the cabinet. This ensures an isolated hot environment inside the oven, without being influenced by the outer environment.
13. **Perforated shelves:** The materials to be sterilised are kept on the shelves. The perforations ensure proper circulation of the hot air inside the oven. The shelves are removable.
14. **Door locking system:** It locks the door tightly to the cabinet.
15. **Circulating fan:** It is a small fan fitted inside the cabinet, which circulates the hot air inside the oven, thereby helping in uniform distribution of temperature throughout the oven.
16. **Digital timer:** It is used to set the required time, after which the oven switches off automatically.
17. **Digital time indicator:** It digitally displays the time left to reach the set (required) time.
18. **Digital temperature controller:** It is a microprocessor based PID digital temperature controller used to set the temperature required. After the set temperature is reached, it automatically maintains the oven at that temperature constantly. The oven maintains the temperature by alternate heating and no-heating cycles. During the heating phase, the heating elements heat the oven. During the no-heating phase, heating by these elements is discontinued and the oven is allowed to cool by radiating heat to the surrounding.
19. **Digital temperature indicator:** It digitally displays the actual temperature inside the oven throughout its period of operation.
20. **Power indicator:** It indicates supply of electric current to the oven by glowing.
21. **Heating indicator:** The heating indicator glows when the heating cycle goes on and the heating elements heat the oven.

Figure 3.3: A modern hot air oven

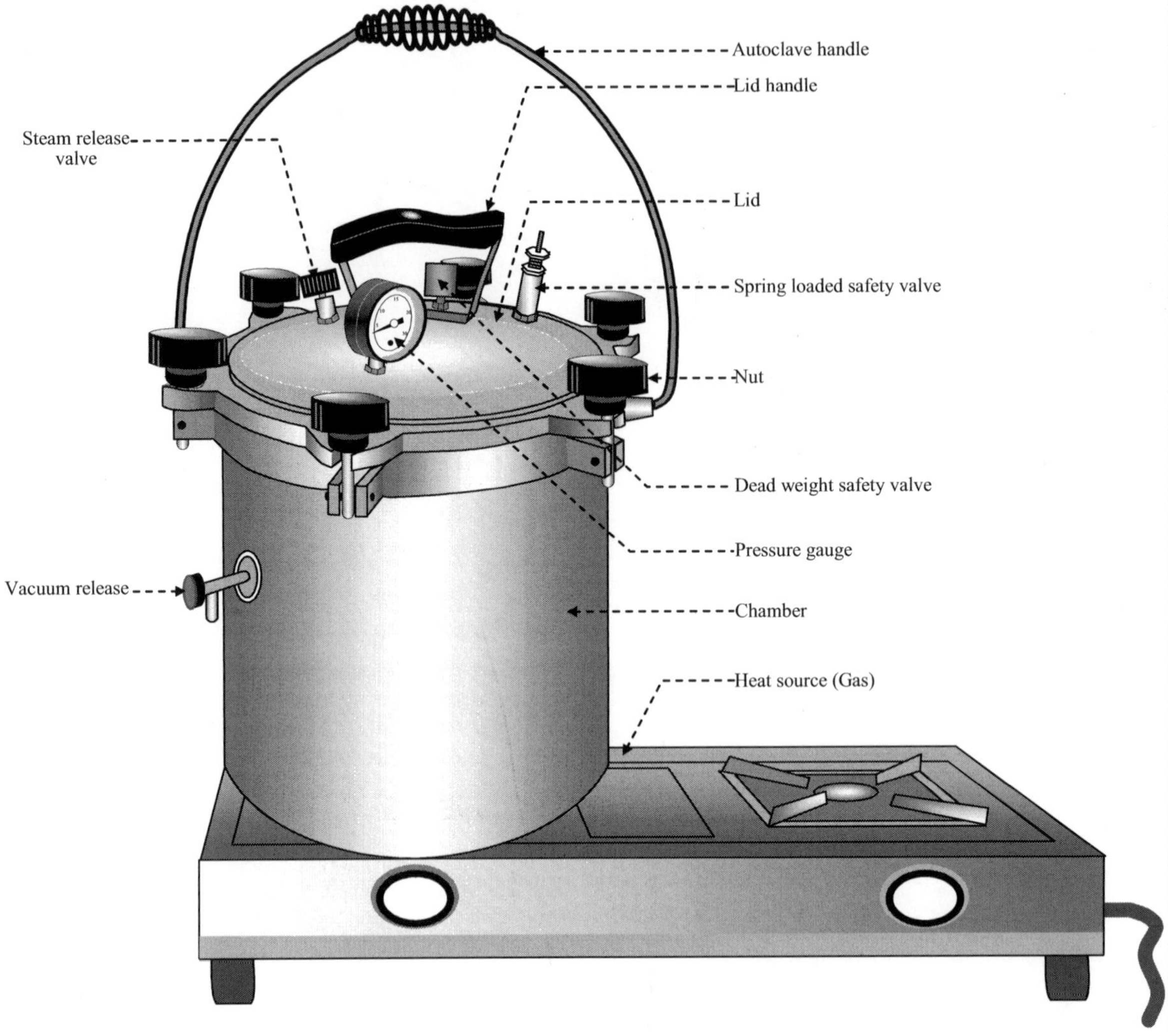

1. **Autoclave handle:** It is a metal rod bent to a half circle and hinged to the top of the chamber. It is used to move the chamber whenever required.
2. **Lid handle:** It is an insulated handle used to lift the lid and separate it from the chamber.
3. **Lid:** It is the cover, which closes the chamber of the autoclave. It is made of heavy gauge aluminium. A neoprene rubber gasket provides airtight seal between the chamber and the lid, thereby preventing leakage of steam to outside from the autoclave.
4. **Spring loaded safety valve:** It allows steam to escape, in case the pressure inside the autoclave becomes very high beyond the limit. Thus, it prevents bursting of the autoclave and thereby, helps in its safety.
5. **Nut:** These help in holding the lid tightly on the chamber so as to make it airtight and prevent leakage of steam from the autoclave to outside. These nuts are tightened manually after keeping the lid in position. Opposite nuts must be tightened simultaneously so as to make the autoclave perfectly airtight.
6. **Dead weight safety valve:** It blows out in case the pressure inside the autoclave becomes very high beyond the limit. Thus, it prevents bursting of the autoclave and thereby helps in the safety of the autoclave. It occurs when the pressure inside the autoclave goes beyond the capacity of the spring loaded safety valve.
7. **Pressure gauge**: It indicates the steam pressure inside the chamber.
8. **Chamber:** It is the main body of the autoclave, in which water is heated by an external heating source (LPG gas or electric heater) to produce steam. In the chamber, the materials to be sterilised are kept and sterilised at a steam pressure of 15 psi (121°C) for 15 minutes. It is made of heavy gauge aluminium. A stand is put at the bottom of the chamber on which the materials are to be kept. Pressure is adjustable from 10-20 psi. For safety reasons, all pressure vessels are tested hydraulically upto 40 psi.
9. **Vacuum release valve (Vacuum breaker):** It breaks the vacuum, if formed, inside the chamber due to condensation of steam when the hot autoclave is allowed to cool to room temperature in closed airtight condition.
10. **Steam release valve:** It is the knob, which is rotated to release steam from the chamber to outside after the sterilisation process. Using this knob, air is also allowed to escape from the chamber before sterilisation so that steam completely fills the chamber.
11. **Heat source:** Usually the external heat source is either gas or electric heater. In some portable autoclaves, in addition, there is an in-built electric heating system. In these autoclaves, a heating element is fixed on the wall of the chamber towards the bottom. It always remains submerged under water and heats it to generate steam.

Figure 3.4: A portable externally-heated autoclave

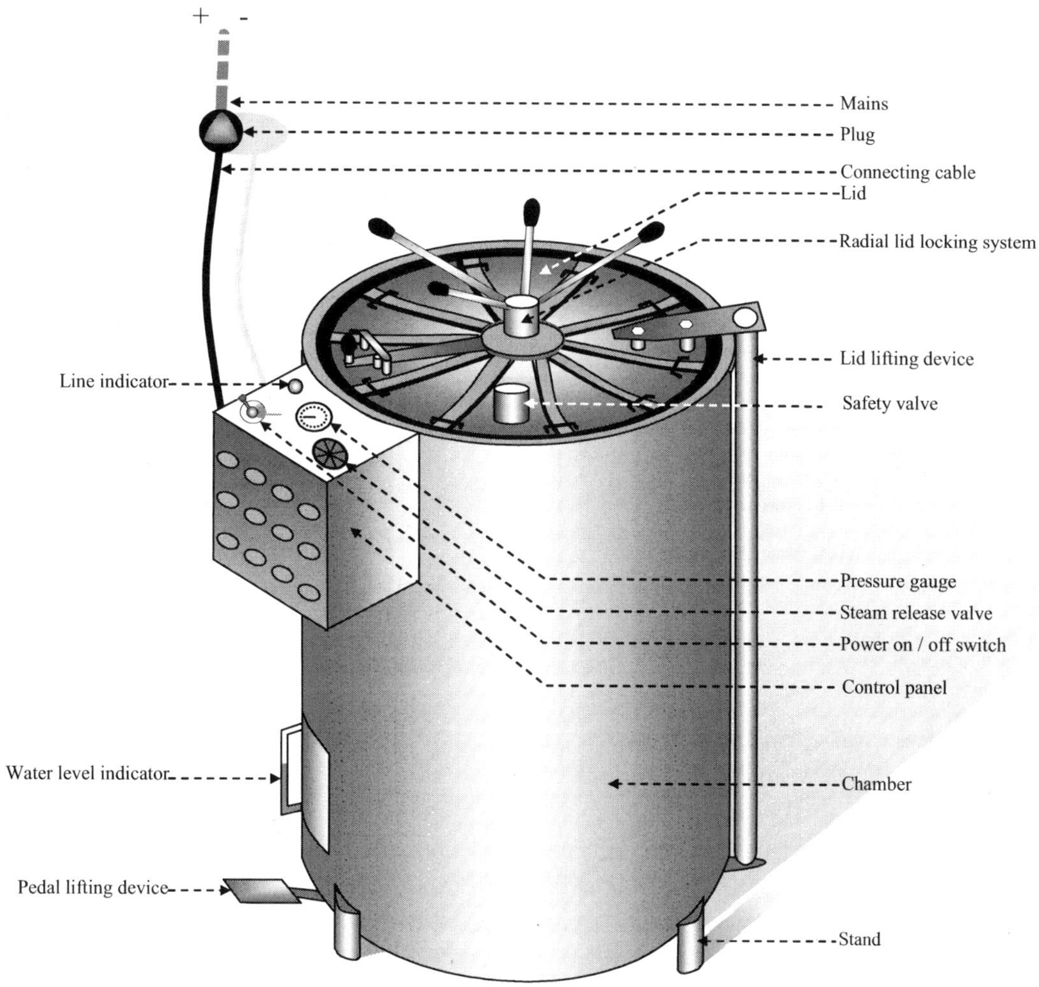

1. **Mains:** It is the source of electric current for the equipment. The autoclave runs using alternating current (AC) supplied through a three-ply cable. The three wires are phase (+), neutral (-) and earthing (E). The earthing helps in the safe operation of the autoclave against electric shock due to any short-circuit in the autoclave.
2. **Plug:** A three-pin plug (15 ampere capacity) provides non-sparking interface between the autoclave and the mains.
3. **Connecting cable:** A three-ply cable connects the mains with the autoclave.
4. **Lid:** It is the heavy gauge stainless steel cover, which closes the chamber of the autoclave. A neoprene rubber gasket provides airtight seal between the chamber and the lid, thereby preventing leakage of steam from the autoclave to outside.
5. **Radial lid locking system:** It locks the lid tightly to the chamber.
6. **Lid lifting device:** It helps in lifting the heavy lid by pressing the paddle on the opposite side.
7. **Safety valve:** It blows out, in case the pressure inside the autoclave becomes very high beyond the limit. Thus, it prevents bursting of the autoclave and thereby, helps in its safety.
8. **Pressure gauge :** It indicates the steam pressure inside the chamber.
9. **Steam release valve :** It is the knob, which is rotated to release steam from the chamber to outside after the sterilisation process. Using this knob air is also allowed to escape from the chamber before sterilisation so that steam completely fills the chamber.
10. **Power on / off switch**: It controls the entry of electric current into the autoclave.
11. **Control panel:** It is the panel or switchboard containing all the switches and indicators, with which the functions of the autoclave can be controlled.
12. **Chamber:** It is the main body of the autoclave consisting of a two-layered cylindrical enclosure. The space between the two layers is filled with glass wool to provide thermal insulation. Water is heated in this chamber by electric heating elements to produce steam. The insulation minimises heat loss from the autoclave and reduces consumption of electric current, thereby working the autoclave efficiently. In the chamber, the materials to be sterilised are kept and sterilised at a steam pressure of 15 psi (121°C) for 15 minutes. It is made of heavy gauge stainless steel. It is made leak proof by argon arc wielding, so as make the autoclave airtight during sterilisation. Pressure is adjustable from 10-20 psi. For safety reasons, all pressure vessels are tested hydraulically upto 40 psi.
13. **Stand:** It supports the total weight of the autoclave along with its contents.
14. **Pedal lifting device:** It is a pedal, which is pressed by leg to lift the heavy lid by the lid lifting device located on the opposite side.
15. **Water level indicator:** The level of water must remain sufficiently above the heating element. If water level goes down too much exposing the heating elements, dry heating damages them. The water level indicator indicates the level of water inside the autoclave, so that water can be poured into the autoclave before the heating elements get exposed
16. **Line indicator:** It indicates supply of electric current to the autoclave by glowing.

Figure 3.5: A conventional vertical autoclave

materials to be sterilised are covered with craft paper and arranged on an aluminum or wooden frame kept on the bottom of the autoclave, otherwise if the materials remain half-submerged or floating, they tumble during boiling and water may enter. The autoclave is closed perfectly airtight only keeping the steam release valve open. Then, it is heated over flame or by the in-built heating element. Air inside the autoclave should be allowed to escape completely through this valve. When water vapour is seen to escape through the valve, it is closed. Temperature and pressure inside goes on increasing. The pressure increase is observed on the pressure dial. Usually sterilisation is done at 121°C (a pressure of 15 pounds per square inch *i.e.* 15 psi) for 15 minutes. The required time is considered from the point, when the required temperature-pressure is attained. Once required temperature-pressure is attained, it is maintained by controlling the heating source. After the specified time (15 minutes), heating is discontinued and steam release valve slightly opened. If fully opened immediately, due to sudden fall in pressure, liquids may spill out from the containers. Gradually, the steam release is opened more and more, so as to allow all steam to escape. The autoclave is opened only after the pressure drops back to normal atmospheric pressure (0 psi). The autoclave should never be opened, when there is still pressure inside. The hot sterilised materials are removed by holding them with a piece of clean cloth or asbestos-coated hand gloves.

In case of a steam-jacketed horizontal autoclave, a boiler produces the steam (Figure 3.6). It is released at a designated pressure, into the outer chamber (jacket). Air is allowed to escape and then its steam release valve is closed. The hot jacket heats the inner chamber, thereby heating the materials to be sterilised. This prevents condensation of steam on the materials. Now, steam under pressure is released from the jacket into the inner chamber and air is allowed to escape from it. Then, its steam release valve is closed. The steam under pressure in the inner chamber reaches temperatures in excess of 100°C, which can sterilise the materials kept inside it. The autoclave also has automatic shutting system *i.e.* unless temperature and pressure comes down near to room conditions, the door cannot be opened. Besides the pressure dial, it also has separate temperature dial to indicate the temperature inside the inner chamber. Moreover, the autoclave maintains the temperature and pressure automatically and switches off after the set time of sterilisation.

4. Microbiological Incubator

Profuse growth of microbes is obtained in the laboratory by growing them at suitable temperatures. This is done by inoculating the desired microbe into a suitable culture medium and then incubating it at the temperature optimum for its growth. Incubation is done in an incubator (Figure 3.7), which maintains a constant temperature specifically suitable for the growth of a specific microbe. As most of the microbes pathogenic to man grow profusely at body temperature of normal human being (*i.e.* 37°C), the usual temperature of incubation is 37°C. The incubator has a thermostat, which maintains a constant temperature, set according to requirement. The temperature reading on the thermostat is approximate. Accurate temperature can be seen on the thermometer fixed on the incubator. Exact temperature, as per requirement, is set by rotating the thermostat knob by trial and error and noting the temperature on the thermometer.

Most of the modern incubators (Figure 3.8) are programmable, which do not need trial and error temperature setting. Here, the operator sets the desired temperature and the required period of time. The incubator automatically maintains it accordingly. Moisture is supplied by placing a beaker of water in the incubator during the growth period. A moist environment retards the dehydration of the media and thereby, avoids spurious experimental results.

5. BOD Incubator (Low Temperature Incubator)

Some microbes are to be grown at lower temperatures for specific purposes. The BOD low temperature incubator (Figure 3.9), which can maintain temperatures from 50°C to as low as 2-3°C is used for incubation in such cases. The constant desired temperature is set by rotating the knob of the

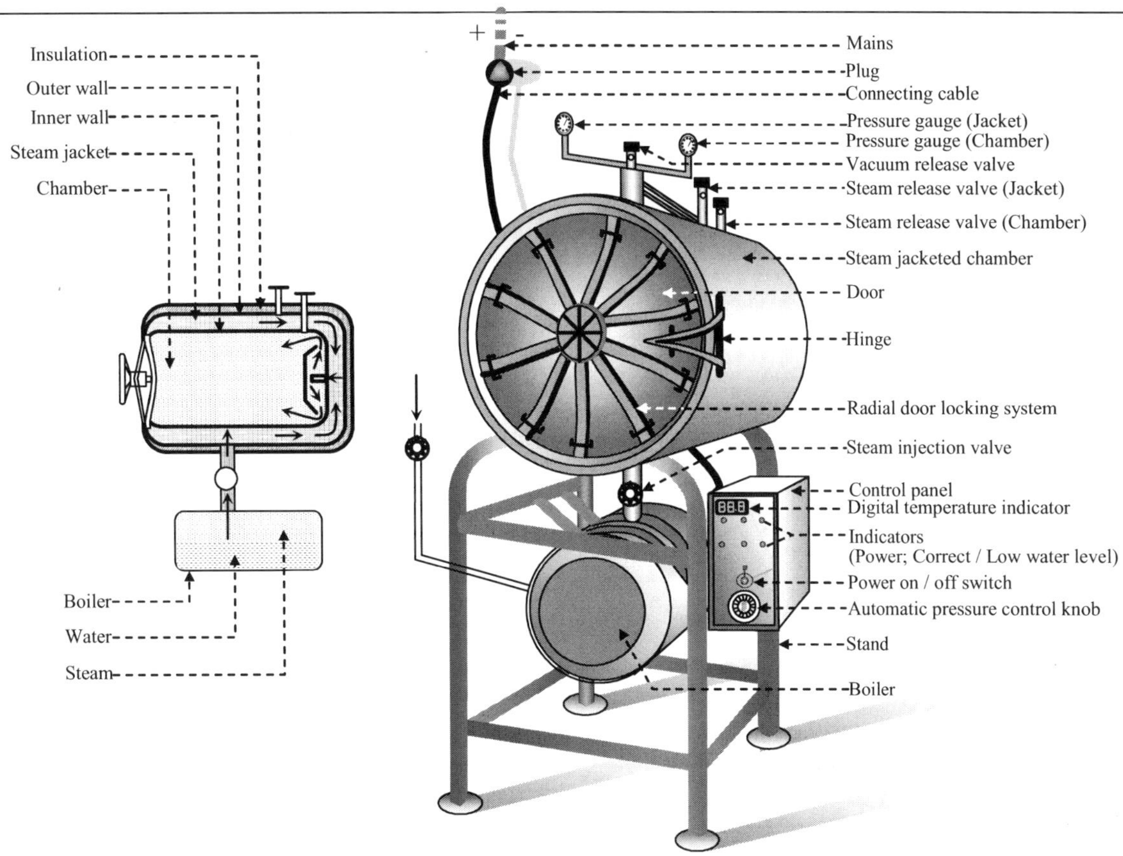

1. **Mains:** It is the source of electric current for the equipment. The autoclave runs using alternating current (AC) supplied through a three-ply cable. The three wires are phase (+), neutral (-) and earthing (E). The earthing helps in the safe operation of the autoclave against electric shock due to any short-circuit in the autoclave.
2. **Plug:** A three-pin plug (15 ampere capacity) provides non-sparking interface between the autoclave and the mains.
3. **Connecting cable:** A three-ply cable connects the mains with the autoclave.
4. **Pressure gauge (Jacket):** It indicates the steam pressure inside the outer chamber (jacket).
5. **Pressure gauge (Chamber):** It indicates the steam pressure inside the chamber.
6. **Vacuum release valve (Vacuum breaker):** It breaks the vacuum inside the chamber, in case vacuum is formed due to condensation of steam.
7. **Steam release valve (Jacket):** Steam that enters from the boiler into the jacket, removes the air present inside it through this valve. After the sterilisation process, steam present in the jacket is also allowed to escape to outside through this valve.
8. **Steam release valve (Chamber):** Steam that enters from the jacket into the chamber, removes the air present inside it through this valve. After the sterilisation process, steam present in the chamber is also allowed to escape to outside through this valve.
9. **Steam-jacketed chamber:** It is the main body of the autoclave, consisting of a double-walled cylindrical enclosure. The outer wall encloses the steam jacket. It is again two-layered and is made of heavy gauge stainless steel. The space between the two layers is filled with glass wool to provide thermal insulation. The insulation minimises heat loss from the autoclave and reduces consumption of electric current, thereby working the autoclave efficiently. The inner wall encloses the chamber, in which the materials to be sterilised are kept and sterilised at a steam pressure of 15 psi (121°C) for 15 minutes. It is made of heavy gauge stainless steel. The chamber and jacket are made leak proof by argon arc wielding, so as make the autoclave airtight during sterilisation. Pressure is adjustable from 10-20 psi. For safety reasons, all pressure vessels are tested hydraulically upto 40 psi.
10. **Door:** It is the heavy gauge stainless steel lid, which closes the chamber of the autoclave. A neoprene rubber door gasket provides airtight seal between the chamber and the door, thereby preventing leakage of steam to outside from the autoclave.
11. **Hinge:** It holds the door to the chamber.
12. **Radial door locking system:** It locks the door tightly to the chamber. It also has an automatic shutting system, which does not allow the door to be opened, unless the temperature and pressure comes down near to room conditions.
13. **Steam injection valve:** Steam enters from the boiler into the steam jacket through this valve.
14. **Control panel:** It is the panel or switchboard containing all the switches and indicators, with which the functions of the autoclave can be controlled.
15. **Digital temperature indicator:** It digitally displays the actual temperature inside the chamber throughout its period of operation.
16. **Indicators:** The power indicator indicates supply of electric current to the autoclave by glowing. The correct / low water level indicators glow according to the level of water in the boiler.
17. **Power on / off switch**: It controls the entry of electric current into the autoclave.
18. **Automatic pressure control knob:** It is used to set the pressure required. After the set pressure is reached, it automatically maintains the autoclave at that steam pressure constantly by alternate closing and opening of the valve, injecting steam into the chambers from the jacket.
19. **Stand:** It supports the total weight of the autoclave along with its contents.
20. **Boiler:** It is an airtight horizontal cylindrical enclosure, in which water is allowed to boil to produce steam. It is located below the steam jacketed chamber. It receives water form the water supply system and heats it by electrical heating elements. The steam produced goes to the steam jacket through the steam injection valve. It is fitted with water level indicator, pressure gauge, low water level cut-off device and automatic pressure control device.

Figure 3.6: A modern steam-jacketed horizontal autoclave

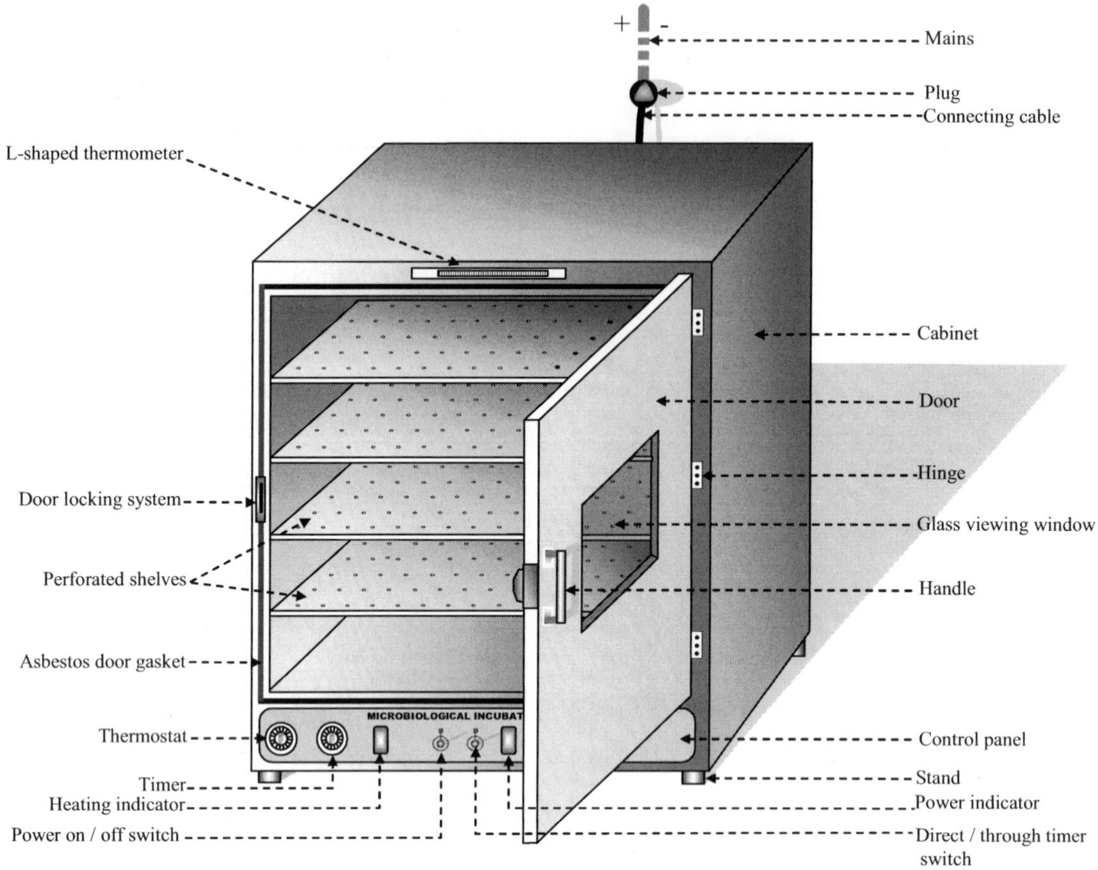

1. **Mains:** It is the source of electric current for the equipment. The incubator runs using alternating current (AC) supplied through a three-ply cable. The three wires are phase (+), neutral (-) and earthing (E). The earthing helps in the safe operation of the incubator against electric shock due to any short-circuit in the incubator.
2. **Plug:** A three-pin plug (15 ampere capacity) provides non-sparking interface between the incubator and the mains.
3. **Connecting cable:** A three-ply cable connects the mains with the incubator.
4. **Cabinet:** It is the main body of the incubator consisting of a double-walled cuboidal enclosure. The outer wall is made of mild steel sheets while the inner wall is made of anodised aluminium or stainless steel. From the inner wall, there are inward projections (battens) to support the sliding shelves. The space between the two walls is filled with glass wool to provide thermal insulation. The insulation minimises heat loss from the incubator and reduces consumption of electric current, thereby working the incubator efficiently.
5. **Door:** It is the insulated wall, which closes the insulated cabinet of the incubator.
6. **Hinge:** It holds the door to the cabinet.
7. **Glass viewing door:** It enables visualisation of the interior of the incubator during incubation without disturbing the interior environment.
8. **Handle:** It is used to open the door by pulling.
9. **Control panel:** It is the panel or switchboard containing all the switches and indicators, with which the functions of the incubator can be controlled.
10. **Stand:** It supports the total weight of the incubator along with its contents.
11. **Power indicator:** It indicates supply of electric current to the incubator by glowing.
12. **Direct / through timer switch:** This switch gives option to operate the oven directly or through the timer. In case of direct operation, the oven has to be switched off after the required time. Through timer option operates the oven through the timer, which starts functioning and switches off the oven after the set time.
13. **Power on / off switch**: It controls the entry of electric current into the incubator.
14. **Heating indicator:** The heating indicator glows when the heating cycle goes on and the heating elements heat the incubator.
15. **Timer:** It is used to set the required time, after which the incubator switches off automatically.
16. **Thermostat:** It is used to set the temperature required. After the set temperature is reached, it automatically maintains the incubator at that temperature constantly by alternate heating and no-heating cycles. During the heating phase, the heating elements heat the incubator. During the no-heating phase, heating by these elements is discontinued and the incubator is allowed to cool by radiating heat to the surrounding.
17. **Asbestos door gasket:** It provides an almost airtight seal between the cabinet and the door, thereby preventing the outside air from entering into the cabinet. This ensures an isolated hot environment inside the incubator without being influenced by the outer environment.
18. **Perforated shelves:** The microbes to be cultured, after inoculation to proper growth media, are kept on the shelves. The perforations ensure proper circulation of the hot air inside the incubator. The shelves are removable.
19. **Door locking system:** It locks the door tightly to the cabinet.
20. **L-shaped thermometer:** It is fitted at the top panel of the oven. One of its two arms, having graduations for temperature reading, remains along the top panel, so that the temperature can be easily read and the other arm, which has the mercury bulb at its end, remains protruded slightly into the chamber of the incubator.

Figure 3.7: A conventional microbiological incubator

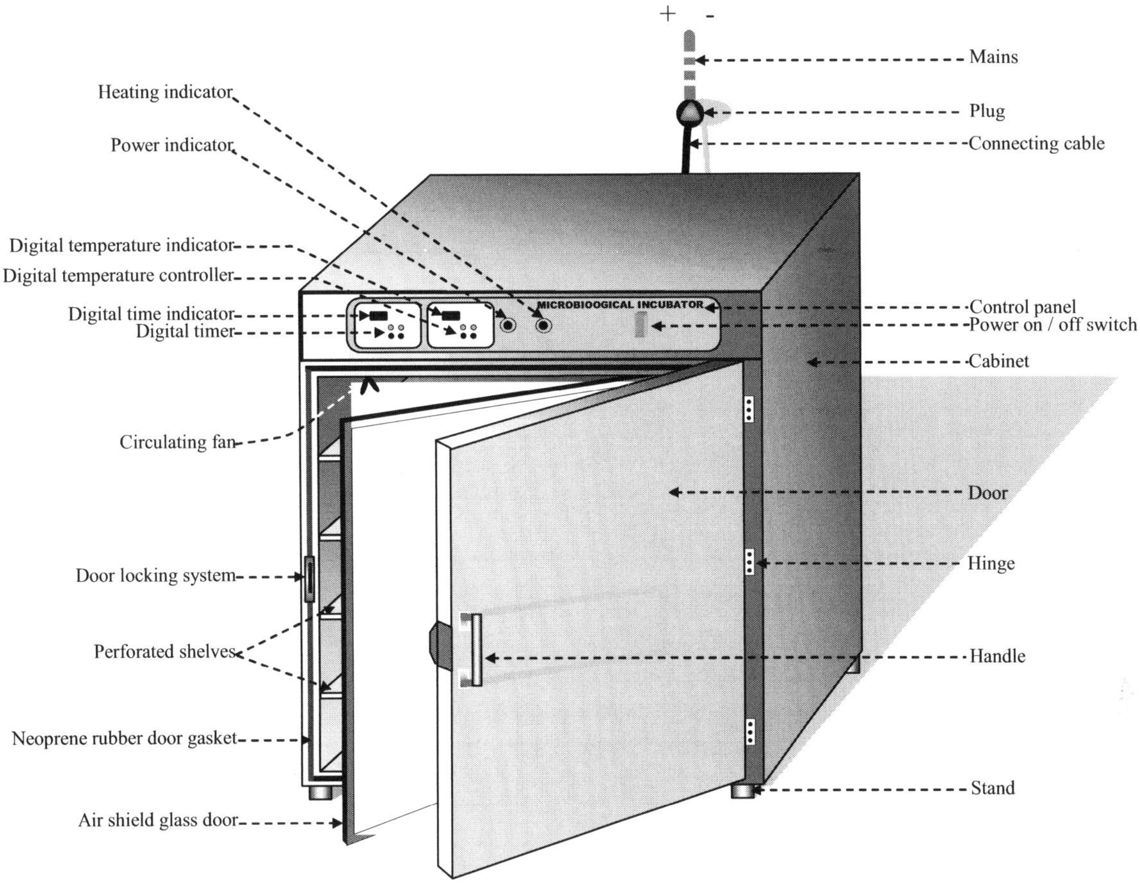

1. **Mains:** It is the source of electric current for the equipment. The incubator runs using alternating current (AC) supplied through a three-ply cable. The three wires are phase (+), neutral (-) and earthing (E). The earthing helps in the safe operation of the incubator against electric shock due to any short-circuit in the incubator.
2. **Plug:** A three-pin plug (15 ampere capacity) provides non-sparking interface between the incubator and the mains.
3. **Connecting cable:** A three-ply cable connects the mains with the incubator.
4. **Control panel:** It is the panel or switchboard containing all the switches and indicators, with which the functions of the incubator can be controlled.
5. **Power on / off switch**: It controls the entry of electric current into the incubator.
6. **Cabinet:** It is the main body of the incubator consisting of a double-walled cuboidal enclosure. The outer wall is made of mild steel sheets, while the inner wall is made of stainless steel. From the inner wall, there are inward projections (battens) to support the sliding shelves. The space between the two walls is filled with glass wool to provide thermal insulation. The insulation minimises heat loss from the incubator and reduces consumption of electric current, thereby working the incubator efficiently.
7. **Door:** It is the insulated wall, which closes the insulated cabinet of the incubator.
8. **Hinge:** It holds the door to the cabinet.
9. **Handle:** It is used to open the door by pulling.
10. **Stand:** It supports the total weight of the incubator along with its contents.
11. **Air shield glass door:** This glass door enables clear visualisation of the interior of the incubator during incubation and at the same time prevents draft of cool outside air from entering in and reducing its temperature below the set temperature.
12. **Neoprene rubber door gasket:** It provides an almost airtight seal between the cabinet and the door, thereby preventing the outside air from entering into the cabinet. This ensures an isolated hot environment inside the incubator without being influenced by the outer environment.
13. **Perforated shelves:** The microbes to be cultured, after inoculation to proper growth media, are kept on the shelves. The perforations ensure proper circulation of the hot air inside the incubator. The shelves are removable.
14. **Door locking system:** It locks the door tightly to the cabinet.
15. **Circulating fan:** It is a small fan fitted inside the cabinet, which circulates the hot air inside the incubator, thereby helping in uniform distribution of temperature throughout the incubator.
16. **Digital timer:** It is used to set the required time, after which the incubator switches off automatically.
17. **Digital time indicator:** It digitally displays the time left to reach the set (required) time.
18. **Digital temperature controller:** It is a microprocessor based PID digital temperature controller used to set the temperature required. After the set temperature is reached, it automatically maintains the incubator at that temperature constantly. The incubator maintains the temperature by alternate heating and no-heating cycles. During the heating phase, the heating elements heat the incubator. During the no-heating phase, heating by these elements is discontinued and the incubator is allowed to cool by radiating heat to the surrounding.
19. **Digital temperature indicator:** It digitally displays the actual temperature inside the incubator throughout its period of operation.
20. **Power indicator:** It indicates supply of electric current to the incubator by glowing.
21. **Heating indicator:** The heating indicator glows when the heating cycle goes on and the heating elements heat the incubator.

Figure 3.8: A modern microbiological incubator

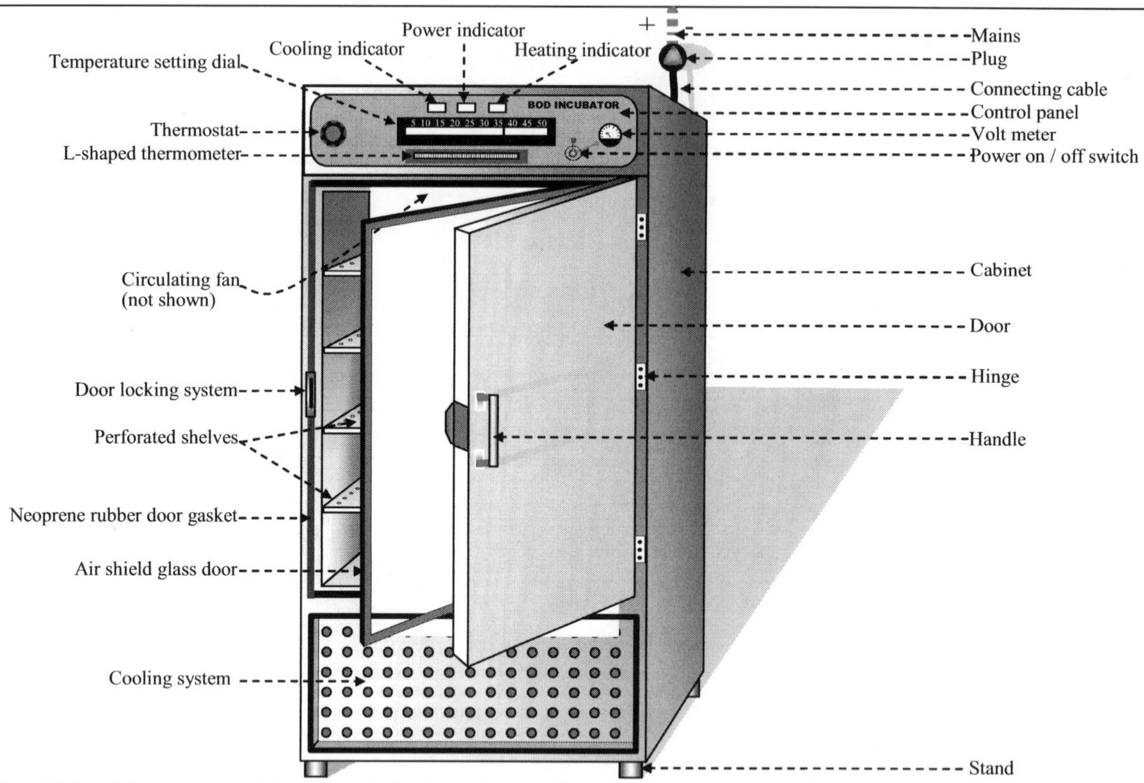

1. **Mains:** It is the source of electric current for the equipment. The BOD low temperature incubator runs using alternating current (AC) supplied through a three-ply cable. The three wires are phase (+), neutral (-) and earthing (E). The earthing helps in the safe operation of the incubator against electric shock due to any short-circuit in the incubator.
2. **Plug:** A three-pin plug (15 ampere capacity) provides non-sparking interface between the low temperature incubator and the mains.
3. **Connecting cable:** A three-ply cable connects the mains with the incubator.
4. **Control panel:** It is the panel or switchboard containing all the switches and indicators, with which the functions of the incubator can be controlled.
5. **Volt meter:** It indicates the voltage of the AC current going into the incubator.
6. **Power on / off switch**: It controls the entry of electric current into the incubator.
7. **Cabinet:** It is the main body of the incubator consisting of a double-walled cuboidal enclosure. The outer wall is made of mild steel sheets, while the inner wall is made of stainless steel. From the inner wall, there are inward projections (battens) to support the sliding shelves. The space between the two walls is filled with glass wool to provide thermal insulation. The insulation minimises heat loss from the incubator and reduces consumption of electric current, thereby working the incubator efficiently.
8. **Door:** It is the insulated wall, which closes the insulated cabinet of the incubator.
9. **Hinge:** It holds the door to the cabinet.
10. **Handle:** It is used to open the door by pulling.
11. **Stand:** It supports the total weight of the incubator along with its contents.
12. **Cooling system:** It reduces the temperature of the incubator, when it has to be maintained below the ambient temperature.
13. **Air shield glass door:** This glass door enables clear visualisation of the interior of the incubator during incubation and at the same time prevents draft of outside air from entering in and changing its temperature away from the set temperature.
14. **Neoprene rubber door gasket:** It provides an almost airtight seal between the cabinet and the door, thereby preventing the outside air from entering into the cabinet. This ensures an isolated environment inside the incubator without being influenced by the outer environment.
15. **Perforated shelves:** The microbes to be cultured, after inoculation to proper growth medium, are kept on the shelves. The perforations ensure proper circulation of the air inside the incubator. The shelves are removable.
16. **Door locking system:** It locks the door tightly to the cabinet.
17. **Circulating fan:** It is a small fan fitted inside the cabinet, which circulates the air inside the incubator, thereby helping in uniform distribution of temperature throughout the incubator.
18. **L-shaped thermometer:** It is fitted at the top panel of the incubator. One of its two arms, having graduations for temperature reading, remains along the top panel, so that the temperature can be easily read and the other arm, which has the mercury bulb at its end, remains protruded slightly into the chamber of the incubator.
19. **Thermostat:** It is used to set the temperature required. After the set temperature is reached, it automatically maintains the incubator at that temperature constantly. If the desired temperature is above the ambient temperature, then the incubator maintains it by alternate heating and no-heating cycles. During the heating phase, the heating elements heat the incubator. During the no-heating phase, heating by these elements is discontinued and the incubator is allowed to cool by radiating heat to the surrounding. On the other hand, if the desired temperature is below the ambient temperature, then the incubator maintains it by alternate refrigeration and no-refrigeration cycles. During the refrigeration phase, the cooling coils cool the incubator. During the no-refrigeration phase, cooling by these cooling coils is discontinued and the incubator is allowed to warm up by absorbing heat from the surrounding.
20. **Temperature setting dial:** When the thermostat is rotated to set the temperature, a needle moves on the temperature setting dial and indicates the set temperature.
21. **Cooling indicator:** The cooling indicator glows, when the refrigeration cycle goes on and the cooling coils cool the incubator.
22. **Power indicator:** It indicates supply of electric current to the incubator by glowing.
23. **Heating indicator:** The heating indicator glows, when the heating cycle goes on and the heating elements heat the incubator.

Figure 3.9: A conventional BOD low temperature incubator

thermostat. Rotation of the thermostat knob moves a needle on a dial showing approximate temperature. Exact required temperature is obtained, by rotating the knob finely by trial and error and noting the temperature on the thermometer fixed on the incubator.

Most of the modern BOD incubators (Figure 3.10) are programmable, which do not need trial and error temperature setting. Here, the operator sets the desired temperature and the required period of time. The incubator automatically maintains it accordingly.

6. Fridge (Refrigerator)

It serves as a repository for thermolabile chemicals, solutions, antibiotics, serums and biochemical reagents at cooler temperatures and even at sub-zero temperatures (at less than 0°C). Stock cultures of bacteria are also stored in it between sub-culturing periods. It is also used for the storage of sterilised media, so as to prevent their dehydration.

*7. Deep-fridge

It is used to store chemicals and preserve samples at very low sub-zero temperatures.

8. Electronic Top-pan Balance

It is used for weighing large quantities of media and other chemicals, where precise weighing is not of much importance.

9. Electronic Analytical Balance

It is used to weigh small quantities of chemicals and samples precisely and quickly.

10. Double-pan Analytical Balance

It is used to weigh chemicals and samples precisely. Weighing takes more time, for which it is used in emergency only.

11. Distilled Water Plant

Water is used in the preparation of media and reagents. If the media are prepared using tap water, the chemical impurities present in it may interfere with the growth of the microorganisms in the media. Moreover, the higher is the bacteria content of the media, the longer is the time required for their sterilisation and greater is the chance of survival of some bacteria. Distilled water, though not bacteria-free, contains less number of bacteria. That is why, it is preferred in the preparation of microbiological media. It is also used in the preparation of reagents, because the chemical impurities present in tap water may interfere with the proper functioning of the reagent chemicals. As manufacture of distilled water by Liebig condenser is a time-taking process, in most laboratories, it is prepared by 'distilled water plants'. Usually a distilled water plant is made of steel or brass. It is also called distilled water still. It has one inlet to be connected to the water tap and two outlets, one for distilled water to drop into a container and the other for the flow out of hot cooling water into the sink. The still is installed on the wall. It is heated by in-built electric heating elements (immersion heater). The still works efficiently, when the water in-flow is so adjusted that, the temperature of the cooling water flowing out from the still into the sink is neither too high nor too low *i.e.* warm water should flow out. The distilled water may contain traces of metals corroded from the steel or brass container. To get metal-free distilled water, glass distillation apparatus is used and still better is quartz distillation apparatus. However, for a microbiology laboratory, a steel or glass distillation apparatus is sufficient. For precision analyses, double- or triple- distilled water is used.

*12. Ultrapure Water Purification System

For precision analytical works, now-a-days, instead of using double- or triple-distilled water, micro-filtered water is used. In case of distilled water, there is chance that, few volatile substances present in the water get volatilised during heating of the water and subsequently get condensed into the distilled

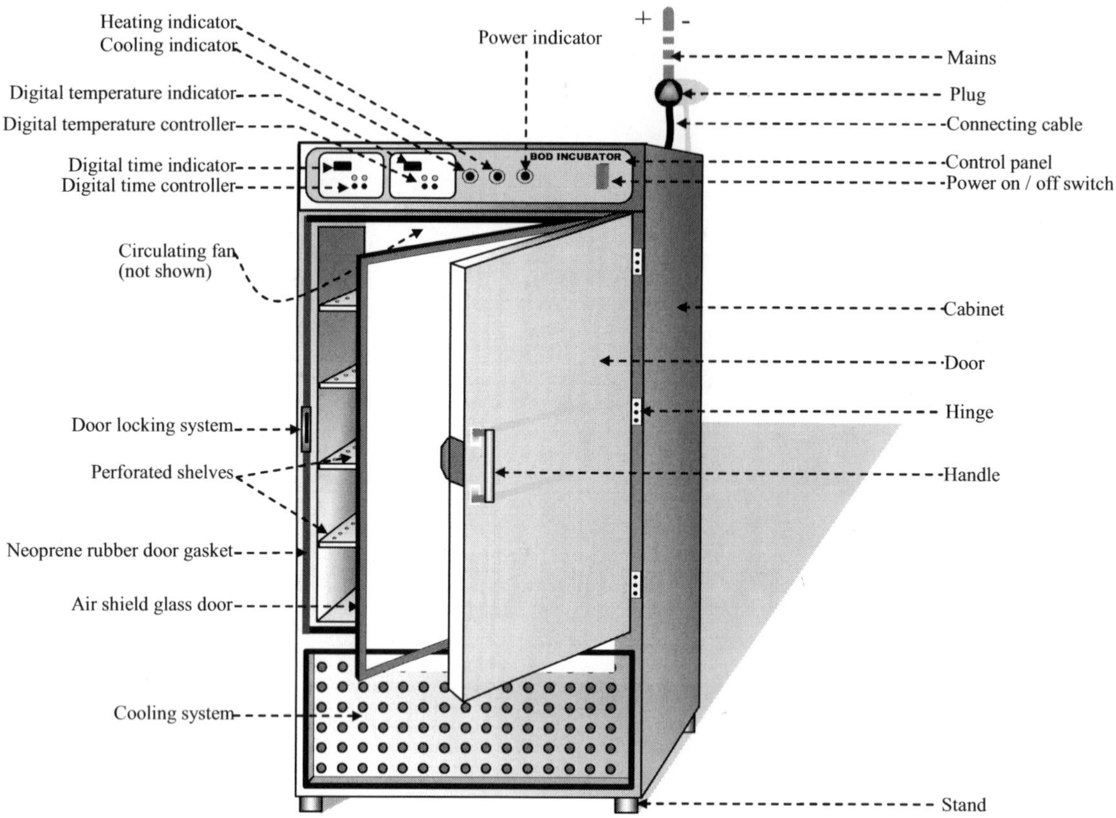

1. **Mains:** It is the source of electric current for the equipment. The BOD low temperature incubator runs using alternating current (AC) supplied through a three-ply cable. The three wires are phase (+), neutral (-) and earthing (E). The earthing helps in the safe operation of the incubator against electric shock due to any short-circuit in the incubator.
2. **Plug:** A three-pin plug (15 ampere capacity) provides non-sparking interface between the low temperature incubator and the mains.
3. **Connecting cable:** A three-ply cable connects the mains with the incubator.
4. **Control panel:** It is the panel or switchboard containing all the switches and indicators, with which the functions of the incubator can be controlled.
5. **Power on / off switch:** It controls the entry of electric current into the incubator.
6. **Cabinet:** It is the main body of the incubator consisting of a double-walled cuboidal enclosure. The outer wall is made of mild steel sheets, while the inner wall is made of stainless steel. From the inner wall, there are inward projections (battens) to support the sliding shelves. The space between the two walls is filled with glass wool to provide thermal insulation. The insulation minimises heat loss from the incubator and reduces consumption of electric current, thereby working the incubator efficiently.
7. **Door:** It is the insulated wall, which closes the insulated cabinet of the incubator.
8. **Hinge:** It holds the door to the cabinet.
9. **Handle:** It is used to open the door by pulling.
10. **Stand:** It supports the total weight of the incubator along with its contents.
11. **Cooling system:** It reduces the temperature of the incubator, when it has to be maintained below the ambient temperature.
12. **Air shield glass door:** This glass door enables clear visualisation of the interior of the incubator during incubation and at the same time prevents draft of outside air from entering in and changing its temperature away from the set temperature.
13. **Neoprene rubber door gasket:** It provides an almost airtight seal between the cabinet and the door, thereby preventing the outside air from entering into the cabinet. This ensures an isolated environment inside the incubator without being influenced by the outer environment.
14. **Perforated shelves:** The microbes to be cultured, after inoculation to proper growth medium, are kept on the shelves. The perforations ensure proper circulation of the air inside the incubator. The shelves are removable.
15. **Door locking system:** It locks the door tightly to the cabinet.
16. **Circulating fan:** It is a small fan fitted inside the cabinet, which circulates the hot air inside the incubator, thereby helping in uniform distribution of temperature throughout the incubator.
17. **Digital timer:** It is used to set the required time after which the incubator switches off automatically.
18. **Digital time indicator:** It digitally displays the time left to reach the set (required) time.
19. **Digital temperature controller:** It is used to set the temperature required. After the set temperature is reached, it automatically maintains the incubator at that temperature constantly. If the desired temperature is above the ambient temperature, then the incubator maintains it by alternate heating and no-heating cycles. During the heating phase, the heating elements heat the incubator. During the no-heating phase, heating by these elements is discontinued and the incubator is allowed to cool by radiating heat to the surrounding. On the other hand, if the desired temperature is below the ambient temperature, then the incubator maintains it by alternate refrigeration and no-refrigeration cycles. During the refrigeration phase, the cooling coils cool the incubator. During the no-refrigeration phase, cooling by these cooling coils is discontinued and the incubator is allowed to warm up by absorbing heat from the surrounding.
20. **Digital temperature indicator:** It digitally displays the actual temperature inside the incubator throughout its period of operation.
21. **Cooling indicator:** The cooling indicator glows, when the refrigeration cycle goes on and the cooling coils cool the incubator.
22. **Heating indicator:** The heating indicator glows, when the heating cycle goes on and the heating elements heat the incubator.
23. **Power indicator:** It indicates supply of electric current to the incubator by glowing.

Figure 3.10: A modern BOD low temperature incubator

water collected. Thus, there may be traces of such substances in the distilled water. To overcome this, ultrapure water is used. Here, water is allowed to pass through very fine microscopic pores, which retain the microscopic suspended particle including the microbes. Then, the water passes through two columns of ion exchange resins. The anion exchange resin adsorbs the cations present in the water, while the cation exchange resin adsorbs the anions. The water that comes out is extremely pure.

13. Homogeniser

For microbiological analysis, liquid samples are directly used, whereas solid samples have to be mixed thoroughly with a diluent (usually physiological saline), so as to get a homogenous suspension of bacteria. This suspension is assumed to contain bacteria homogenously. The mixing of solid samples and diluents is done by a homogeniser, in which a motor rotates an impeller with sharp blades at high speed inside the closed homogeniser cup containing the sample and the diluent. It has a speed regulator for controlling the speed of rotation of the impeller. In some laboratories mixing is done manually by sterilised pestle and mortar. In modern laboratories, a disposable bag is used, inside which the solid sample and liquid diluent are put aseptically and mixed mechanically by peristaltic action of a machine on the bag. This machine is called stomacher.

14. pH Meter

A pH meter is an instrument for determining the pH of liquid media, liquid samples and buffers. It has a glass pH electrode. When not in use, it should be kept half immersed in water contained in a small beaker and preferably be covered by a bell jar to avoid dust accumulation in the water and loss of water through evaporation. Before use, the meter is calibrated using two standard buffers of known pH. Usually buffers of pH 4.0, 7.0 and 9.2 are available commercially. The instrument is switched on and left for 30 minutes to warm up. The temperature calibration knob is rotated to the temperature of the solutions whose pH is to the measured. Then, the electrode is dipped into the buffer (pH 7.0). If the reading is not 7.00, the pH calibration knob is rotated till the reading is 7.00. Then, the electrode is dipped in another buffer (pH 4.0 or 9.2). If the reading is same as the pH of the buffer used, the instrument is working properly. Otherwise, the electrode is activated by dipping in 0.1 N HC1 for 24 hours. After calibration, the pH of samples is determined by dipping the electrode into them and noting the reading. Every time, before dipping into any solution, the electrode should be rinsed with distilled water. The samples should not contain any suspended sticky materials, which may form a coating on the tip of the electrode and reduce its sensitivity. The old model pH meters have double electrodes (one of them acting as reference electrode), while new models have single combined electrode. Moreover, to overcome the problem of temperature correction, now pH meters with automatic temperature correction are available. Here, another 'temperature electrode' is also put into the solution along with the pH electrode, which measures the temperature of the solution and automatically corrects the influence of temperature variations. Sophisticated pH meters have single gel electrode. Such electrodes have very little chance of breakage, as they are almost completely enclosed in a hard plastic casing except at the tip. The tip has both pH and temperature sensors. Moreover, they are easy to maintain, as they do not require constant dipping in distilled water, because the electrode tip is closed with a plastic cap containing saturated solution of potassium chloride, when not in use. However, in preparation of microbiological media, pH is determined by narrow-range pH papers and is adjusted to the required pH by adding acids or alkalis as required.

15. Hot Plate

Hot plate is used to heat chemicals and reagents. The hot plate is made of an iron plate, which gets heated by an electric heating element from below. The required degree of heating is obtained by a regulator.

16. Shaking Water Bath

Sometimes, heating at very precise temperatures is required. Such precise temperatures cannot be obtained in an incubator or oven, in which temperature fluctuates, though slightly. However, precise temperatures can be maintained in a water bath, which provides a stable temperature. A water bath consists of a container containing water, which is heated by electric heating elements. The required water temperature is obtained by increasing or decreasing the rate of heating by rotating the thermostat by trial and error. In a shaking water bath, the substance is heated at the required temperature and at the same time, it is shaken constantly. Shaking is done by a motor, which rotates and moves the containers to and fro in each rotation. The rate of shaking is again controlled by a regulator. Shaking agitates the substance and enhances the rate of the process. Most modern water baths are programmable and do not need trial and error temperature setting. A desired water temperature can be maintained over a desired period of time by programming accordingly. It is used for cultivation of bacteria in broth medium at a specific temperature.

17. Quebec Colony Counter

In enumeration of bacteria in samples, it is assumed that a single bacterium gives rise to a single visible colony, when grown on a plate of solidified nutrient medium. Thus, by counting the number of colonies, the number of bacteria in a sample can be estimated. Sometimes, colonies are very small and too much crowded making it difficult to count. Counting becomes easy, when a mechanical hand counter, called Quebec colony counter (Figure 3.11), is used. It divides the plate into several square divisions and the colonies are magnified 1.5 times by a magnifying glass, which makes counting easy.

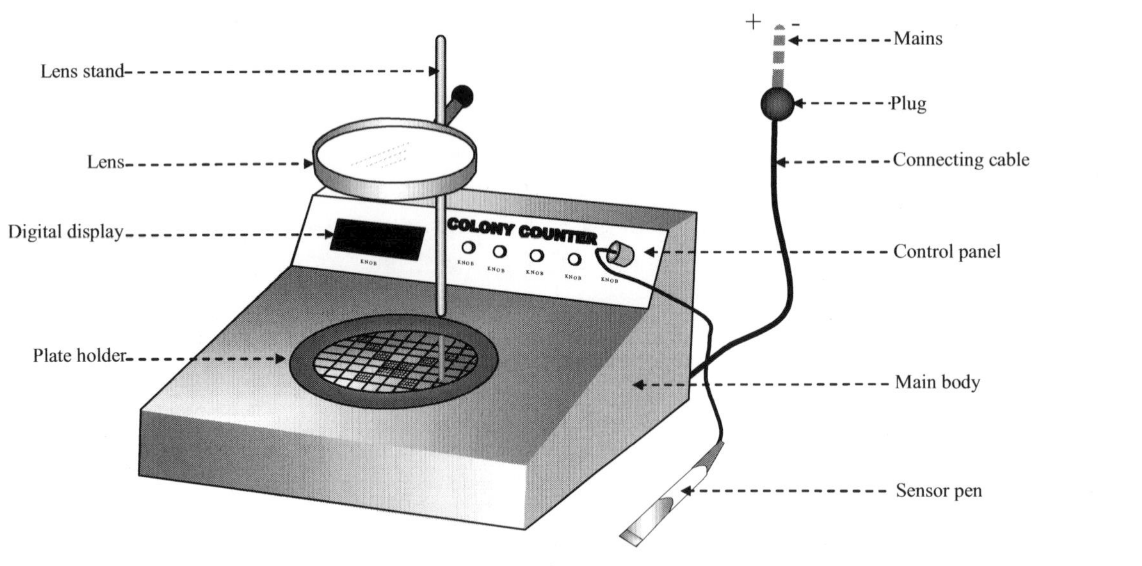

1. **Mains:** It is the source of electric current for the colony counter. The equipment runs using alternating current (AC) supplied through a three-ply cable. The three wires are phase (+), neutral (-) and earthing (E). The earthing helps in the safe operation of the equipment against electric shock due to any short-circuit.
2. **Plug:** A three-pin plug (5 ampere capacity) provides non-sparking interface between the equipment and the mains.
3. **Connecting cable:** A three-ply cable connects the mains with the equipment.
4. **Control panel**: It is the panel or switchboard containing all the switches and indicators with which the functions of the colony counter can be controlled.
5. **Main body:** It encloses the parts of the equipment. It is made of metal sheets.
6. **Sensor pen:** It is an electronic sensor, which passes an electric impulse to the equipment, each time its tip touches the surface of the petri dish containing colonies of bacteria. Its tip is touched once on each colony. The inking tip marks the counted colonies, thereby helping in proper counting.
7. **Plate holder:** It is a circular area, which tightly holds the plate containing colonies of bacteria. The plate is kept here upside down so that the colonies can be seen and marked on the glass surface by the sensor pen. The area can be illuminated from below for clear visibility of the colonies. The area is also divided into several small squares to help in the counting process.
8. **Digital display:** It displays the number of colonies. Each time the tip of the sensor pen touches the surface of the plate, it increases by one.
9. **Lens:** A convex lens fitted above the plate holder magnifies the area 1.5 times thereby helping in counting very small colonies.
10. **Lens stand:** It holds the lens in position. The height of the lens above the plate can be adjusted.

Figure 3.11: A Quebec colony counter

18. Electronic Colony Counter

Electronic colony counter is of two types: (1) Hand-held electronic colony counter and (2) Table-top electronic colony counter. The hand-held electronic colony counter is a pen-style colony counter with an inking felt-tip marker. For counting of colonies of bacteria grown in a petri dish, it is kept in an inverted position, so that the colonies are visible through the bottom surface of the petri dish. The colonies are marked by touching the glass surface of the petri dish with the felt-tip of the colony counter. Thus, each colony is marked by a dot made by the ink of the felt-tip on the bottom surface of the petri dish. In a single motion, the electronic colony counter marks, counts and confirms with a beep sound. The cumulative count of colonies is displayed on a four-digit LED display. In case of table-top electronic colony counter, the petri dish containing the colonies of bacteria is placed on an illuminated stage and the count bar is depressed. The precise number of colonies is instantly displayed on a digital read out.

*19. Magnetic Stirrer

In the preparation of solutions, certain chemicals require stirring for long time, to be dissolved in certain solvents. Magnetic stirrer is used to dissolve such substances easily and quickly. A small teflon-coated magnet, called 'stirring bar', is put into a container containing the solvent and the solute. Then, the container is placed on the platform of the magnetic stirrer, below which a magnet rotates at high speed by a motor. Attracted by the rotating magnet, the teflon-coated magnet rotates inside the container and stirs the contents. Now, the solute dissolves quickly. The teflon coating prevents the magnet from reacting with the solution, which comes in contact with it. After complete dissolution, the teflon-coated magnet is removed from the solution by mean of a long retriever, called 'stirring bar retriever'.

*20. Sonicator

It is used to rupture cells using high frequency waves.

21. Vortex Mixer

It is an instrument used for thorough mixing of liquids in test tubes. It has a rotor, whose speed can be controlled. On the tip of the rotor is a foam-rubber top. When the bottom of a test tube is pressed upon this foam-rubber top, the rotor starts rotating, thereby rotating the bottom of the test tube at high speed. Due to centripetal force, the solution gets mixed thoroughly. It is particularly helpful during serial dilution in enumeration of bacteria, which needs homogenous suspension of bacteria cells.

21. Laminar Flow Chamber

It is a chamber (Figure 3.12) used for aseptic transfer of sterilised materials, as well as for inoculation of microbes. Dust particles floating in the air harbour microbes. These microbe-laden dust particles may enter into the sterilised media and contaminate them, when they are opened for short periods of time during inoculation of microbe or transfer from one container to another. To overcome this, when inoculation is done in open air, the air of the small inoculating area is sterilised by the flame of a bunsen burner. The heated air becomes light and moves upwards, thereby preventing the dust particles from falling on the media during the short opening process. To further reduce the chance of contamination by the microbe-laden air, a laminar flow chamber is used. It is a glass-fitted cuboidal chamber. An air blower blows air from the surrounding and passes it through a HEPA filter (High Efficiency Particulate Air filter), so as to make it dust free (microbe-free). This microbe-free air passes through the chamber in a laminar manner and comes out from the chamber through the open front door. This laminar flow of microbe-free air from the chamber to outside through the open door prevents the outside air from entering into the chamber. Thus, the chamber does not get contaminated with the microbes present in the outside air, though the door is kept opened during inoculation or transfer of media. An UV lamp fitted inside the chamber sterilises the chamber before operation. It has a stainless steel platform with provision for gas pipe connection for a bunsen burner. Before use, the platform is cleaned and disinfected with lysol, the bunsen burner is connected and then the glass door is closed. The UV light is switched

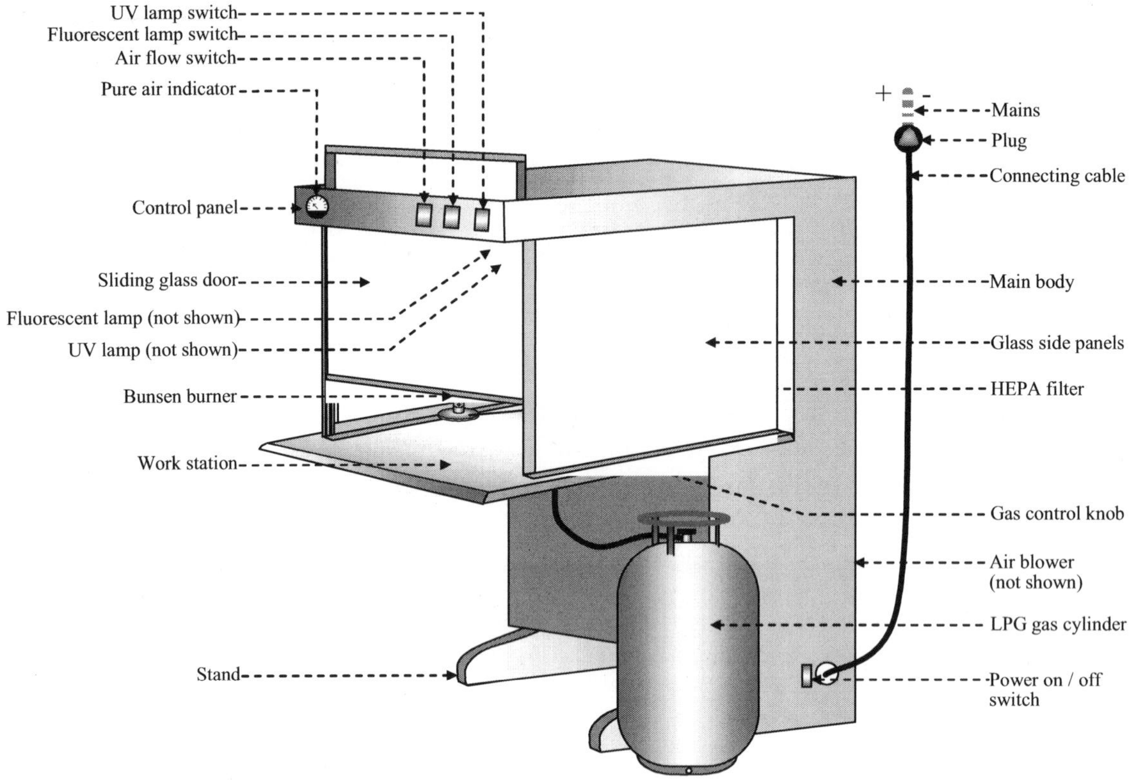

1. **Mains:** It is the source of electric current for the laminar flow chamber. The equipment runs using alternating current (AC) supplied through a three-ply cable. The three wires are phase (+), neutral (-) and earthing (E). The earthing helps in the safe operation of the equipment against electric shock due to any short-circuit.
2. **Plug:** A three-pin plug (15 ampere capacity) provides non-sparking interface between the equipment and the mains.
3. **Connecting cable:** A three-ply cable connects the mains with the equipment.
4. **Main body:** It encloses the parts of the equipment. It is made of metal sheets or laminated wood.
5. **Glass side panels:** The two glass side panels help in viewing the interior of the chamber.
6. **HEPA filter:** The high efficiency particulate air filter (HEPA filter), fixed at the backside of the chamber, filters out the dust particles, thereby allowing dust-free air to enter into the chamber in a laminar manner from the rear side towards the front door.
7. **Gas control knob:** It is fixed to the workstation and controls the flow of gas from the cylinder to the burner.
8. **Air blower:** It blows the air at high speed, which passes through the HEPA filter to produce a laminar flow.
9. **LPG gas cylinder:** It provides gas to the burner.
10. **Power on / off switch:** : It controls the entry of electric current into the equipment.
11. **Stand:** It supports the total weight of the autoclave along with its contents.
12. **Work station:** It is the rectangular bottom of the chamber on which the things required during aseptic transfer are kept.
13. **Bunsen burner:** It provides the flame for the flame-sterilisation of needles and loops as well as of mouths of containers.
14. **UV lamp:** It is fitted to the top panel. It is switched on for 10 minutes after closing the front sliding door to sterilise the interior of the chamber.
15. **Fluorescent lamp:** It is fitted to the top panel. It lightens the interior of the chamber.
16. **Sliding glass door:** It closes the chamber when not in operation.
17. **Control panel**: It is the panel or switchboard containing all the switches and indicators, with which the functions of the laminar flow chamber can be controlled.
18. **Pure air indicator:** It indicates the purity of the air entering into the chamber through the HEPA filter, based on which the filter is removed and cleaned periodically.
19. **Air flow switch:** It controls the entry of electric current into the air blower.
20. **Fluorescent lamp switch:** It controls the entry of electric current into the fluorescent lamp.
21. **UV lamp switch:** It controls the entry of electric current into the UV lamp.

Figure 3.12: A laminar flow chamber

on for 10 minutes to sterilise the environment inside the chamber and then switched off. The glass door should never be opened when the UV light is on, because UV light has detrimental effect on skin and vision. The blower is switched on and then the glass door is opened. Now, the bunsen burner is lighted and media transfer or inoculation is carried out in the chamber aseptically (*See* page 115). If extremely hazardous microbes are to be handled, a laminar flow chamber with gloves projecting into the chamber from the front glass door is used, as inoculation has to be done keeping the front door closed.

*22. Electronic Cell Counter

It is used to directly count the number of bacteria in a given liquid sample. An example of electronic cell counter is the 'Coulter counter'. In this equipment, a suspension of bacteria cells is allowed to pass through a minute orifice, across which an electric current flows. The resistance at the orifice is electronically recorded. When a cell passes through the orifice, being non-conductor, it increases resistance momentarily. The number of times resistance increases momentarily is recorded electronically, which indicates the number of bacteria present in the liquid sample.

23. Membrane Filtration Apparatus

Certain substances like urea disintegrate and lose their original properties, if sterilised by heat. Such substances are sterilised by membrane filtration apparatus. In this apparatus, the solution of the substance to be sterilised is filtered through a membrane filter, which does not allow bacteria cells to pass down. Filtration is done under suction pressure to increase the rate of filtration (Figure 2.19, page 30).

24. Microscopes

Different types of microscopes are used for visual observation of morphology, motility, staining and fluorescent reactions of bacteria. (*See* Chapter 4 on Microscopes at page 64).

*25. Computers

Computers are generally used for analysis of results. They are also used for identification of bacteria easily within few hours. Otherwise, identification of bacteria is a tedious process and takes days together to identify one bacteria species. The computers used for identification of bacteria are Apple II, IBM PC and TRS-80 and their modern variants. Each research personnel of the laboratory should be provided with a computer, along with internet facility.

*26. Spectrophotometer

It is an instrument for measuring the differences in colour intensities of solutions. A beam of light of a particular wavelength is passed through the test solution and the amount of light absorbed (or transmitted) is measured electronically. A simple visible spectrophotometer can pass light with wavelengths within visible range, whereas a UV-cum-visible spectrophotometer can pass light with wavelengths in ultraviolet as well as in visible range. In microbiology lab, it is used for direct counting of bacteria in suspension as well as for other purposes.

27 Electrical Devices

Fluctuations of electric voltage in the laboratory is one of the most important reasons, which reduces the longevity of the equipments and sometimes damage them. Therefore, all the voltage-sensitive equipments should be provided with voltage protection devices like stabilisers, servo stabilisers or constant voltage transformers (CVT) as per the recommendations of the manufacturers of the equipments. Computers, balances and some sophisticated equipments should be connected through uninterrupted power supply (UPS), as any breakdown in the electric power supply during their operation may severely damage some of their sensitive components. The laboratory should have a high capacity generator to supply electric current to the whole laboratory in case of power failure. This is because, power failure not only brings the activities of the laboratory to a stand still, it also brings about undesirable irreversible changes in the samples stored in the deep-fridges and refrigerators.

*28. Automatic Bacteria Identification System

It is an instrument used for automatic computer-assisted identification of bacteria (Figures 3.13 and 3.14). The conventional method of identification of bacteria is very lengthy and cumbersome. It mainly involves staining, motility test, cultural characteristics, a series of biochemical tests and finally searching the name of the bacteria in 'Bergey's Manual of Determinative Bacteriology' by matching the results with those available in the manual. The automatic bacteria identification system automatically identifies the bacteria in very short time. The system, like VITEK 2 (Figure 3.14) uses disposable cards. One card is required for the identification of one bacteria. The system can accommodate a series of cards, which can be arranged on a cassette, thus enabling the identification of several bacteria at a time. Each card has several rows of wells. Usually there are 8 rows of 8 wells each (8 X 8 =64 wells). The wells contain different dehydrated media required for different biochemical tests. A capillary tube is

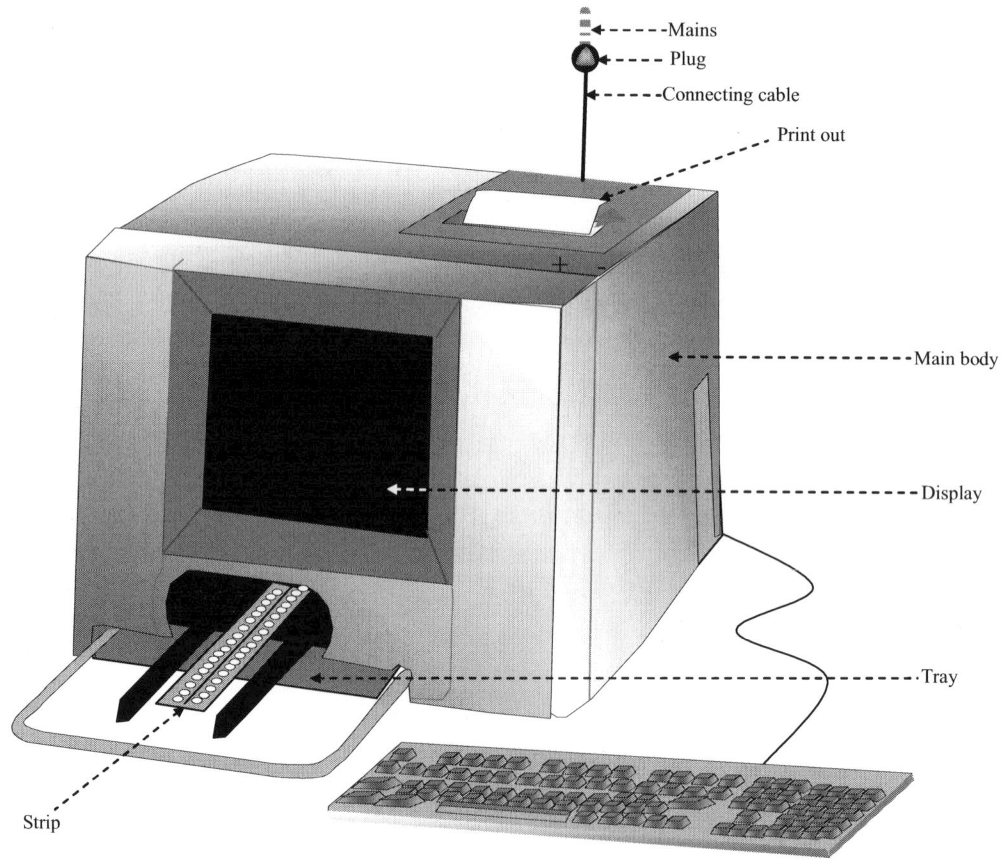

1. **Mains:** It is the source of electric current for the equipment. The equipment runs using alternating current (AC) supplied through a three-ply cable. The three wires are phase (+), neutral (-) and earthing (E). The earthing helps in the safe operation of the equipment against electric shock due to any short-circuit.
2. **Plug:** A three-pin plug provides non-sparking interface between the equipment and the mains.
3. **Connecting cable:** A three-ply cable connects the mains with the equipment.
4. **Print out:** It gives the print out of the results and other relevant information regarding the genus and species of the unknown bacteria.
5. **Main body:** It encloses the parts of the equipment. It is made of metal sheets. It houses the colour reader, which reads the colour changes in the test strips. The results of colour changes are compared automatically in the system, with those available in its library. Finally, the name of the unknown bacteria upto genus and species level is displayed.
6. **Display:** It displays the input data and the output results of identification, as well as other relevant informations.
7. **Tray:** It carries the inoculated and incubated strips into the system for colour reading and further comparison, leading to identification.
8. **Strip:** Identification of each bacteria needs a disposable strip. Each strip has a series of cupules (usually 32 numbers), each containing a definite medium required for a biochemical test. The unknown bacteria culture to be identified is first made into a suspension of a particular density as read by a densitometer. This suspension is then inoculated manually into all the cupules. The inoculated test strip is incubated at a prescribed temperature for a prescribed period of time in an incubator. The bacteria grows in the media in the cupules and produces colour changes, which are characteristic of that bacteria. Then the strip is put on the tray, which carries it into the system for colour reading and further comparison leading to the identification of the bacteria.

Figure 3.13: Automatic bacteria identification system (MINI API)

fixed to each card, which sucks the suspension of bacteria to be identified and dispenses into all the wells. The dehydrated media in the wells become hydrated by the suspension liquid, thereby allowing growth of the bacteria. After a prescribed period of incubation, the colour changes in all the wells are recorded automatically in the system. The results of the colour changes go to a computer attached to the system. The computer automatically compares the results with those available in its library for different bacteria and finally gives the name of the bacteria with a definite probability.

For identification, the given bacteria, grown as isolated colony on a plate or as pure culture grown on a slant is taken. A loopful of the bacteria is transferred aseptically into sterile saline solution in a test tube and a suspension of the bacteria is made. The suspension should contain a prescribed density of bacteria, as determined by a densitometer. The test tube is fixed to the cassette and a card is fixed near it, such that the tip of the suction capillary tube of the card remains deeply submerged in the suspension. Several such test tubes and cards are fixed to each cassette, depending on the number of bacteria to be identified. The cassette is put in the vacuum chamber of the system. A high vacuum is created inside the chamber, which forces the bacteria suspension to be sucked into the capillary tubes and dispensed into the wells of the cards. The cassette is taken out and put inside the incubation and analysis chamber. Here, the capillary tubes are cut and the cut ends sealed automatically. Then, the incubation process starts at a prescribed temperature for a prescribed period of time, which is programmed by the control panel. During incubation, in every 15 minutes, each card automatically goes to the colour reader, which reads the colour changes in the wells and records them. The recorded results go to the computer, which automatically compares them with those available in its library for different bacteria. Finally, it gives the names of the bacteria with definite probabilities. The used cards fall into the waste disposal chamber of the system for removal and final disposal after sterilisation. The renowned automatic bacteria identification systems are VITEK 2 and API. While VITEK 2 works on the above principle, the API (Analytical Profile Indexing) system (Figure 3.13) uses a slightly different method for the automatic identification of bacteria, which involves manual inoculation and external incubation.

***29. PCR Thermocycler, Refrigerated Centrifuge, Ultra-centrifuge, Gas Chromatography (GC), High Performance Liquid Chromatography (HPLC), Thin Layer Chromatography (TLC), Paper Chromatography, Column Chromatography and Electrophoresis Unit**

These are instruments used for isolation, purification and identification of biochemical substances, such as bacterial DNA, plasmids, microbial toxins etc. Polymerase chain reaction (PCR) is an important tool in nucleic acid based methods. It is a workhorse in modern microbiology and biotechnology laboratories.

C. Glasswares and Labwares

Experiment 3

Aim: **To get acquainted with the different glasswares and labwares used in the microbiology laboratory.**

A number of glasswares and labwares are required in the microbiology laboratory. Some of them, which are required in bulk quantity, are given below.

1. Petri dishes
2. Test tubes
3. Pipettes (2,10 and 1.1ml)
4. Slides
5. Cover slips
6. Cavity slides
7. Durham tubes
9. Craft paper
8. Non-absorbent cotton
10. Thread or rubber bands

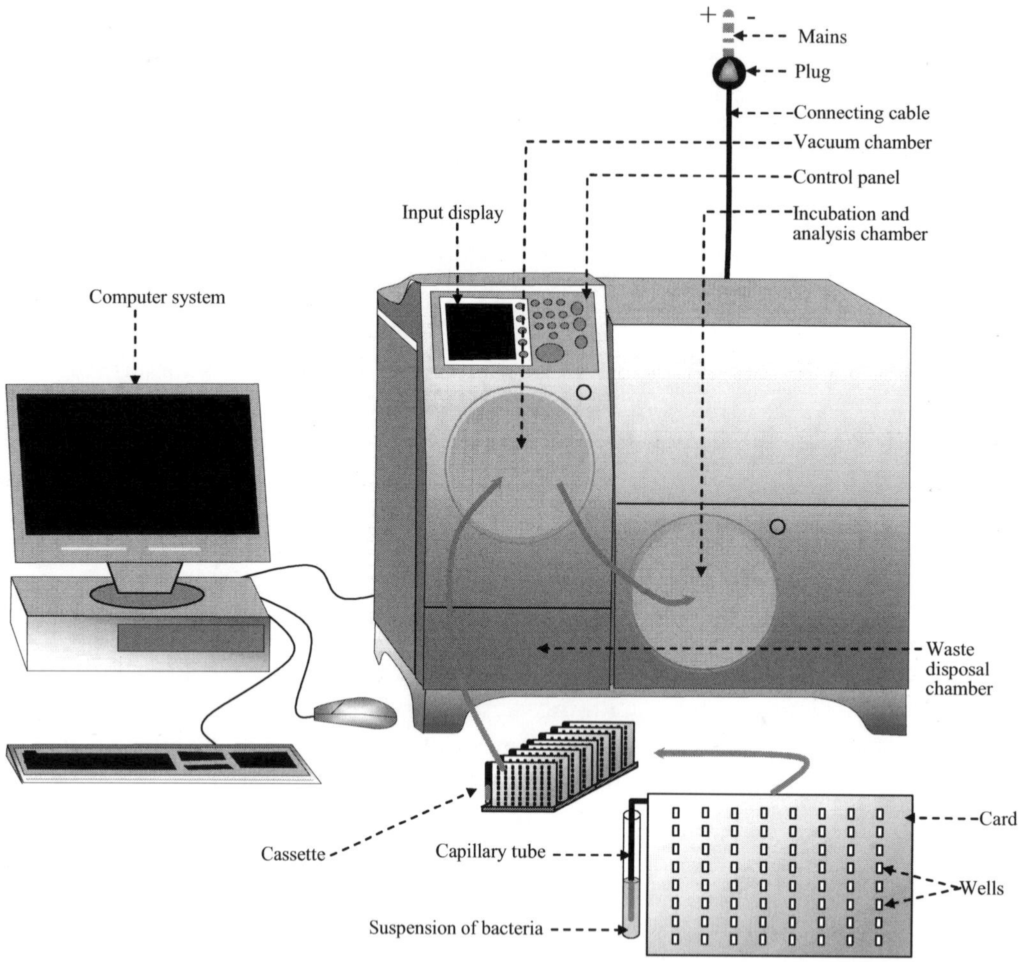

1. **Mains:** It is the source of electric current for the equipment. The equipment runs using alternating current (AC) supplied through a three-ply cable. The three wires are phase (+), neutral (-) and earthing (E). The earthing helps in the safe operation of the equipment against electric shock due to any short-circuit.
2. **Plug:** A three-pin plug provides non-sparking interface between the equipment and the mains.
3. **Connecting cable:** A three-ply cable connects the mains with the equipment.
4. **Control panel:** It is the panel or switchboard containing all the switches, with which the functions of the system can be controlled. The different parameters like temperature and time of incubation required for the operation of the system can be programmed on the panel.
5. **Vacuum chamber:** It is the chamber, into which the cassette containing the cards and the bacteria suspensions to be identified is put. A high vacuum is created inside the chamber, which forces the bacteria suspensions to be sucked into the capillary tubes and dispensed into the wells of the cards.
6. **Incubation and analysis chamber:** In this chamber, incubation and colour reading takes place simultaneously. The cassette containing the cards dispensed with the bacteria suspensions is put into it. After scanning the bar codes on the cards, the capillary tubes are cut and the cut ends sealed automatically. Then, the cards are positioned onto a carosol (a wheel-like structure), which moves in such a way that, in every 15 minutes each card comes in front of the colour reader. The colour reader reads the changes in colour at three different wavelengths. The changes in colour of the media in the wells of each card are recorded and sent to the computer for comparison of the results with the database and display of the names of the bacteria in terms of genus and species
7. **Waste disposal chamber:** After analysis, the used cards automatically get collected in the waste disposal chamber for further disposal to outside after sterilisation.
8. **Card:** The identification of each unknown bacteria requires one disposable card. There are few types of cards each specific for a particular group of bacteria. The type of card to be used for a particular unknown bacteria is determined by a preliminary test like gram staining.
9. **Wells:** Each card has several rows of well. Usually there are 8 rows of 8 well each (8 X 8 =64 wells). The wells contain different dehydrated media for different biochemical tests required for the identification of bacteria. When bacteria suspension is dispensed into all the wells, the dehydrated media become hydrated by the suspension liquid. The hydrated media allow the bacteria to grow. The growth of the bacteria in the wells results in the change in the colour of the media in a particular way, which is characteristic for each bacteria species.
10. **Suspension of bacteria:** The unknown bacteria, grown as isolated colony on a plate or as pure culture grown on a slant is taken. A loopful of the bacteria is transferred aseptically into sterile saline solution in a test tube and a suspension of the bacteria is made. The suspension should contain a prescribed density of bacteria as determined by a densitometer.
11. **Capillary tube:** A capillary tube is fixed to each card, which sucks the suspension of bacteria and dispenses into all the wells.
12. **Cassette:** It can hold a series of cards along with their respective test tubes containing bacteria suspensions. The test tubes and cards are fixed in such a way that the tips of the suction capillary tubes of the cards remain deeply submerged in the suspensions.
13. **Computer system:** The results of colour changes recorded by the analysis chamber go to the computer, which automatically compares them with those available in its library (database) for different bacteria. Finally, it gives the names of the bacteria with definite probabilities.
14. **Input display:** It displays the input programme required for operation of the system.

Figure 3.14: Automatic bacteria identification system (VITEK 2)

Some other glasswares and labwares that are required in small quantities include the following.

1. Loops and needles with detachable handle[2]
2. Conical flasks or Erlenmeyer flasks (100, 250, 500, 1000 ml)
3. Measuring cylinders (10, 100, 500, 1000 ml)
4. Reagent bottles (125, 250, 500 ml)
5. Volumetric flasks (100, 250, 500, 1000 ml)
6. Beakers (100, 250, 500 ml)
7. Glass rods (4 mm diameter for making spreader)[3]
8. Wash bottles
9. Dispose jars
10. Dropping bottles
11. Ocular micrometers
12. Stage micrometers
13. Tripod stands
14. Wire gauges with asbestos center
15. Pipette stands
16. Pipette cases (Stainless steel)[4]
17. Test tube baskets
18. Foam pads
19. Funnels
20. Desiccators
21. Bunsen burners
22. Rubber pipes
23. Vacuum pumps (glass)
24. Marker pens and stickers

D. Chemicals and Media

Experiment 4

***Aim*: To get acquainted with the different chemicals and media used in the microbiology laboratory.**

In the laboratory, bacteria are grown on nutrient-rich substances called 'media'. A variety of media are also required for specific uses. The components of the media are weighed in a given proportion, mixed in the required amount of water and sterilised in autoclave. Bacteria is inoculated into it and allowed to grow. Weighing the ingredients of media is a tedious job and some ingredients may be missed unknowingly. To overcome this difficulty, now-a-days ready-made media in powder form are available. These media contain all the ingredients in the prescribed proportions. To a definite quantity

2 Wire loops are made by cutting a long platinum or nichrome wire into pieces of 6 cm (approximately) and forming a loop of 3 mm diameter at one end. Then, the other end is pushed into the loop holder and is tightened by a nut. Similarly, needles are prepared by pushing the pieces of wire without loop into the loop holder and then tightening the nut.

3 Glass spreader is a bent glass rod used for spreading a suspension of bacteria sample on an agar plate. It is obtained by heating a piece of glass rod on flame (preferably on a fish tail burner) and bending with slight pressure at the point of heating.

4 Stainless steel pipette cases are used to store sterilised pipettes aseptically for use in lab. Pipettes are kept in these cases, sterilised in oven and kept in the lab for future use.

of the powder media (as mentioned on the label of the pack), specified amount of water is added and sterilised. Culture media are of the following types.

I. Chemically Defined Media

Chemically defined media or synthetic media are the media, in which all the specific chemicals (molecules and atoms) and their concentrations can be determined. The chemicals may include H_2O, NaCl, Na_2SO_4, KCl and agar. Examples: inorganic synthetic broth, glucose salt broth.

II. Complex Media

Complex media are the media, in which all the specific chemicals (molecules and atoms) and their concentrations cannot be determined. For fastidious bacteria, few complex substances, like beef extract, yeast extract and peptone are used in the media, whose exact chemical composition (molecules and atoms) vary considerably and is not known. These media are mainly used for profuse growth of bacteria. Examples: nutrient broth and nutrient agar.

III. Specialised Media

These media are used for specific purposes, rather than only for the growth of bacteria. Based on the purpose of use, they are of the following types.

1. Selective Media

They are the media containing a specific composition of ingredients, which supports the growth of some target bacteria and inhibits the growth of the others. They are used to isolate specific groups of bacteria. When a particular group of bacteria grows in a selective medium, it manifests typical colony characteristics, which help in its detection and enumeration in various samples. The particular bacteria of interest, found as isolated colonies are taken for further tests for confirmed identification. Sometimes, selective media are also used as differential media. The examples of selective media are given below.

(a) MacConkey Agar

It is used to grow gram-negative species of bacteria. The crystal violet used in the medium inhibits the growth of gram-positive bacteria, while allowing the gram-negative species to grow.

(b) EMB Agar

Eosine methylene blue agar (EMB agar) is used to grow gram-negative species of bacteria. It partially inhibits the growth of gram-positive bacteria, due to which the gram-negative species of bacteria grow in it more profusely. It is also used in the identification of the enteric coliform *Escherichia coli*, which grows on it as blue-black colonies with a metallic green sheen. Other enteric coliforms, such as *Enterobacter aerogenes*, grow on it as thick, mucoid, pink colonies. Besides these lactose-fermenters, lactose-non-fermenters also grow on it, but as colourless colonies, for which they take up the purple colour of the medium.

(c) Mannitol Salt Agar

It is used to grow *Staphylococcus* spp. The high salt concentration (7.5% NaCl) present in the medium inhibits the growth of most other bacteria. It also differentiates *Staphylococcus* into mannitol-fermenting *Staphylococcus*, which grows with yellow zones surrounding the colonies and mannitol-non-fermenting *Staphylococcus*, which grows with no change in colouration.

2. Differential Media

They are the media, on which different bacteria grow as colonies, with different visual characteristics. The examples of differential media are given below.

(a) MacConkey Agar

On this medium, the non-pathogenic normal intestinal bacteria, which are lactose-fermenters, grow as red colonies, whereas the pathogenic intestinal bacteria, which are lactose-non-fermenters, grow as colourless colonies.

(b) Blood Agar

Blood is the important constituent of this medium. It is an enrichment ingredient for the fastidious bacteria like *Streptococcus* spp. It is used to differentiate the properties of streptococci to produce different types of haemolysis of blood as follows.

(*i*) *α-haemolysis*: Here, partial destruction of RBC occurs, resulting in green colour zones around colonies due to reduction of haemoglobin to methaemoglobin.

(*ii*) *β-haemolysis*: Here, complete haemolysis of RBC occurs, resulting in clear zone around colonies. This haemolysis is brought about two types of haemolysins, namely 'streptolysin O', which is an antigenic oxygen-labile enzyme and 'streptolysin S', which is a non-antigenic oxygen-stable lysin.

(*iii*) *γ-haemolysis*: Here, no haemolysis occurs, resulting in no zone around colonies.

3. Transport Media

They are the media used for short transport of bacteria, during which growth is undesirable. Such media contain only buffer and salt. The media do not contain any source of C, N and other growth factors. It prevents microbial growth.

4. Enrichment Media

They are the media, in which the relative proportion of the target bacteria is enriched, as they contain the nutrients for the target bacteria, whereas none for the others. For example, fecal matter contains very low number of *Salmonella* and *Shigella*. To isolate them, they are first cultured in selenite broth or GN (gram-negative) broth, in which only *Salmonella* and *Shigella* will grow profusely, while others will not grow and will remain in lag phase. Then, this is streaked on solid media to obtain colonies of *Salmonella* and *Shigella*.

5. Enriched Media

They are the media used to support the growth of maximum types of bacteria.

6. Biochemical Media

These media are used for testing biochemical activities of bacteria, which help in their identification (*See* 'Biochemical Tests' at page 131). A list of important biochemical media used in the biochemical tests performed for the identification of different bacteria is given below.

Sl.No.	*Biochemical Tests*	*Biochemical Media*
1.	Indole test	Indole broth
2.	Methyl red test	MR-VP broth
3.	Voges-Proskauer test	MR-VP broth
4.	Citrate utilisation test	Simmons citrate agar
5.	Oxidation-fermentation test (O/F Test)	Hugh-Leifson glucose broth
6.	Amino acid decarboxylase test	Amino acid decarboxylase broth
7.	Urease test	Urea agar
8.	Nitrate reduction test	Nitrate broth
9.	Triple sugar iron (TSI) test	Triple sugar iron agar (TSI agar)
10.	Gelatinase test	Fraizer's gelatin agar
11.	Starch hydrolysis test	Starch agar
12.	Lipid hydrolysis test	Tributyrin agar
13.	Deoxyribonuclease (DNase) test	DNase agar
14.	Phenylalanine deaminase test	Phenylalanine agar
15.	Ortho-nitrophenyl galactoside test (ONPG test)	Triple sugar iron agar (TSI agar)
16.	Hydrogen sulphide test	Triple sugar iron agar (TSI agar)/Cysteine broth
17.	Carbohydrate fermentation test	Carbohydrate broth
18.	Litmus milk test	Litmus milk broth

Besides media, several other chemicals are also required in the microbiology laboratory. Lists of media and chemicals required in the microbiology laboratory have been given in the Appendix I and II respectively.

E. Care and Maintenance

Experiment 5

Aim: **To acquaint with the different care and maintenance steps to be taken in the microbiology laboratory.**

The following care and maintenance steps should be adopted in the microbiology laboratory.

1. Extreme cleanliness should be maintained in the laboratory. Everyday, it should be cleaned properly, preferably using a disinfectant solution such as phenyl.
2. Each person working in the lab should wear an apron before entering into the lab. It protects clothing from contamination, accidental discolouration or acid charring. It should be removed, whenever going out from the lab. All such laboratory clothing should be sterilised before washing.
3. Long hair should be tied back or covered with a head scarf, so as to minimise contamination.
4. Books and other paraphernalia should never be kept on the laboratory tables. They should be kept in a specified place (property counter).
5. Eating, drinking and smoking in the laboratory should be strictly prohibited.
6. Before starting and after finishing each laboratory session, the laboratory table-tops should be cleaned with a germicidal solution (*e.g.* hypochlorite solution containing at least 200 ppm available chlorine or phenyl solution) using a foam pad.
7. In the laboratory, nothing should be done hastily.
8. All microbes cultured in the laboratory should be treated as potential pathogens. Therefore, extreme care should be taken in handling them. Removal of cultures from the laboratory without proper precautionary measures should be strictly prohibited.
9. Cultures in test tubes should always be kept in test tube racks on tables and should be moved along with the racks, when required.
10. Broth cultures should never be pipetted by mouth.
11. The cultures should not spill out during transfer or when flaming the loop. In case it occurs, the whole area should be covered with a cloth soaked in germicidal solution. After 15 minutes, the place should be wiped with that cloth. Then the cloth is autoclaved.
12. In any experiment, the cultures or media should never be contaminated. That is why, during inoculation of bacteria or transfer of media, after removing the cap or cotton plug, the mouth of the containers containing media or cultures is shown over flame.
13. On completion of each experiment, all the plate cultures, slant cultures and broth cultures to be discarded, should be kept in the place labeled 'wastes to be sterilised'. As they contain large number of bacteria and all bacteria are potential pathogens, the materials are sterilised in autoclave before discarding.
14. To keep the instruments in good working condition, they should be covered properly and should be operated or at least be kept 'on' for sometime everyday.
15. After prolonged use, the inside of ovens, incubators, fridges and all such cabinets should be sterilised. For this, a little amount of potassium permanganate is taken in a watch glass and a few drops of formaldehyde solution is poured into it. As soon as fumes start coming out, it is kept inside the cabinet to be sterilised and its door closed. After few hours the door can be opened and the equipment used.

16. While sterilising some materials, due to incorrect readings on the pressure gauge, temperature dial or thermometer, the materials may not get sterilised properly. To ensure sterility of the materials, 'sterility test' should be performed. In this test, usually commercially available sterility test strips are incorporated along with the material to be sterilised. The strips change color, if conditions lethal to bacteria could be maintained inside the autoclave or oven, so as to sterilise the materials completely.
17. Used pipettes should be dipped in germicidal solution contained in a dispose jar. After each laboratory session, these pipettes are cleaned using detergent. Then, they are rinsed with distilled water and air-dried. They are put in bulk inside stainless steel pipette cases and sterilised in oven.
18. Glasswares should be cleaned properly. If water drops adhere to the surface of the glasswares, then they are not perfectly clean. If they do not get cleaned even after washing with detergent solution, they should be soaked in chromic acid solution (4.5 g $K_2Cr_2O_7$ + 100 ml distilled water + 100 ml concentrated sulphuric acid) overnight and then cleaned.
19. After an experiment is over, all media, chemicals and glasswares should be kept back in their original position.
20. After the experiment is over, hands should be washed with soap or liquid detergent before leaving the laboratory.

4

Microscopes

Microorganisms are usually not visible to naked human eye. They can be made visible, only when they are magnified under microscopes. Microscopes are instruments, which can produce enlarged images of very small objects, making it possible to view them, which, otherwise, cannot be seen distinctly by naked human eye. Different types of microscopes are used by the microbiologists for specific purposes. Microscopes are of the following types (Figure 4.1).

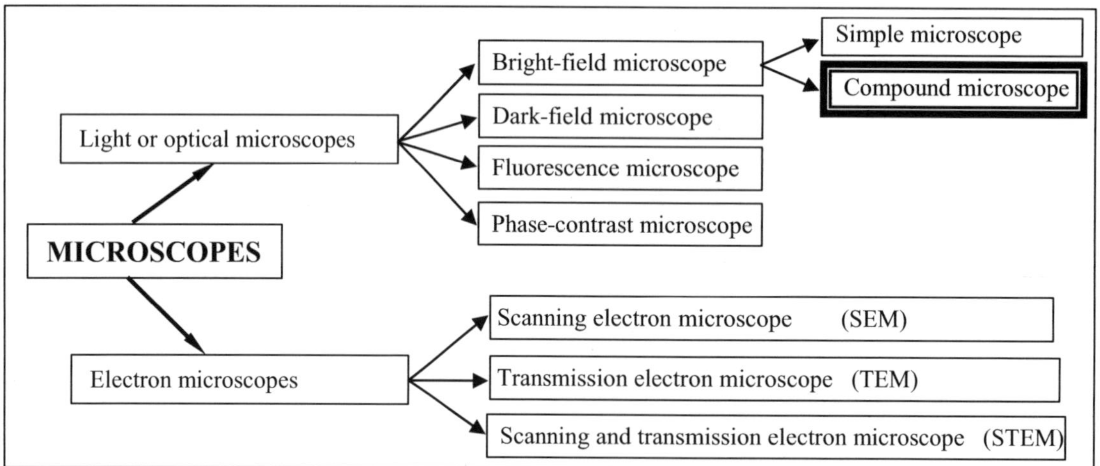

Figure 4.1: Types of microscopes

A. Light or Optical Microscopes

In light or optical microscopes, 'light waves' are used to produce the enlarged images of very small objects and magnification is obtained by a system of 'optical lenses'. Ordinarily, microbes do not absorb much light, but staining them with dyes greatly increases their light absorbing ability, resulting in greater contrast and color differentiation. Light microscopes are of four types as described below.

(1) Bright-field Microscope

In a bright-field microscope, the microscopic field (the circular area visible under microscope) is brightly illuminated and the microbes (or biological specimen) appear darker, as they absorb some of the light passing through them. It is of two types as follows.

(*a*) Simple Microscope

A simple microscope is used to obtain small magnifications. A single biconvex lens magnifies the size of the object to get an enlarged virtual image.

(b) Compound Microscope

The most commonly used microscope for general purposes is the standard compound microscope. It magnifies the size of the object by a complex system of lens arrangement. It has a series of two lenses; the objective lens and the ocular lens, to magnify the size of the object.

2. Dark-field Microscope

In a dark-field microscope, the object is brilliantly illuminated against a dark background.

3. Fluorescence Microscope

It is used to view fluorescent microbes and microbes stained with fluorescent dyes for specific purposes.

4. Phase-contrast Microscope

With a phase-contrast microscope, the differences among various cells with different refractive indices or thickness can be seen in unstained condition. Unstained structures within cells, not discernible by most other microscopes can also be observed, due to the slight differences in their refractive indices or thickness. It is a compound microscope fitted with a phase-contrast condenser and a phase-contrast objective.

B. Electron Microscopes

In electron microscopes, 'electron beams' are used to produce the image of the object and magnification is obtained by a system of 'electromagnetic fields', unlike in light microscopes, in which 'light waves' are used to produce the image of the object and magnification is obtained by a system of 'optical lenses'. The resolving power of electron microscopes is 200 times greater than that of light microscopes. They can produce useful magnifications upto X 400,000, as compared to X 2000 in light microscopes. Thus, the useful magnifications is 200 times greater in electron microscopes than in light microscopes. Electron microscopes are of three types as described below.

1. Transmission Electron Microscope (TEM)

In this microscope, electron beam is transmitted through an ultra-thin section of the object and the image is magnified by the electromagnetic fields. It is used to observe finer details of internal structures of microscopic objects like bacteria and other cells.

2. Scanning Electron Microscope (SEM)

This microscope uses an electron beam to scan the surface of the object, thereby inducing it to release a shower of electrons, which are collected by a detector to generate the image. It is used to observe the surface structure of microscopic objects.

3. Scanning and Transmission Electron Microscope (STEM)

It has both transmission and scanning electron microscope functions.

A. Light or Optical Microscopes

(1) Bright-Field Microscope

Experiment 6

(a) Simple Microscope (Dissecting Microscope)

***Aim*: To study the working principle and parts of a simple microscope.**

Working Principle

A simple microscope is used to obtain small magnifications. It is usually used for study of microscopic algae, fungi and biological specimen. Light from a light source (mirror) passes through a thin transparent object (Figure 4.2). A biconvex lens magnifies the size of the object to get an enlarged virtual image. The image is viewed from the other side.

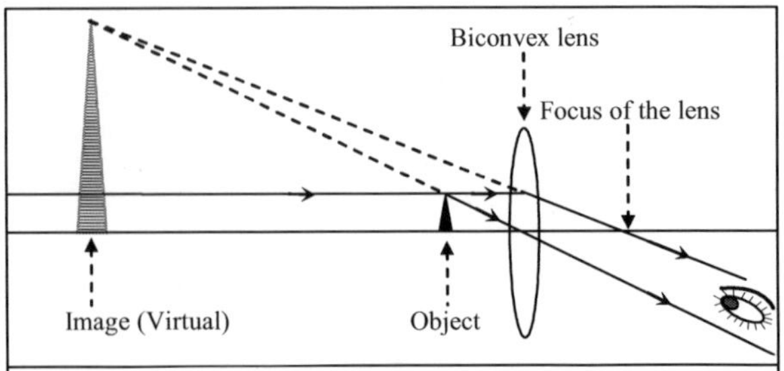

Figure 4.2: Ray diagram of a simple microscope

Parts of a Simple Microscope

The parts of a simple microscope are of two categories as follows.

(*i*) Mechanical parts

(*ii*) Optical parts

(i) Mechanical parts

These parts support the optical parts and help in their adjustment for focusing the object. They include the following components (Figure 4.3).

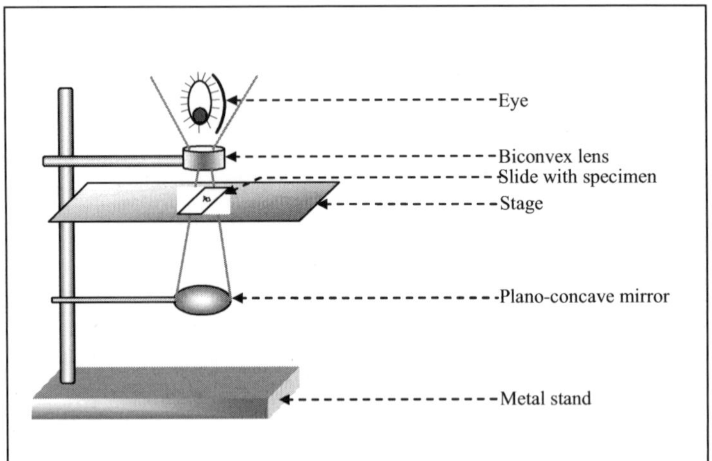

Figure 4.3: A simple microscope

1. *Metal Stand:* It has a heavy base plate and a vertical rod fitted to it, which provide support and stability to other parts of the microscope.
2. *Stage:* It is a rectangular metal plate fitted to the vertical rod. It has a central hole for light to pass from below. Slide with specimen to be observed is kept on the stage, in such a way that, the specimen remains just on the central hole. Some microscopes have a pair of slanting wings projecting from the both the sides of the stage. They provide support to hand for manipulating the object.

(ii) Optical parts

These parts are involved in passing the light through the object (specimen) and magnifying its size. The components of the optical parts are as follows.

1. *Mirror:* A plano-convex mirror is fitted below the stage to the vertical rod by means of a frame. It focuses the surrounding light on the object to be observed.
2. *Lens:* A biconvex lens is fitted above the stage, to the vertical rod, by means of a frame. It magnifies the size of the object and the enlarged virtual image formed is observed by keeping the eye above it. For proper focusing, the lens can be moved up and down by the frame.

Experiment 7

(b) Compound Microscope

***Aim*: To study the working principle and parts of a compound microscope.**

Working Principle

The most commonly used microscope for general purposes is the standard compound microscope. It magnifies the size of the object by a complex system of lens arrangement. It has a series of two lenses; (*i*) the objective lens close to the object to be observed and (*ii*) the ocular lens or eyepiece, through which the image is viewed by eye. Light from a light source (mirror or electric lamp) passes through a thin transparent object (Figure 4.4). The objective lens produces a magnified 'real image' (first image) of the object. This image is again magnified by the ocular lens (eyepiece) to obtain a magnified 'virtual image'

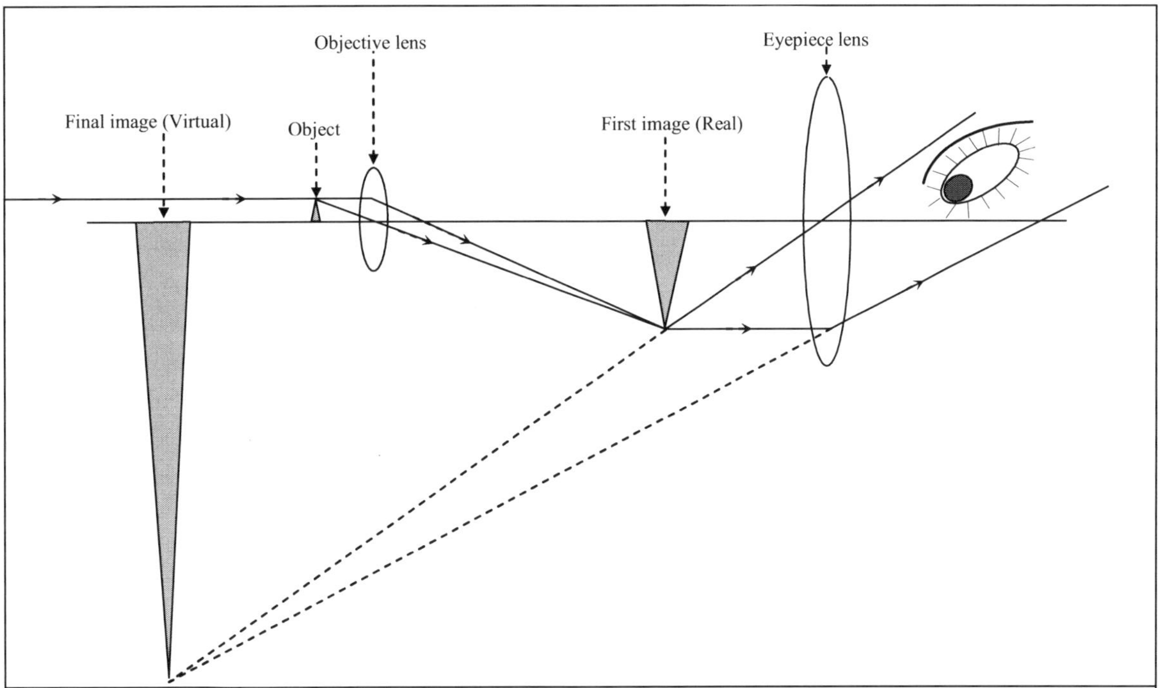

Figure 4.4: Ray diagram of a compound microscope

(final image), which can be seen by eye through the eyepiece. As light passes directly from the source to the eye through the two lenses, the field of vision is brightly illuminated. That is why, it is a bright-field microscope.

Parts of a Compound Microscope

The parts of a compound microscope are of two categories as given below.

(i) Mechanical Parts

These are the parts, which support the optical parts and help in their adjustment for focusing the object (Figures 4.5 and 4.6). The components of mechanical parts are as follows.

1. *Base or Metal Stand:* The whole microscope rests on this base. Mirror, if present, is fitted to it.
2. *Pillars:* It is a pair of elevations on the base, by which the body of the microscope is held to the base
3. *Inclination joint:* It is a movable joint, through which the body of the microscope is held to the base by the pillars. The body can be bent at this joint into any inclined position, as desired by

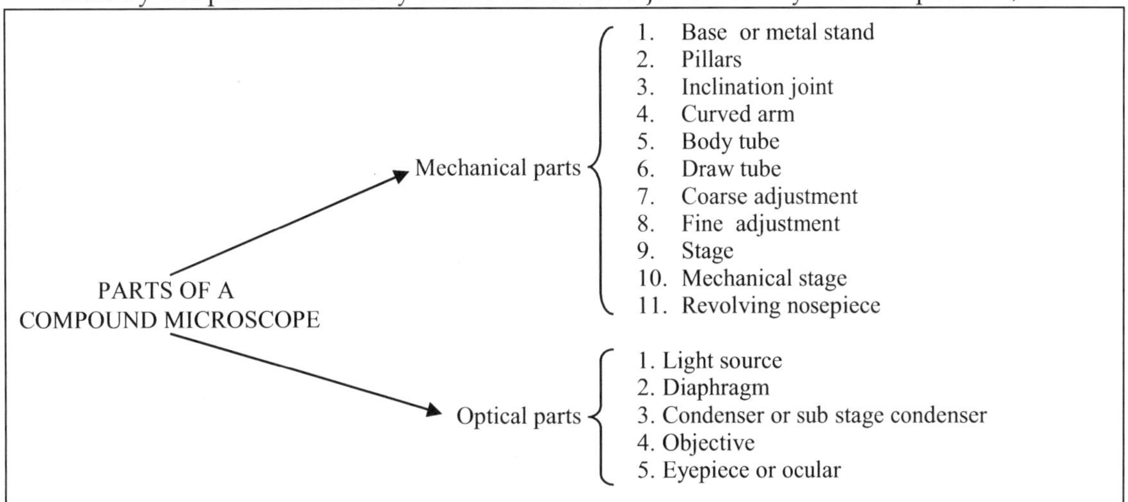

Figure 4.5: Parts of a compound microscope

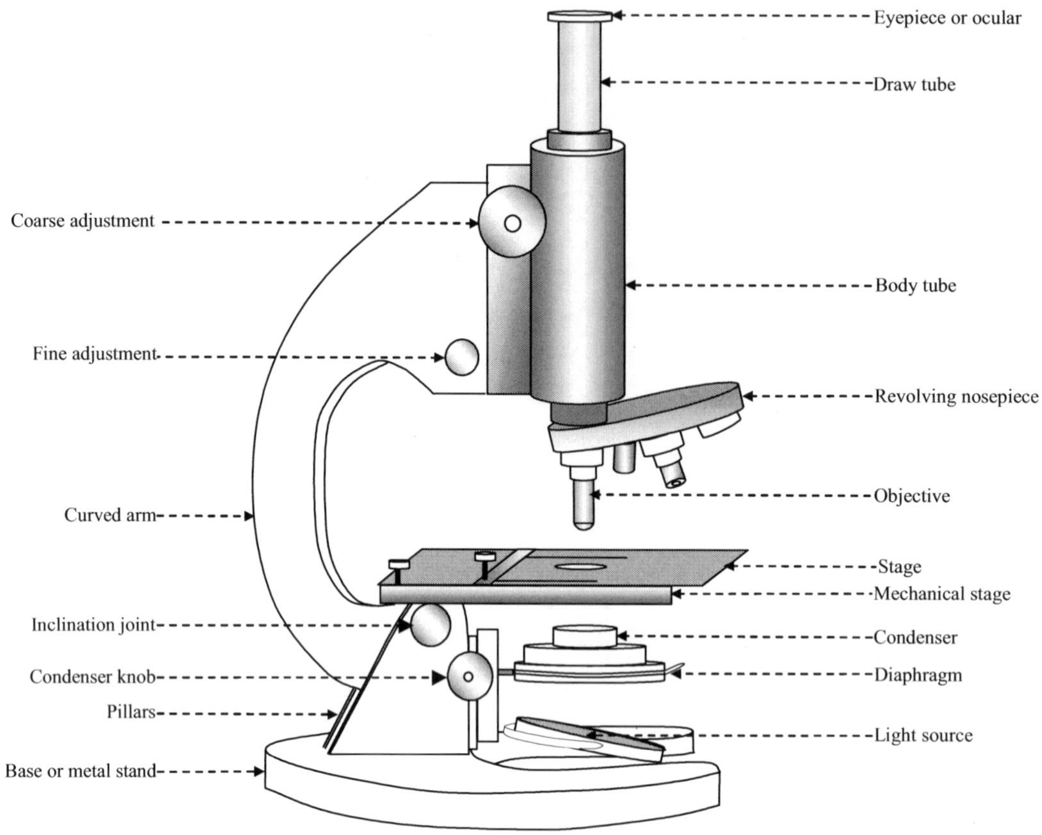

Figure 4.6: A compound microscope

the observer, for easier observation. In new models, the body is permanently fixed to the base in an inclined position, thus needing no pillar or joint.

4. *Curved Arm:* It is a curved structure held by the pillars. It holds the stage, body tube, fine adjustment and coarse adjustment.
5. *Body Tube:* It is usually a vertical tube holding the eyepiece at the top and the revolving nosepiece with the objectives at the bottom. The length of the draw tube is called 'mechanical tube length' and is usually 140-180 mm (mostly 160 mm).
6. *Draw Tube:* It is the upper part of the body tube, slightly narrower, into which the eyepiece is slipped during observation.
7. *Coarse Adjustment:* It is a knob with rack and pinion mechanism to move the body tube up and down for focusing the object in the visible field. As rotation of the knob through a small angle moves the body tube through a long distance relative to the object, it can perform coarse adjustment. In modern microscopes, it moves the stage up and down and the body tube is fixed to the arm.
8. *Fine Adjustment:* It is a relatively smaller knob. Its rotation through a large angle can move the body tube only through a small vertical distance. It is used for fine adjustment to get the final clear image. In modern microscopes, fine adjustment is done by moving the stage up and down by the fine adjustment.
9. *Stage:* It is a horizontal platform projecting from the curved arm. It has a hole at the center, upon which the object to be viewed is placed on a slide. Light from the light source below the stage passes through the object into the objective.

10. *Mechanical Stage (Slide Mover):* Mechanical stage consists of two knobs with rack and pinion mechanism. The slide containing the object is clipped to it and moved on the stage in two dimensions by rotating the knobs, so as to focus the required portion of the object.
11. *Revolving Nosepiece:* It is a rotatable disc at the bottom of the body tube with three or four objectives screwed to it. The objectives have different magnifying powers. Based on the required magnification, the nosepiece is rotated, so that only the objective specified for the required magnification remains in line with the light path.

(ii) Optical Parts

These parts are involved in passing the light through the object and magnifying its size. The components of optical parts include the following.

1. *Light Source:* Modern microscopes have in-built electric light source in the base. The source is connected to the mains through a regulator, which controls the brightness of the field. But in old models, a mirror is used as the light source. It is fixed to the base by a binnacle, through which it can be rotated, so as to converge light on the object. The mirror is plane on one side and concave on the other. It should be used in the following manner:
   (*a*) *Condenser Present:* Only plane side of the mirror should be used, as the condenser converges the light rays.
   (*b*) *Condenser Absent*:
      (*i*) Daylight: Plane or concave (plane is easier)
      (*ii*) Small artificial light:
         High power objective: Plane side
         Low power objective: Concave side
2. *Diaphragm:* If light coming from the light source is brilliant and all the light is allowed to pass to the object through the condenser, the object gets brilliantly illuminated and cannot be visualised properly. Therefore, an iris diaphragm is fixed below the condenser to control the amount of light entering into the condenser.
3. *Condenser:* The condenser or substage condenser is located between the light source and the stage. It has a series of lenses to converge on the object, light rays coming from the light source. After passing through the object, the light rays enter into the objective. The 'light condensing', 'light converging' or 'light gathering' capacity of a condenser is called 'numerical aperture of the condenser'. Similarly, the 'light gathering' capacity of an objective is called 'numerical aperture of the objective'. If the condenser converges light in a wide angle, its numerical aperture is greater and vice versa. If the condenser has such numerical aperture that it sends light through the object with an angle sufficiently large to fill the aperture back lens of the objective, the objective shows its highest numerical aperture (Figure 4.7). Most common condensers have numerical aperture 1.25.

   If the numerical aperture of the condenser is smaller than that of the objective, the peripheral portions of the back lens of the objective is not illuminated and the image has poor visibility. On the other hand, if the numerical aperture of condenser is greater than that of the objective, the back lens may receive too much light resulting in a decrease in contrast.

   There are three types of condensers as follows.
   (*a*) Abbe condenser (Numerical aperture=1.25): It is extensively used.
   (*b*) Variable focus condenser (Numerical aperture =1.25)
   (*c*) Achromatic condenser (Numerical aperture =1.40): It has been corrected for both spherical and chromatic aberration and is used in research microscopes and photomicrographs.

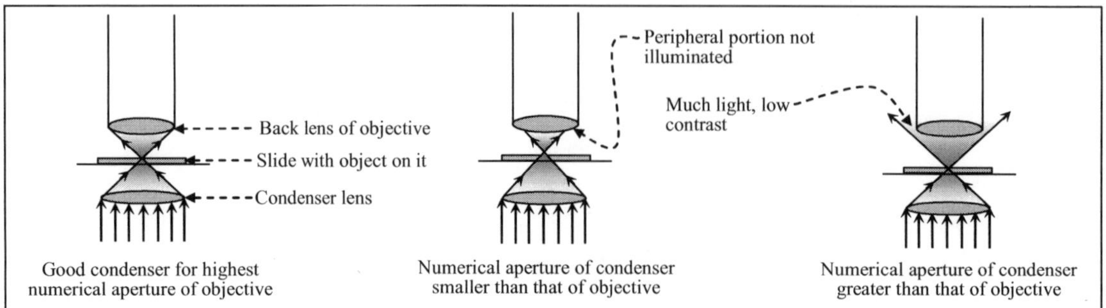

Figure 4.7: Numerical aperture of condensers

4. *Objective:* It is the most important lens in a microscope. Usually three objectives with different magnifying powers are screwed to the revolving nosepiece. The objectives are
   (*a*) Low power objective (X 10): It produces ten times magnification of the object.
   (*b*) High dry objective (X 40): It gives a magnification of forty times.
   (*c*) Oil-immersion objective (X 100): It gives a magnification of hundred times, when immersion oil fills the space between the object and the objective

   The scanning objective (X 4) is optional. The primary magnification (X4, X10, X40 or X100) provided by each objective is engraved on its barrel. The oil-immersion objective has a ring engraved on it towards the tip of the barrel.

   Resolving Power of Objective: It is the ability of the objective to resolve each point on the minute object into widely spaced points, so that the points in the image can be seen as distinct and separate from one another, so as to get a clear unblurred image.

   It may appear that very high magnification can be obtained by using more number of high power lenses. Though possible, the highly magnified image obtained in this way is a blurred one. That means, each point in the object cannot be found as widely spaced distinct and separate point on the image. Mere increase in size (greater magnification) without the ability to distinguish structural details (greater resolution) is of little value. Therefore, the basic limitation in light microscopes is one not of magnification, but of resolving power, the ability to distinguish two adjacent points as distinct and separate, *i.e.* to resolve small components in the object into finer details on the image. Resolving power is a function of two factors as given below.

   (*a*) Numerical aperture (n.a.)
   (*b*) Wavelength of the light (λ)

   (*a*) *Numerical aperture*: Numerical aperture is a numerical value concerned with the diameter of the objective lens in relation to its focal length. Thus, it is related to the size of the lower aperture of the objective, through which light enters into it. In a microscope, light is focused on the object as a narrow pencil of light, from where it enters into the objective as a diverging pencil (Figure 4.8). The angle θ subtended by the optical axis (the line joining the centers of all the lenses) and the outermost ray still covered by the objective is a measure of the aperture called 'half aperture angle'.

   A wide pencil of light passing through the object 'resolves' the points in the object into widely spaced points on the lens, so that the lens can produce these points as distinct and separate on the image. Here, the lens gathers more light. On the other hand, a narrow pencil of light cannot 'resolve' the points in the object into widely spaced points on the lens, so that the lens produces a blurred image. Here, the lens gathers less light. Thus, the greater is the width of the pencil of light entering into the objective (2θ), the higher is its 'resolving power'.

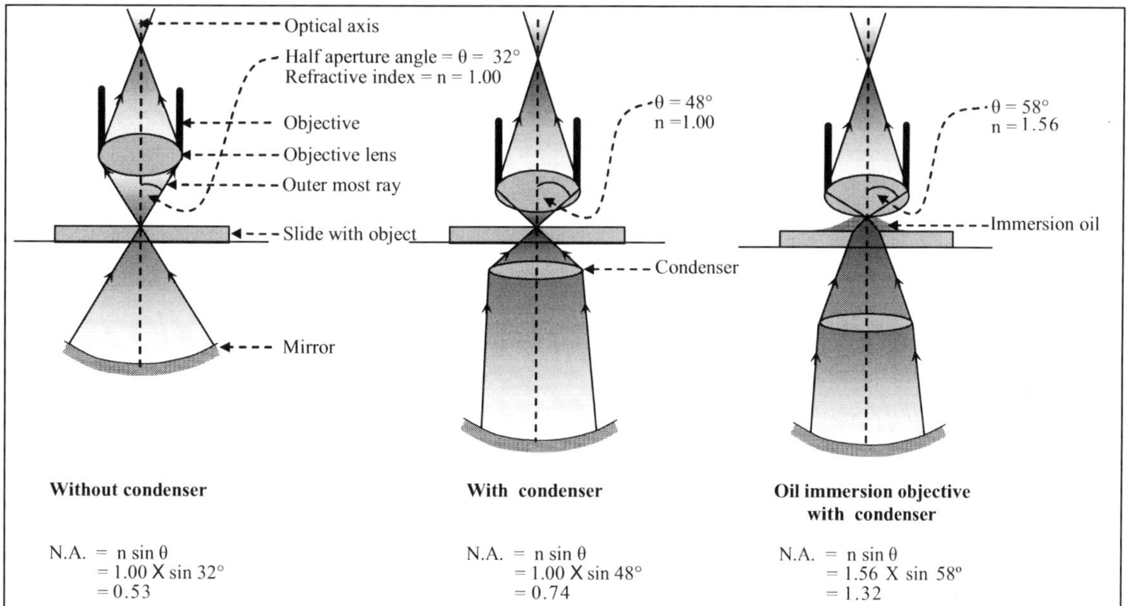

Figure 4.8: Numerical aperture of objectives

The numerical aperture of an objective is its light gathering capacity, which depends on the sine of the angle θ and the refractive index of the medium existing between the object and the objective.

$$\text{Numerical aperture (n.a.)} = n \sin \theta$$

where,

n = Refractive index of the medium between the object and the objective and

θ = Half aperture angle

For air, the value of 'n' is 1.00. When the space between the lower tip of the objective and the slide carrying the object is air, the rays emerging through the glass slide into this air are bent or refracted, so that some portion of it do not pass into the objective. Thus, loss of some light rays reduces numerical aperture and decreases the resolving power. However, when this space is filled with an immersion oil, which has greater refractive index (n=1.56) than that of air (n=1.00), light rays are refracted or bent more towards the objective. Thus, more light rays enter into the objective and greater resolution is obtained. In oil immersion objective, which provides the highest magnification, the size of the aperture is very small. Therefore, it needs bending of more rays into the aperture, so that the object can be distinctly resolved. That is why, immersion oils, such as cedar wood oil and liquid paraffin are used to fill the gap between the object and the objective, while using oil-immersion objective.

(b) Wavelength of light (λ): The smaller is the wavelength of light (λ), the greater is its ability to resolve the points on the object into distinctly visible finer details in the image. Thus, the smaller is the wavelength of light, the greater is its resolving power.

Limit of resolution of objective (d): The limit of resolution of an objective (d) is the distance between any two closest points on the microscopic object, which can be resolved into two separate and distinct points on the enlarged image. Points with their in-between distance less than 'd' or objects smaller than 'd' cannot be resolved into separate points on the image. If the resolving power is high, points very close to each other can be seen as clear and distinct. Thus, the limit of resolution (the distance between the two resolvable points) is smaller. Therefore, smaller objects or finer details can be seen, when 'd' is smaller. Smaller 'd' is obtained by increasing the resolving power, which in turn is obtained by using shorter wavelength of light (λ) and greater numerical aperture.

$$\text{Limit of resolution} = d = \frac{\lambda}{2\ \text{n.a.}}$$

where,

λ = Wave length of light and

n.a. = Numerical aperture of the objective.

If $\lambda_{green} = 0.55\ \mu$ and n.a. = 1.30, then $d = \frac{\lambda}{2\ \text{n.a.}} = \frac{0.55}{2 \times 1.30} = 0.21\mu$. Therefore, the smallest details that can be seen by a typical light microscope is having the dimension of approximately 0.2 μ. Smaller objects or finer details than this cannot be resolved in a compound microscope.

5. *Eyepiece:* The eyepiece is a drum, which fits loosely into the draw tube. It magnifies the magnified real image formed by the objective to a still greatly magnified virtual image to be seen by the eye (Figure 4.9). Usually, each microscope is provided with two types of eyepieces with different magnifying powers (X10 and X25). Depending upon the required magnification, one of the two eyepieces is inserted into the draw tube before viewing. Three varieties of eyepieces are usually available. They are the Huygenian, the hyper plane and the compensating. Among them, the Huygenian is very widely used and efficient for low magnification. In this eyepiece, two simple plano-convex lenses are fixed, one above and the other below the image plane of the real image formed by the objective. The convex surfaces of both the lenses face downward. The lens towards the objective is called 'field lens' and that towards eye, 'eye lens'. The rays after passing through the eye lens, come out through a small circular area known as Ramsden disc or eye point, where the image is viewed by the eye.

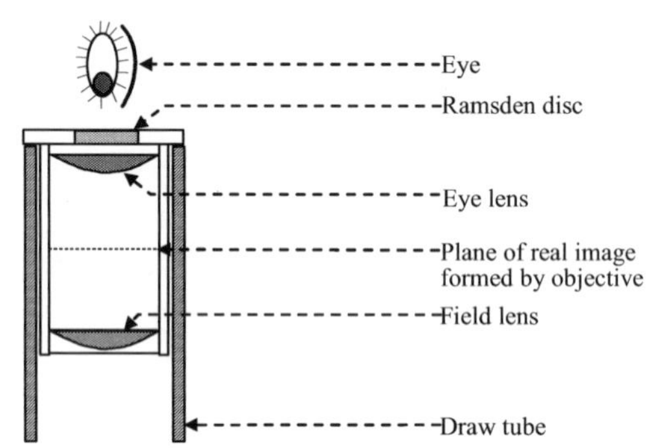

Figure 4.9: Eyepiece (Ocular)

Total magnification: The total magnification obtained in a compound microscope is the product of objective magnification and ocular magnification.

$$M_t = M_{ob} \times M_{oc}$$

where,

M_t = Total magnification,

M_{ob} = Objective magnification and

M_{oc} = Ocular magnification

If the magnification obtained by the objective (M_{ob}) is 100 and that by the ocular (M_{oc}) is 10, then total magnification (M_t) = $M_{ob} \times M_{oc}$ =100 X 10 =1000. Thus, an object of 1μ will appear as 1000 μ.

Useful magnification: It is the magnification that makes visible the smallest resolvable particle. The useful magnification in a light microscope is between X1000 and X2000. Any magnification beyond X2000 makes the image blurred.

Experiment 8

(2) Dark-field Microscope

***Aim*: To study the working principle of a dark-field microscope.**

Working Principle

In a dark-field microscope, the object is brilliantly illuminated against a dark background (Figure 4.10). This is accomplished by equipping a light microscope with a special kind of condenser. It is a condenser with a dark-field stop, which is an opaque disc obstructing the path of light from the light source centrally, but allowing a peripheral ring of light. Thus, the condenser transmits a hollow cone of light from the light source. This cone of light converges on the object and diverges from there again as an inverted hollow cone. Thus, no light enters into the objective, as it remains in the dark cone and the field essentially appears dark in absence of any object. However, if some objects such as microbial cells are present, some of the light rays are scattered (diffracted) by them. These diffracted rays enter into the objective and reach the eye. Thus, the object (microbial cells) appears bright in an otherwise dark microscopic field. Dark-field microscopy is particularly valuable for examination of unstained microbes suspended in fluids (hanging drop preparation and wet mount), where live cells are to be viewed (*See* page 81-86).

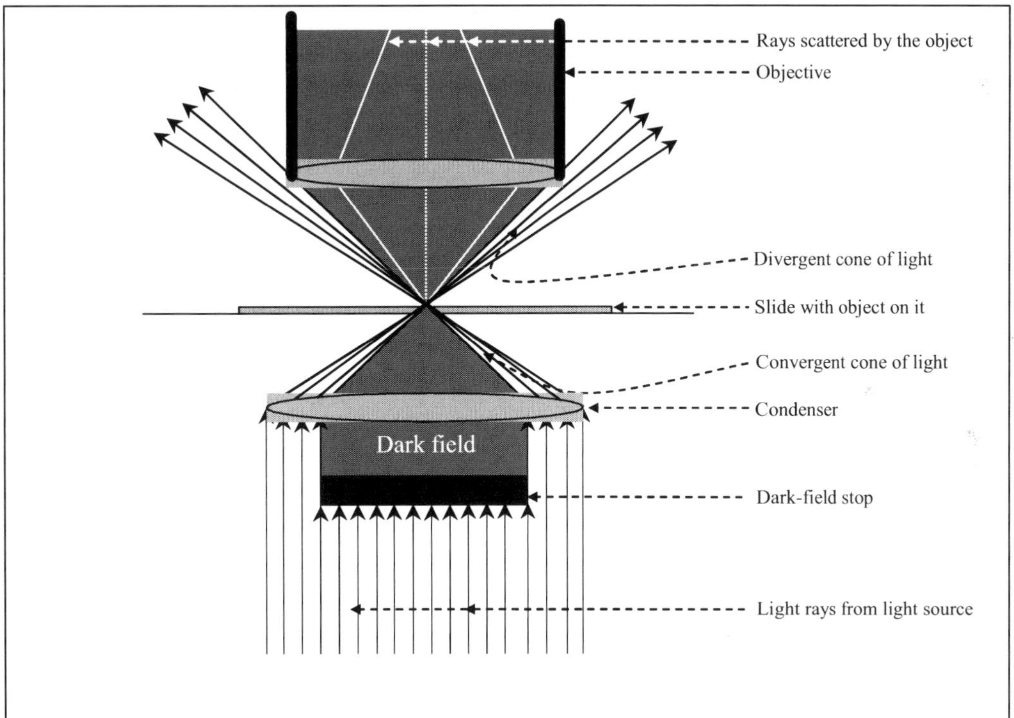

Figure 4.10: Ray diagram of a dark-field microscope

Experiment 9

(3) Fluorescence Microscope

***Aim*: To study the working principle of a fluorescence microscope.**

Working Principle

Many substances absorb light. However some of them, after absorbing light of a particular wavelength and energy, emit light of a longer wavelength and lesser energy. Such substances are called 'fluorescent substances'. Application of this phenomenon is the basis of fluorescence microscope. In practice, microbes are stained with a fluorescent dye and then illuminated with blue light. The dye absorbs blue light (shorter wavelength) and emits green light (longer wavelength).

In a fluorescence microscope, a high intensity mercury arc lamp is used as the light source (Figure 4.11). It emits white light, which is passed through an 'exciter filter'. It allows only the blue component of the white light (the white light consists of seven colors, which in the decreasing order of wavelength are violet, indigo, blue, green, yellow, orange and red) to pass through it and blocks out all other color components. A dichroic mirror, which reflects blue light, but allows green light, is used on the path of the blue light. The mirror is fixed at such an angle that the blue light is reflected downward to the specimen. The specimen is previously stained with a fluorescent dye, such as acridine orange NO, acridine yellow, acriflavine, thioflavine S, thioflavine T or titan yellow G. Certain portions of the specimen retain the dye, while others do not. The portions, which retain the fluorescent dye, absorb blue light and emit green light. The emitted green light goes upward and passes through the dichroic mirror. It reflects back blue light, if any, and allows only green light to pass through. Then, the light reaches a 'barrier filter'. It allows green light to pass to eye and blocks out any residual blue light from the specimen, which might not have been completely reflected by the dichroic mirror. Thus, the eye perceives the stained portions of the specimen as glowing green object against a jet-black background, whereas the unstained portions of the specimen remain invisible.

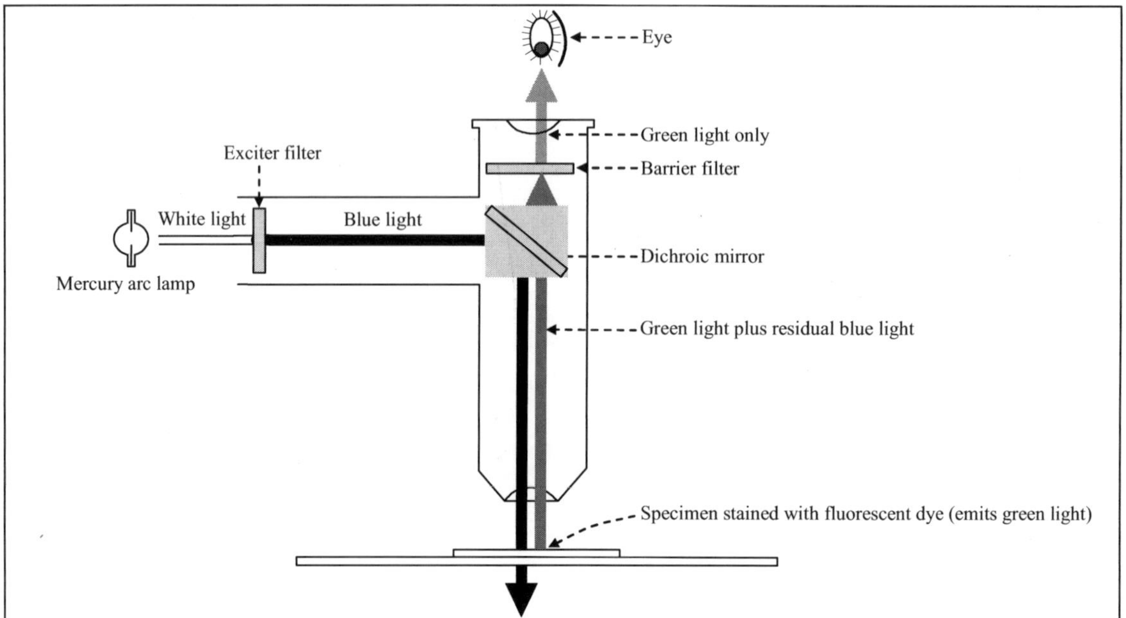

Figure 4.11: Ray diagram of a fluorescence microscope

Experiment 10

(4) Phase-contrast Microscope

***Aim*: To study the working principle of a phase-contrast microscope.**

Working Principle

Light passing from one object into another object of a slightly different refractive index or thickness undergoes a change in phase. In a phase-contrast microscope, this difference in phase is translated into variation in brightness of the image and hence is detectable by eye. With a phase-contrast microscope, the differences among various cells with different refractive indices or thickness can be seen in unstained condition. Microscopic objects can be seen in unstained condition, due to the difference in the refractive index of the object and its surrounding medium. Unstained structures within cells, not discernible by other microscopic methods can also be observed due to the slight differences in their refractive indices or thickness.

A phase-contrast microscope is a compound microscope fitted with a phase-contrast condenser and a phase-contrast objective (Figure 4.12). An annular aperture in the diaphragm placed in the focal

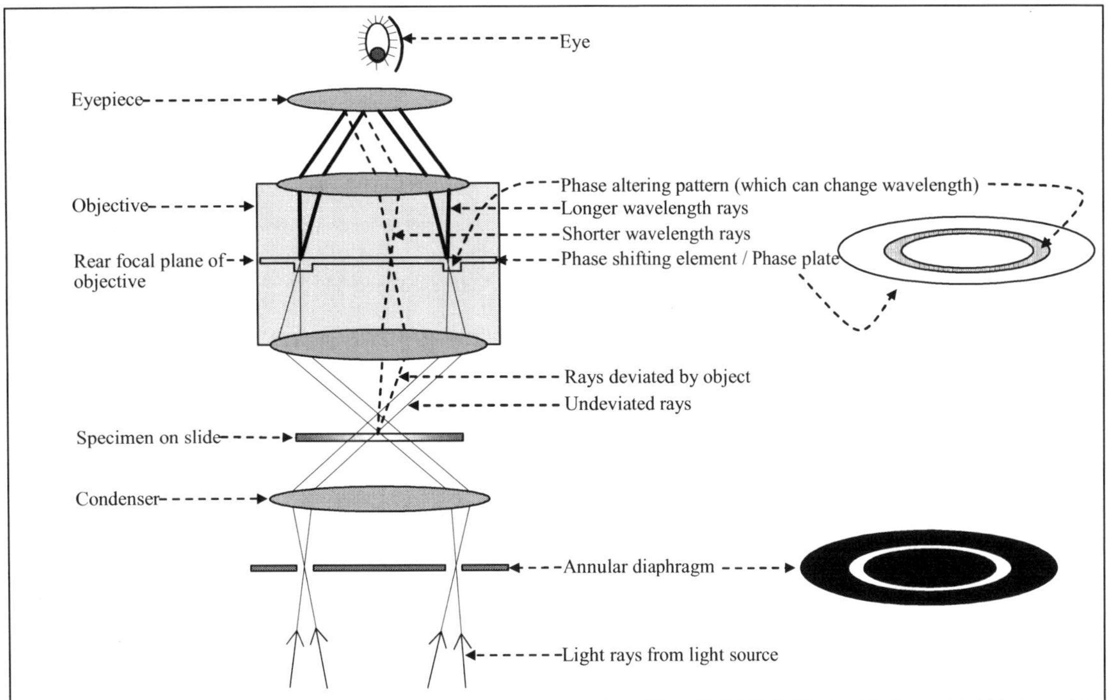

Figure 4.12: Ray diagram of a phase-contrast microscope

plane of the substage condenser controls the illumination of the object. The image of the aperture is formed at the rear focal plane of the objective. In this plane, there is a phase-shifting element or phase-plate. The phase plate also has an annular ring of phase altering pattern, which can increase the wavelength of light passing through it.

Light coming through the annular aperture of condenser passes through the object. Those rays, which are not deviated by the object (solid lines in figure), pass through the phase-altering pattern of the phase plate and acquire longer wavelength. Those rays, which are deviated by the object structures (broken lines in figure), due to different refractive index, pass through the phase-plate not covered by the phase altering pattern. Thus, their wavelength remains unchanged. The difference in phase (wavelength) gives the contrast for clear visibility of the object.

Experiment 11

B. Electron Microscopes

***Aim*: To study the working principle of electron microscopes.**

Working Principle

An electron microscope uses an 'electron beam' to produce the image of the object and magnification is obtained by 'electromagnetic fields'; unlike light or optical microscopes, in which 'light waves' are used to produce the image and magnification is obtained by a system of 'optical lenses'. It has already been discussed that, the smaller is the wavelength of light, the greater is its resolving power (*See* page 71). The wavelength of green light (=0.55μ) is 1,10,000 times longer than that of electron beam (=0.000005μ or 0.05 Å; 1μ = 10,000 Å). That is why, despite its smaller numerical aperture, an electron microscope can resolve objects as small as 0.001μ (=10 Å), as compared to 0.2μ by a light microscope. Thus, the resolving power of an electron microscope is 200 times greater than that of a light microscope. It produces useful magnification upto X 400,000, as compared to X 2000 in a light microscope. Thus, the useful magnification is 200 times greater in an electron microscope than that in a light microscope.

There are three types of electron microscopes as described below.

(1) Transmission Electron Microscope (TEM)

In this microscope, an electron beam from an electron gun, is transmitted through an ultra-thin section of the microscopic object and the image is magnified by the electromagnetic fields. It is used to observe finer details of internal structures of microscopic objects like bacteria and other cells. The specimen to be examined is prepared as an extremely thin dry film or as an ultra-thin section on a small screen and is introduced into the microscope at a point between the magnetic condenser and the magnetic objective (Figure 4.13) The point is comparable to the stage of a light microscope. The magnified image may be viewed on a fluorescent screen through an airtight window or recorded on a photographic plate by an in-built camera. Modern variants have facility to record the photograph by digital camera.

(2) Scanning Electron Microscope (SEM)

In a scanning electron microscope, the specimen is exposed to a narrow electron beam from an electron gun, which rapidly moves over or scans the surface of the specimen (Figure 4.13). This causes the release of a shower of secondary electrons and other types of radiations from the specimen surface. The intensity of these secondary electrons depends upon the shape and the chemical composition of the irradiated object. These electrons are collected by a detector, which generates electronic signals. These signals are scanned in the manner of a television system to produce an image on a cathode ray tube (CRT). The image is recorded by capturing it from the CRT. Modern variants have facility to record the photograph by digital camera. This microscope is used to observe the surface structure of microscopic objects.

(3) Scanning and Transmission Electron Microscope (STEM)

It has both transmission and scanning electron microscope functions.

Limitations of Electron Microscopes

The limitations of electron microscopes are as follows.

(*a*) Live specimen cannot be observed.

(*b*) As the penetration power of electron beam is very low, the object should be ultra-thin. For this, the specimen is dried and cut into ultra-thin sections before observation.

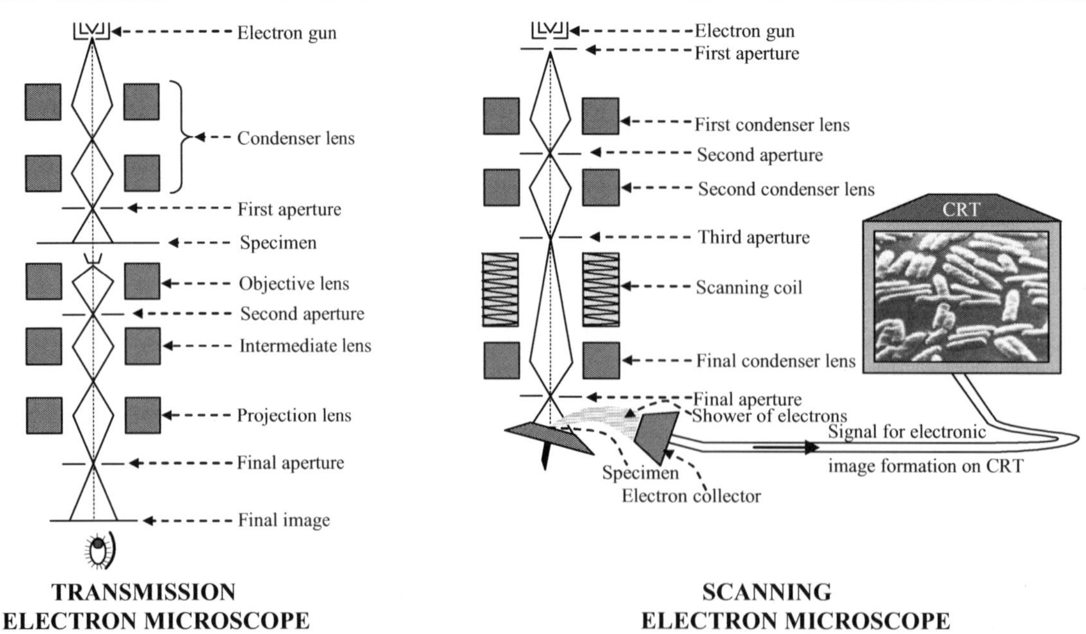

Figure 4.13: Ray diagram of a transmission electron microscope and a scanning electron microscope

Experiment 12

C. Use and Care of Microscopes

***Aim*: To learn how to use and take care of light microscopes.**

The following steps should be followed in use and care of light microscopes.

1. As microscopes are costly instruments, most of them are housed in special cabinets. For use, the cabinet is opened and the microscope is removed by holding its curved arm firmly with right hand.
2. It is taken to the laboratory table very carefully, holding the curved arm firmly with right hand and the base with left hand.
3. The microscope is placed on the laboratory table.
4. When the light source is a plano-concave mirror, it is located at the base of the microscope. If it has not been fitted to the microscope, the bifurcation of the binnacle tip is opened slightly, so that it fits tightly into the hole between the base legs and does not slip out. The microscope is kept on the laboratory table near the window, so that natural light falls on the mirror. The scanning objective (X4) or low power objective (X10) is clicked to position by rotating the nosepiece. Without putting the eyepiece, the microscope is viewed through the draw tube and the mirror rotated, so that a bright field is obtained by reflection on the plane surface of the mirror. When objectives of higher power are brought to position, the concave side of the mirror is used.

   In modern microscopes, usually the light source is an in-built tungsten lamp fitted to the base. For using such microscopes, the connecting wire is connected to the mains through a voltage regulator with its knob at its lowest voltage position. Then, the light is switched on and viewed through the draw tube. Adjustment is made till a bright clear field is obtained. During final observation, the knob is rotated to higher voltage position, so that a clear image is obtained.
5. Based on the magnification required, either the low power eyepiece (X10) or the high power eyepiece (X25) is slipped into the draw tube.
6. The opening of the iris diaphragm is regulated as required. As objectives with greater power are used, the opening is gradually increased and for oil-immersion objective (highest magnification), it is fully opened.
7. The condenser is moved vertically, as required, by rotating the condenser knob. As objectives with greater power are used, the condenser is elevated gradually till it comes just below the stage, in case of oil-immersion objective.
8. The slide with the object to be observed is placed on the stage and clipped to the mechanical stage. Looking from the side, the slide is moved on the stage by the mechanical stage, so that the specimen remains above the central hole of the stage and light from the light source gets focused on it.
9. Looking from the side, the body tube is lowered by the coarse adjustment, so that the scanning objective or the low power objective, whichever is used, remains very close to the object. In modern microscopes, the stage is elevated by the coarse adjustment to bring the object close to the objective. Then, looking through the eyepiece, the objective is moved upward (or the stage downward in modern microscopes) by the coarse adjustment, till a clear image of the object is obtained. The body tube should never be lowered (the stage should never be elevated in modern microscope), while looking through the eyepiece, as it may sometimes touch the object and break the cover slip and slide. If the object is not visible, the slide should be moved on the stage by the mechanical stage.
10. The object is brought to sharp focus using fine adjustment.

11. The condenser and the diaphragm opening are adjusted, if required, to get optimum illumination.
12. If higher magnification of certain object is required, it is brought to the center of the field. The high power objective is clicked to position by rotating the nosepiece. The condenser is elevated and diaphragm opened wider. Then, with coarse adjustment and fine adjustment, the object is brought to sharp focus as described above.
13. If certain object, for still greater magnification, is to be observed under oil-immersion objective, it is brought to the center of the field and a drop of immersion oil (cedar wood oil or liquid paraffin) is put directly on the area to be viewed. The oil-immersion objective is brought to position. Looking from side, the body tube is lowered (or stage elevated) till the tip of the objective touches the oil drop. The condenser is moved to its highest position and diaphragm is fully opened. Looking through the eyepiece, the body tube is elevated very slowly by fine adjustment till a clear image is observed. In no case, should the tip of oil-immersion objective come out from the oil drop.
14. If several areas of the object are to be viewed, the slide is scanned by moving it horizontally with the help of mechanical stage, without adding oil further, till the tip remains immersed in the oil.
15. For final observation with greater illumination, the voltage to the light source is increased by rotating the knob of the voltage regulator. However, such voltage should be supplied only for a very short duration, otherwise the microscope becomes very hot and the specimen gets dried up.
16. After use, if it has electric light source, the light is switched off and wire removed from the mains. All lenses are cleaned with dry clean lens paper. The parts, which come in direct contact with immersion oil, are cleaned with xylol. The xylol is then removed by a tissue paper soaked in 95% ethyl alcohol.
17. The low power objective is brought to position and body tube lowered completely.
18. Mechanical stage is centered.
19. Microscope is kept in the cabinet carefully and the cabinet is closed.
20. While moving the microscope, great care should be taken to see that the eyepiece, which just slips into the draw tube, does not fall on the ground and gets damaged.
21. In case of projection microscope, the projection head is slipped on the draw tube and tightened by a screw. Now, the image can be observed on the screen of the head. Image appears very clear if observed in a dark room. Here, the main problem is getting a completely illuminated screen. Sometimes, the filament of the bulb (light source) comes on the screen. The illuminated screen is obtained by adjustment at the light source.
22. If temperature and humidity are suitable, fungus grows on the lenses. It has to be cleaned with lens paper. Clothes or similar materials, which may leave even very fine filaments on the lens should never be used, because smallest bit of dust, oil or lint decreases the efficiency of the microscope and interferes with observation of the object. The fungal growth on eyepiece can be detected by rotating it in the draw tube, while focused without any object. Fungal growth, if any, can clearly be seen to rotate. Such fungal growth on eyepiece, very often gives wrong idea about the true image of the object. If any particle is observed while focused without any object, the eyepiece has to be cleaned. The fungal growth on objectives, though reduces efficiency of microscopes, cannot be detected easily. Therefore, when the microscope is not used for long time, the objectives and eyepieces are kept in a desiccator.

5

Microscopic Techniques

Any microscopic object is observed under a microscope with a specific purpose. Based on the purpose, the specimen is processed prior to its microscopic observation. The techniques used in the processing and observation of specimen under microscopes for specific purposes are called 'microscopic techniques'. The techniques are broadly of two types as described below (Figure 5.1).

A. Electron microscopic techniques

B. Light microscopic techniques

Experiment 13

A. Electron Microscopic Techniques

Aim: **To learn the principle of different electron microscopic techniques.**

There are a number of techniques, which are adopted for observation of objects under electron microscopes. These have been described below.

(1) Shadow-casting

In shadow-casting, the microscopic object is dried in a special grid placed inside a vacuum jar. An extremely thin layer of metal (*e.g.* platinum) is deposited on the object from a highly heated filament at an oblique angle, so that the object produces a shadow on the uncoated side. Examination of the shadowed image provides information as to the shape of the object (topographic features of the surface of the object), which can be observed by scanning electron microscope.

(2) Negative Staining

This technique is followed to observe minute details of very small objects, such as viruses and bacterial flagella. An electron-opaque material like phosphotungstic acid or its salt is allowed to form a coat of thick deposit on the surface of the object, without entering into it. When electrons from the electron gun of the electron microscope cannot pass through these coated surfaces, these structures become clearly visible.

(3) Ultra-thin Sectioning

An intact microbial cell is too thick to allow visualisation of its internal fine structures under electron microscope. For observation of the intracellular fine structures, the cell is embedded in a block of plastic material and cut into ultra-thin sections (as thin as 60 nm). The exact structure is interpreted by observing several ultra-thin slices sectioned at different levels and at different angles. Improvement in contrast of structures is possible through the use of special stains, such as uranium and lanthanum salts.

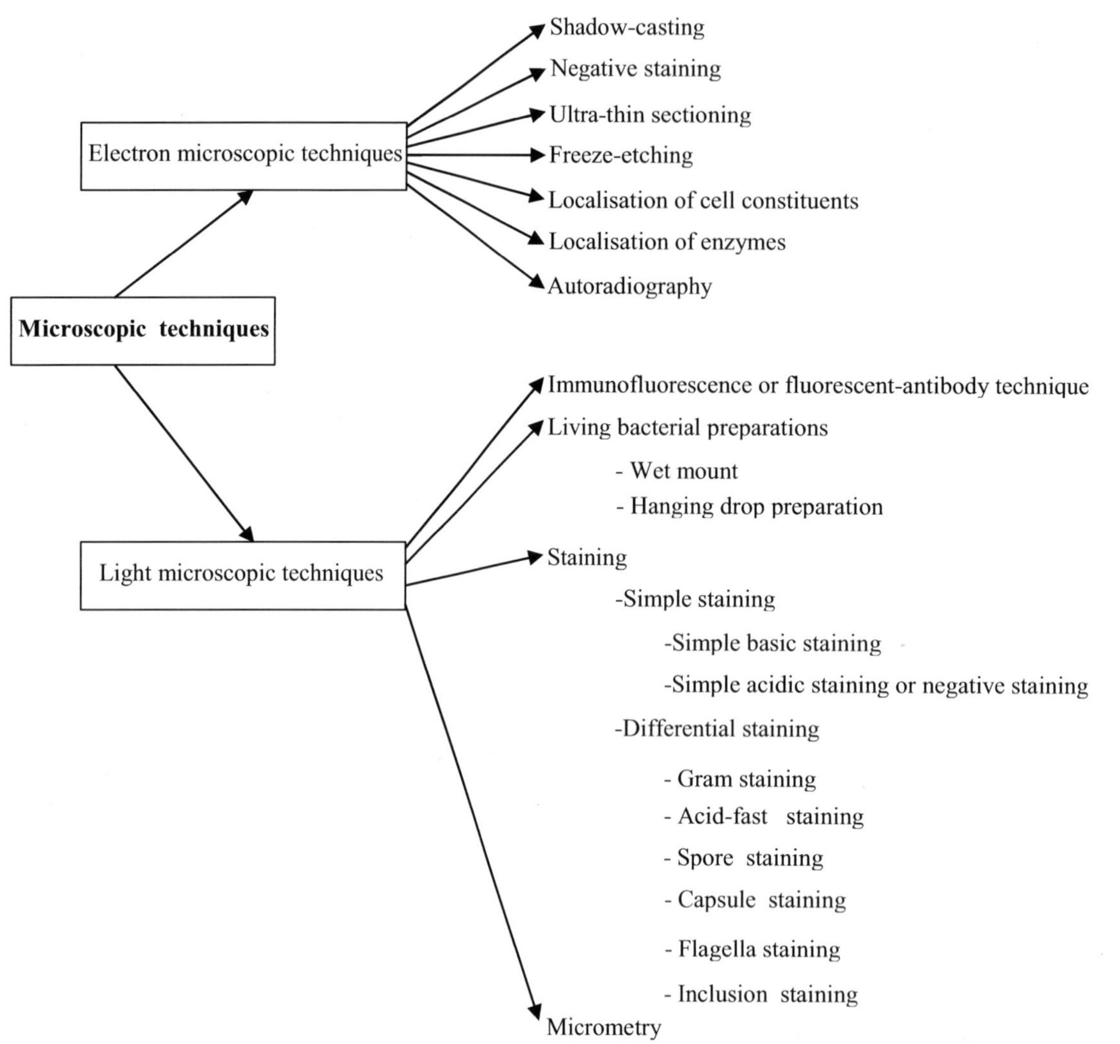

Figure 5.1. Microscopic techniques

(4) Freeze-etching

To obtain ultra-thin sections of an object, it has to be fixed by chemical treatments. Such chemical treatments result in artifacts. These artifacts are overcome by freeze-etching. In freeze etching, the specimen is frozen inside a block and is sectioned, while still contained inside it in frozen condition.

(5) Localisation of Cell Constituents

It is a special technique performed to locate chemical constituents of cells. For example, to locate an antigen in a cell, an ultra-thin section of the cell is treated with a ferritin-labeled antibody, which binds to the antigen to form ferritin-labeled antibody-antigen complex. As ferritin is an iron-containing substance of high density, the antibody-antigen complex markedly affects the passage of an electron beam, thereby producing a high contrast for clear observation under an electron microscope.

(6) Localisation of Enzymes

This technique is used to locate the position of enzymes within cells. For example, in detecting the enzyme isocitrate dehydrogenase, ultra-thin sections of bacteria cells are prepared. Then, colloidal gold is affixed specifically to the enzyme, following an immunochemical technique. The colloidal gold-fixed enzyme can be observed under electron microscope.

(7) Autoradiography

It is a cytochemical technique, in which the location of a particular chemical constituent in an object is determined by observing the site, at which a radioactive material becomes positioned. The object is first exposed to the radioactive substance to permit its uptake. Then, it is covered with a layer of photographic emulsion and kept in darkness for few hours. The ionising radiation emitted during the decay of the substance produces latent images in the emulsion. After photographic processing, the developed images are seen under electron microscope as grains of silver in the preparation.

B. Light Microscopic Techniques

These are the techniques used for observation of objects under light microscopes. These techniques are described below.

Experiment 14

(1) Fluorescence-antibody Technique

Aim: **To learn the principle of immunofluorescence or fluorescence-antibody technique for detection of particular bacteria in a sample.**

Principle

Fluorescence-antibody or immunofluorescence technique is a rapid and reliable procedure for the detection of a particular bacteria in a sample. A number of antibodies, labeled with fluorescent dyes, such as fluorescein isocyanate or isothiocyanate, each specific to a particular bacteria, are available. One of these labeled antibodies, specific to the particular bacteria to be detected, is added in drops to a heat-fixed smear of the unknown sample of bacteria on a slide and spread gently over the surface of the smear. A moistened filter paper is placed inside a petri dish. Then, the slide is placed inside it on a U-shaped glass rod and incubated at 25°C for 35 minutes. Excess antibody on the smear is washed away with 1% phosphate-buffered saline. The slide is immersed into a Coplin jar containing 1% phosphate-buffered saline at 25°C for 10 minutes. The slide is dried by bibulous paper. One drop of glycerol is added to the smear. It is covered with a cover slip and examined under a fluorescence microscope.

If the bacteria specific to the labeled antibody used is present in the unknown sample of bacteria, an antigen-antibody complex is formed (here bacteria is the antigen). As the antibody is tagged with a fluorescent substance, the antigen-antibody complex emits fluorescence, when observed under fluorescence microscope. If bacteria specific to the antibody is absent, the fluorescent antibody is washed away and fluorescence is not observed.

(2) Living Bacteria Preparations

The refractive index of bacteria cells is very close to that of water, in which they are suspended during observation and to that of the glass slides, on which they are observed under microscope. Therefore, it is very difficult to observe them clearly. To overcome this difficulty, the cells are coloured by stains, which impart deep colour to the cells and a light colour to the surrounding medium, in which they are suspended. Thus, the deep-coloured cells get a clear contrast against the light-coloured background and can be observed clearly. But in most of the staining processes, the cells are subjected to heat-fixation for adhering the cells to the glass slide and are treated with chemicals, such as stains, acid and alcohol. All these kill the bacteria cells and disrupt their natural shape, size and motility. That is why, to observe the natural shape, size and motility of bacteria, they are to be observed in living state. This is done in two ways as follows:

(*i*) Wet mount

(*ii*) Hanging drop preparation

For observation of unstained living bacteria, dark-field microscope or phase-contrast microscope should be preferred over compound microscope.

Experiment 15

(*i*) Wet Mount of Bacteria

***Aim*: To prepare wet mount of a bacteria, for observing its natural shape, size and arrangement in living condition.**

Purpose

Bacteria cells can be seen easily and clearly, when coloured by stains, but in most of the staining processes, the cells die and lose their natural shape and size due to heat-fixation as well as due to exposure to chemicals (stains, acid and alcohol). The aim of this experiment is to observe the natural shape, size and arrangement of bacteria in living condition. Motility cannot be observed in wet mount, as the cells are pressed between the slide and the cover slip.

Principle

In wet mount, a drop of the bacteria suspension is placed on a slide, covered with a cover slip and observed under a compound microscope or preferably under a dark-field or phase-contrast microscope using oil-immersion objective.

Materials Required

Glass slide, cover slip, petroleum jelly, immersion oil (cedar wool oil or liquid paraffin), bacteria culture (on solid medium or in liquid suspension), loop and microscope (compound, dark-field or phase-contrast).

Procedure

1. A slide is cleaned properly under tap water, such that water does not remain as drops on its surface (Figure 5.2).
2. The slide is dried by wiping with bibulous paper and subsequently moving over flame or keeping in the sun.
3. If the bacteria has been grown on a solid medium (as slant culture or plate culture), a drop of distilled water is put at the center of the slide. A loop is sterilised by heating it over a flame to red hot. It is cooled to room temperature. Then, aseptically a small portion of bacteria culture is scraped by the loop and transferred to the drop of water. A suspension of bacteria is made by gently mixing the loop of bacteria in the water drop, in such a way that, the drop does not spread. If grown in a liquid medium as suspension, aseptically a drop of the bacteria suspension is placed at the center of the slide directly, using a flame-sterilised loop.
4. Petroleum jelly or similar material is applied surrounding the drop, so that, when the cover slip covers the drop, evaporation and effect of air current is minimised.
5. A cover slip is kept in a slanting position near the drop of bacteria suspension with one edge touching the slide.
6. Slowly the cover slip is lowered, till it touches the surface of the drop.
7. Then, the cover slip is released, so that the drop of bacteria suspension spreads in all directions under the cover slip. Care should be taken, so that no air bubble is formed in the suspension.
8. The slide is clipped on the stage of a compound microscope and observed using low power and high dry objectives. Then, a drop of immersion oil is put on the cover slip and observed using oil-immersion objective of the microscope (*See* point 13 at page 78). Preferably, a phase-contrast or dark-field microscope should be used for clear observation.

Observations (Under Oil-immersion Objective)

1. *Shape of bacteria:* Spherical (coccus)
   Rod-shaped (bacilli)

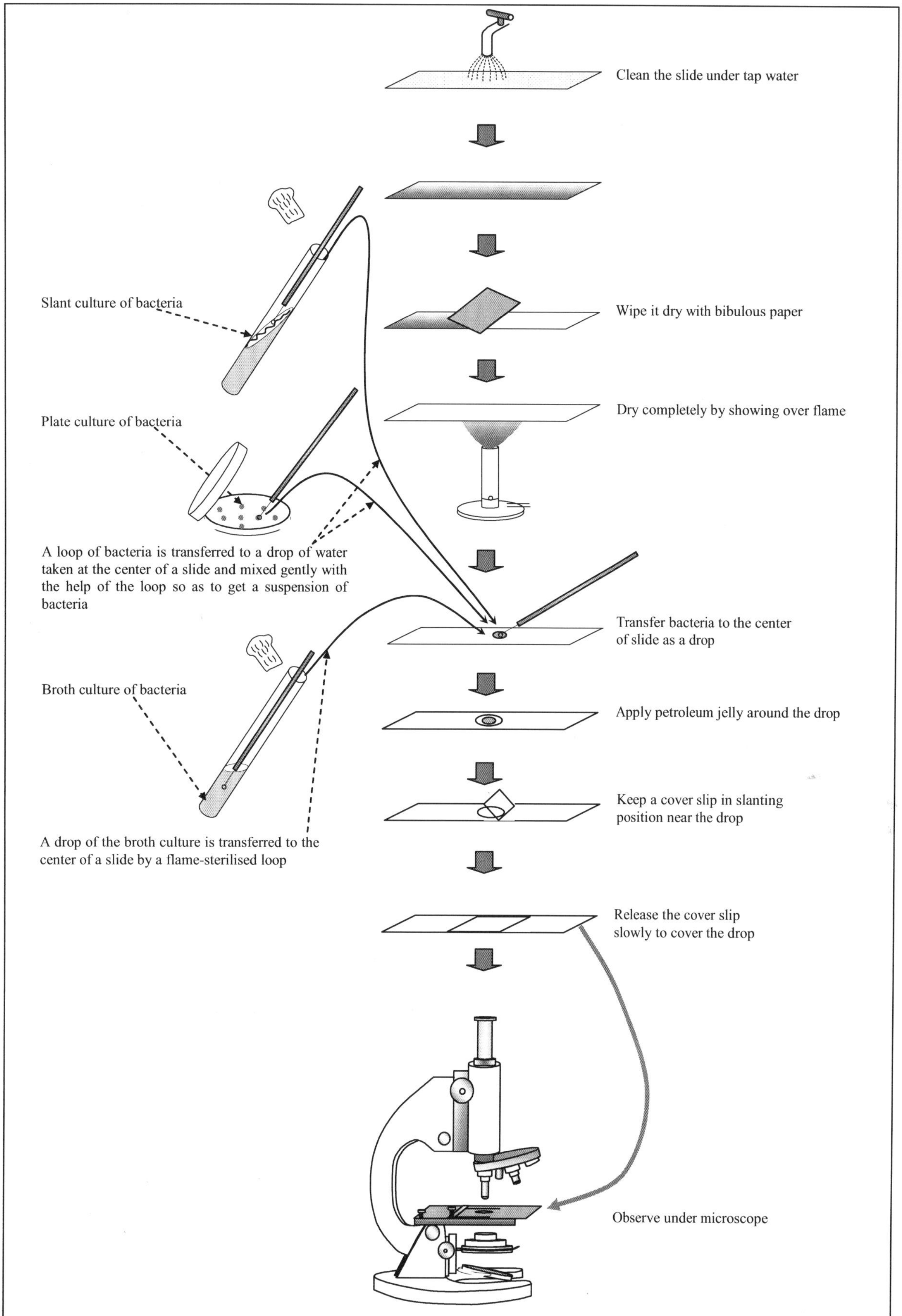

Figure 5.2: Wet mount of bacteria

	Comma-like (vibrio)
	Spiral (spirochetes)
2. *Arrangement of bacteria*:	Pairs (diplobacillus/diplococcus)
	In fours (tetrads)
	In chains (streptococcus/streptobacillus)
	Grape-like clusters (staphylococcus)
	Cuboidal (sarcinae or octet)
3. *Size of bacteria*:	By eye estimation, make drawing of the field under oil-immersion objective.

Experiment 16

(*ii*) Hanging Drop Preparation (Motility Test)

***Aim*: To perform motility test of a bacteria, by hanging drop preparation, to find out whether it is motile or non-motile.**

Purpose

Motility means ability of movement by own power. Based on motility, bacteria can be divided into two groups as follows.

(1) Motile Bacteria

A bacteria, which has the intrinsic ability of movement in the surrounding medium, in which it remains suspended, is a motile bacteria.

(2) Non-motile Bacteria

A bacteria, which does not have the intrinsic ability of movement in the surrounding medium, in which it remains suspended, is a non-motile bacteria. Non-motile bacteria may show apparent motility, resulting from their brownian movement caused by the bombardment of the water molecules in the surrounding medium, on the bacteria cells.

In wet mount, though the shape and size of bacteria can be observed, motility may be hampered, as the suspension is pressed between the slide and the cover slip. That is why, hanging drop preparation or motility test is performed for clear observation of the motility of bacteria, besides their shape and size. It is useful in the identification of bacteria (*See* pages 188 and 189).

Principle

A very small drop of bacteria suspension is hung from the center of a cover slip into the cavity of a cavity slide. The hanging drop is observed under a microscope using oil-immersion objective. If the bacteria is motile, its cells can be seen to have erratic movement in the surrounding medium. In contrast, if it is non-motile, its cells remain static in the medium without any movement or may show brownian movement resulting from the bombardment by the water molecules in the medium, on the bacteria cells.

Materials Required

Cavity slide, cover slip, petroleum jelly or vaseline, immersion oil, 24-hour old broth culture of bacteria, loop and microscope (compound, dark-field or phase-contrast).

Procedure

1. A cavity slide is cleaned properly under tap water, such that water does not remain as drops on its surface. A cavity slide is a glass slide with a small round depression at the center, into which a small drop of bacteria suspension can hang (Figure 5.3).

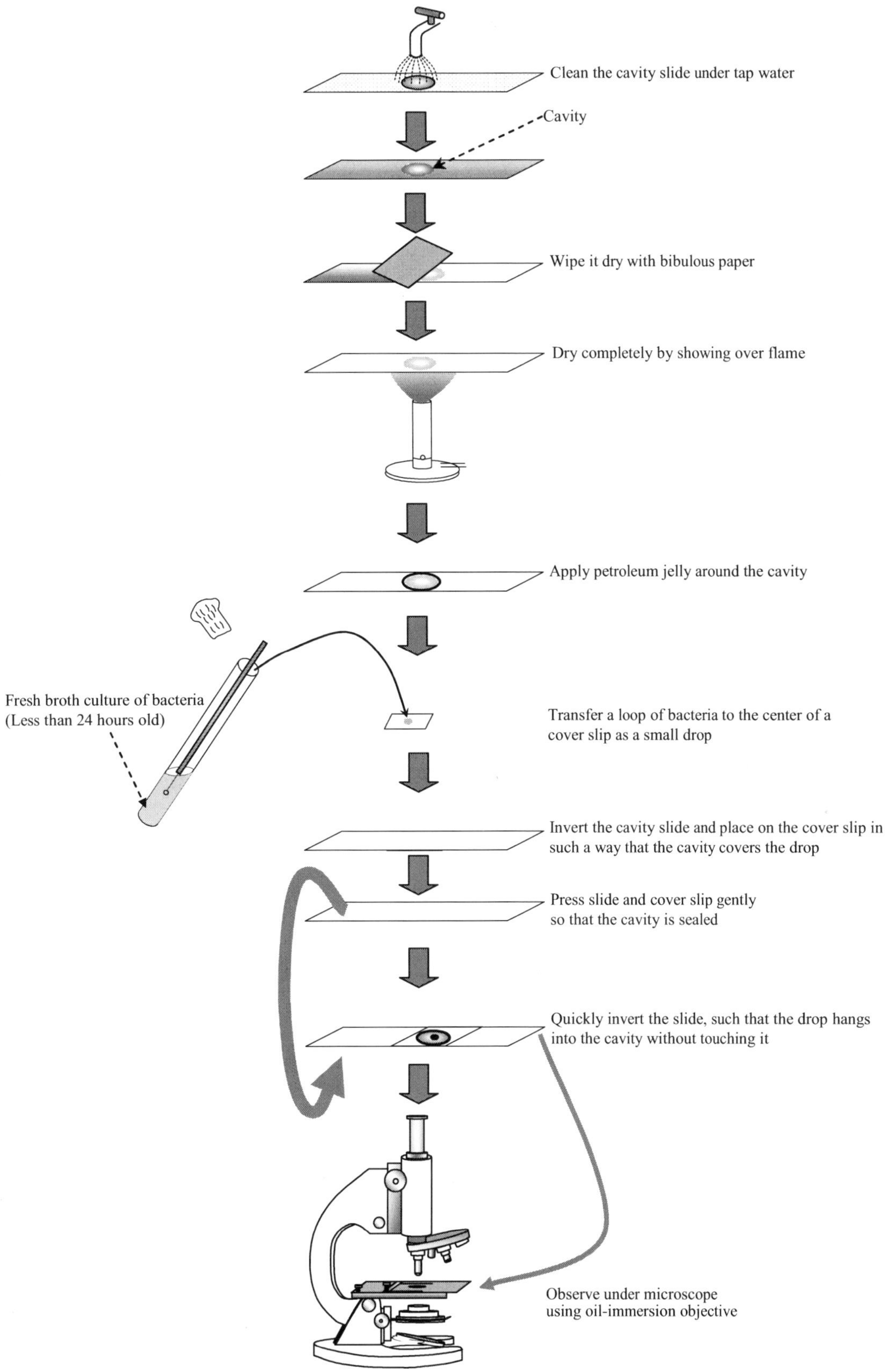

Figure 5.3: Hanging drop preparation (Motility test) of bacteria

2. The slide is dried by wiping with bibulous paper and subsequently, moving it over flame or keeping it in the sun.
3. A ring of petroleum jelly (or vaseline) is applied around the cavity.
4. A loop is sterilised over flame and cooled. A loopful of bacteria suspension is taken from the 24-hour old broth culture[1] aseptically. A small drop of the suspension is placed at the center of a cover slip. The broth culture should not be more than 24 hours old, because bacteria may lose their motility, as they grow older.
5. The cavity slide is inverted and placed on the cover slip, in such a way that, the cavity covers the drop.
6. The slide and cover slip are pressed together gently, so that the cavity is sealed. Care should be taken to see that no part of the cavity touches the drop.
7. The slide is inverted quickly, such that the drop hangs into the cavity without touching it.
8. The slide is clipped to stage of the microscope.
9. The edge of the drop is focused under low power objective. The reasons for focusing the edge of the drop are as follows.
   (*a*) Better contrast is obtained due to difference in the refractive index of the drop and the cover slip.
   (*b*) As the drop hangs, it thins towards the edge, for which the edge contains less number of bacteria to be observed clearly for motility.
   (*c*) Usually aerobic bacteria come towards the edge to get more oxygen for respiration, for which they can be observed on the edge.
10. A drop of immersion oil is put on the cover slip just above the hanging drop and the edge of the hanging drop is observed under oil-immersion objective of the microscope (*See* point 13 at page 78). Preferably, a phase-contrast or dark-field microscope should be used for clear observation.

Observations (Under Oil-immersion Objective)

1. *Motility*:	Motile or non-motile
2. *Shape of bacteria*:	Spherical (coccus)
	Rod-shaped (bacilli)
	Comma-like (vibrio)
	Spiral (spirochetes)
3. *Arrangement of bacteria*:	Pairs (diplobacillus/diplococcus)
	In fours (tetrads)
	In chains (streptococcus/streptobacillus)
	Grape-like clusters (staphylococcus)
	Cuboidal (sarcinae or octet).
4. *Size of bacteria*:	By eye estimation, make drawing of the field under oil-immersion objective.

1 A broth culture is prepared by taking nutrient broth in a test tube, sterilising it in autoclave at 121°C (15 psi pressure) for 15 minutes and inoculating into it, a colony of bacteria to be identified. (For demonstration, some material suspected to contain high load of bacteria *e.g.* curd, cow dung, sewage water may be inoculating into the broth). The inoculated broth is incubated at 37°C in a microbiological incubator for about 24 hours till a turbid suspension of bacteria can be seen. Bacteria grown on solid agar plates or slants cannot be used for hanging drop preparation, as bacteria may lose their motility, when grown on plates or slants.

(3) Staining

Purpose of Staining

The refractive index of bacteria cells is very close to that of water, in which they are suspended during observation and also to that of the glass slide, on which they are observed under microscope. Therefore, it is very difficult to observe them clearly. To overcome this difficulty, the cells are coloured by stains, which impart deep colour to the cells and light colour to the surrounding medium, in which they are suspended. The deep-coloured cells get a clear contrast against the light-coloured background and can be observed clearly. Thus, staining is a method of imparting colour to the otherwise colourless transparent microorganisms with the help of various biological dyes called 'stains' for their microscopic observation.

Chemistry of Stains

Colouring agents are of three types as follows.

1. *Dyes*: They are used for general purpose colouring such as, for colouring textile materials and for colouring walls.
2. *Stains*: They are used for colouring biological or microbiological specimen. These are more accurate and exacting.
3. *Indicators*: They are chemicals, which change colour with change in hydrogen ion concentration (pH).

Though 'stain' is the appropriate term, the term 'dye' is used widely in microbiology to mean colouring agents. In the past, natural dyes were prepared from various plants. They have been widely replaced by synthetic dyes. As the first synthetic dye was prepared from aniline, all synthetic dyes are called 'aniline dyes'. However, most of these dyes are now produced from coal-tar for which they are now called 'coal-tar dyes'. The coal-tar dyes are benzene derivatives. A dye molecule consists of three components (Figure 5.4) as given below.

(*a*) A benzene ring
(*b*) A chromophore group
(*c*) An auxochrome group

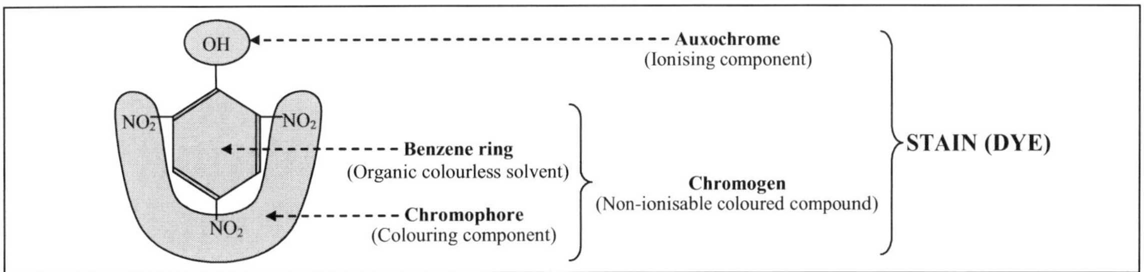

Figure 5.4: Structure of a typical dye molecule

Benzene is an organic colourless solvent, whereas the chromophore is the colouring component of the dye. Benzene combines with the chromophore to form chromogen (Figure 5.5). As chromogen does not possess the property to dissociate, it cannot combine with the cells and is washed away easily. When a chromogen combines with an auxochrome, a dye or stain is formed. The auxochrome imparts the electrolytic dissociation property (salt forming property) to the dye. Thus, chemically a stain is defined as an organic compound containing a benzene ring, a chromophore group and an auxochrome group.

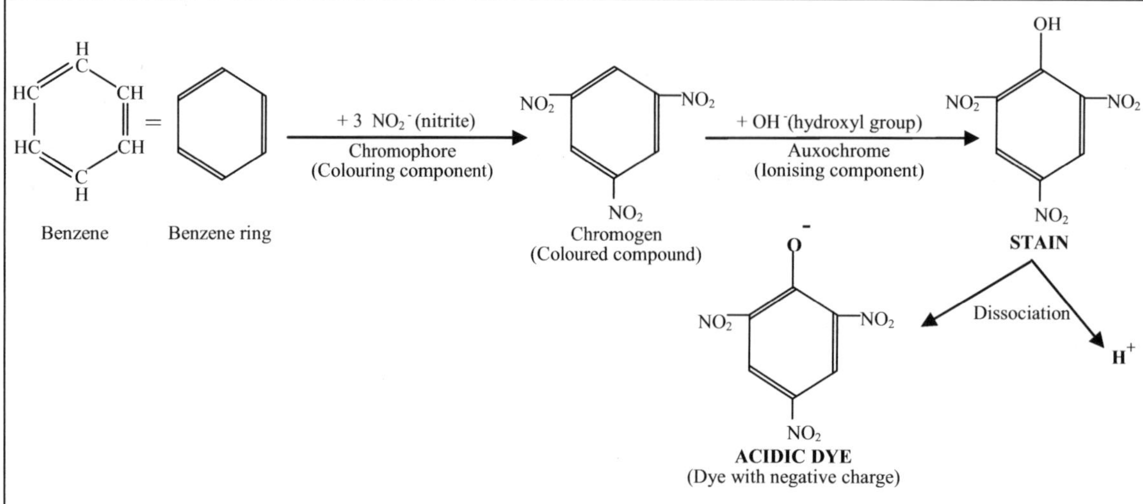

Figure 5.5: Formation of a typical dye (Picric acid)

Types of Staining

Staining of bacteria is of different types as described below (Figure 5.6).

I. Simple Staining

Here, only one stain is used. This staining is used to observe shape (cocci, bacilli, vibrio, spirilli) and arrangement (single, pair, tetrad, chain, cluster) of bacteria. It is of two types as follows.

A. *Basic Staining*

In basic staining, a basic stain, like methylene blue, crystal violet or carbol fuchsin, is used to stain the bacteria cells. The stain binds tightly to the bacteria cells and imparts a deep colour of the stain to the cells, while the surrounding medium gets a light colour of the stain.

B. *Acidic Staining*

In acidic staining, an acidic stain, like eosin or nigrosin, is used to stain the bacteria cells negatively. The stain makes the surrounding coloured, while the bacteria cell remain colourless.

II. Differential Staining

Here, more than one stains are used. It is performed for the following purposes.

A. *Separation into Groups*

These differential staining methods are performed to differentiate bacteria into different groups based on their staining characteristics. These methods include the following.

(*a*) *Gram Staining*: This staining method is performed to differentiate between gram-positive and gram-negative bacteria.

(*b*) *Acid-fast Staining*: It is performed to differentiate between acid-fast and non-acid-fast bacteria.

B. *Visualisation of Specific Structures of Bacteria*

These differential staining methods are performed to visualise specific structural components of bacteria cells. These methods include the following.

(*a*) *Spore Staining*: This staining method is used to stain endospore of spore-forming bacteria.

(*b*) *Capsule Staining*: This method is used to stain the capsule, which surrounds capsulated bacteria.

(*c*) *Flagella Staining*: It is performed to visualise flagella of flagellated bacteria.

(*d*) *Inclusion Staining*: This staining method is performed to stain the cell inclusions of bacteria cells like volutin granules, glycogen granules and PBH granules.

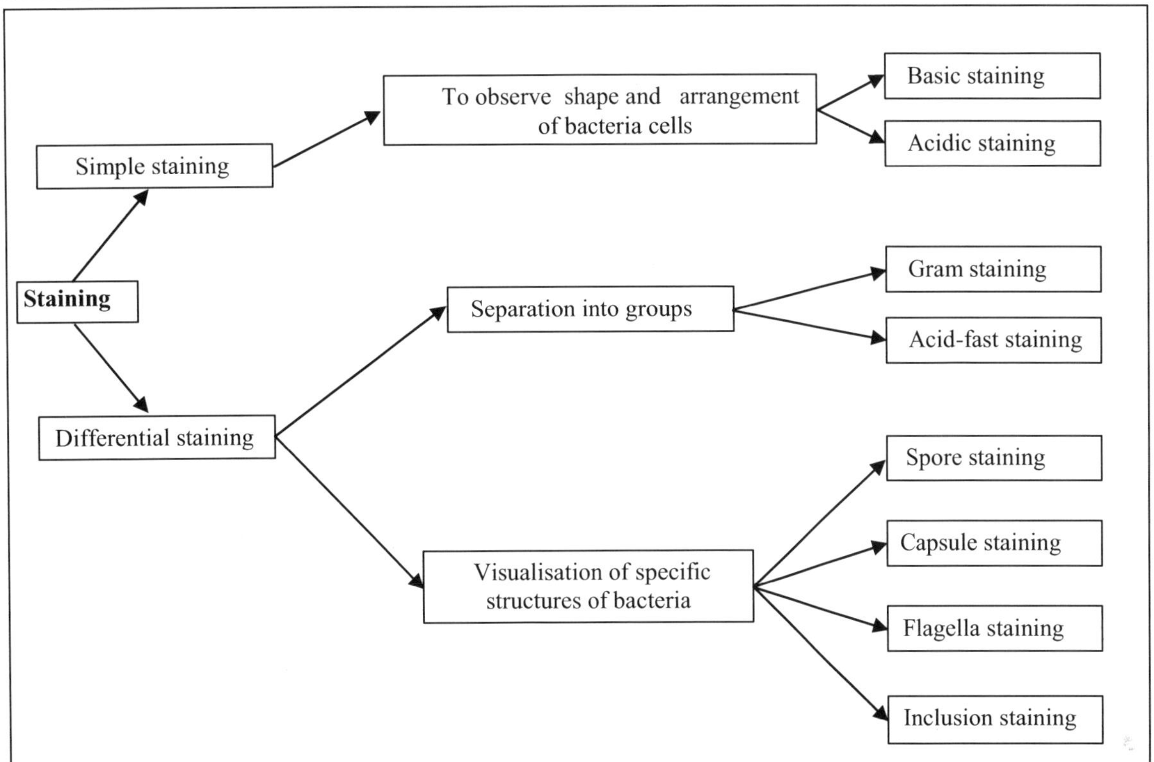

Figure 5.6: Types of staining of bacteria

Experiment 17

(*i*) Simple Basic Staining

***Aim*: To perform simple basic staining of a bacteria, to observe its shape, size and arrangement.**

Purpose

In the process of identification of bacteria, the first step is to observe its shape, arrangement and motility. Bacteria are transparent and their refractive index is close to that of the water, in which they are suspended as well as to that of the glass slide, on which they are observed under microscope. Therefore, it is difficult to observe their shape (cocci, bacilli, vibrios, spirilli) and arrangement (single, pair, tetrad, cluster). Simple basic staining is performed for clear observation of their shape and arrangement. In this method, the stain binds tightly to the bacteria cells and imparts a deep colour of the stain to the cells, whereas the surrounding medium gets a light colour of the stain. This provides the necessary contrast for clear observation of bacteria. However, as staining kills bacteria, motility cannot be tested in this method. Motility test is done by hanging drop preparation.

Principle

The process of basic staining is an ion-exchange reaction between the basic stain and the active sites on the surface of and within the bacteria cells (Figure 5.7). It has been found that bacteria cells are always surrounded by cations (positively charged ions), such as K^+ and Na^+. This implies that, the cells carry negative charges. Such negative charges result from the negative charges of bacterial nucleic acids within the cells and certain cell wall components on the surface. As a basic stain ionises into a cationic chromogen (positively charged dye ion) and an anion, the chromogen ions replace the Na^+ and K^+ ions and bind to the negative charges on the cell surface and within the cells. This imparts deep colour to the cells, as compared to the light colour of the surrounding medium.

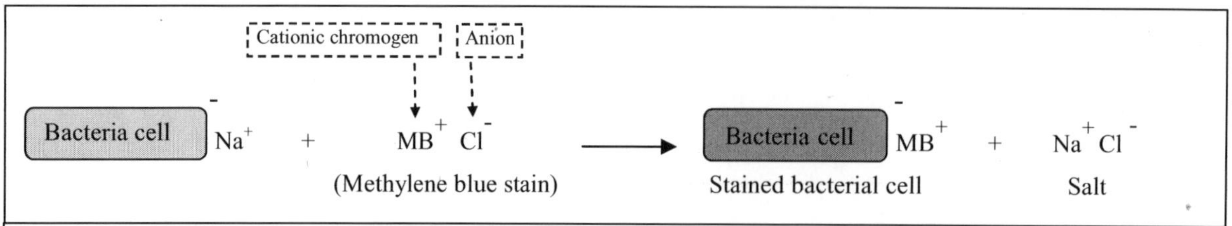

Figure 5.7: Principle of simple basic staining

Materials Required

Glass slide, loop, basic stain (methylene blue/crystal violet/carbol fuchsin) (*See* Appendix II at page 251), broth/plate/slant culture of bacteria, microscope, immersion oil.

Procedure

1. A slide is cleaned properly under tap water, such that water does not remain as drops on its surface (Figure 5.8).
2. The slide is dried by wiping with bibulous paper and subsequently, moving over flame or keeping in the sun.
3. A smear of bacteria is prepared at the center of the slide in two methods as follows.
   (*a*) If bacteria grown on agar plate or agar slant is to be observed, a drop of water is put at the center of the slide and a loop of bacteria from the plate or slant is transferred to it by a loop sterilised over flame. Then, by slow rotation of the loop in the drop, a bacteria suspension is made and it is spread till a smear is obtained.
   (*b*) If bacteria grown in liquid broth is to be observed, a drop of the bacteria suspension is directly placed at the center of the slide by a flame-sterilised loop and a smear is made by spreading.
4. The smear is air-dried.
5. The smear is fixed by heating. Heating results in coagulation of the cellular proteins, due to which the cells stick to the slide surface and do not get washed away during staining. Heat-fixation is done by quickly passing the slide high above a flame 2-3 times, with the smear surface facing upward, so that the smear does not get heated up.
6. The slide is kept on a staining tray and flooded with the solution of the basic stain, such as methylene blue, crystal violet or carbol fuchsin.
7. After the specified time (2 minutes for methylene blue, 1 minute for crystal violet and 30 seconds for carbol fuchsin), excess stain is completely washed away from the smear under gently-flowing tap water, in such a way that, water does not fall directly on the smear.
8. The slide is blotted dry with bibulous paper.
9. The slide is clipped to the stage of the microscope and the smear observed under low power and high dry objectives.
10. A drop of immersion oil is put on the smear.
11. The smear is observed under oil-immersion objective (*See* point 13 at page 78).

Observations (Under Oil-immersion Objective)

1. *Colour of bacteria*: Blue/violet/red
2. *Shape of bacteria*: Spherical (coccus)
   Rod-shaped (bacilli)
   Comma-like (vibrio)
   Spiral (spirochetes)

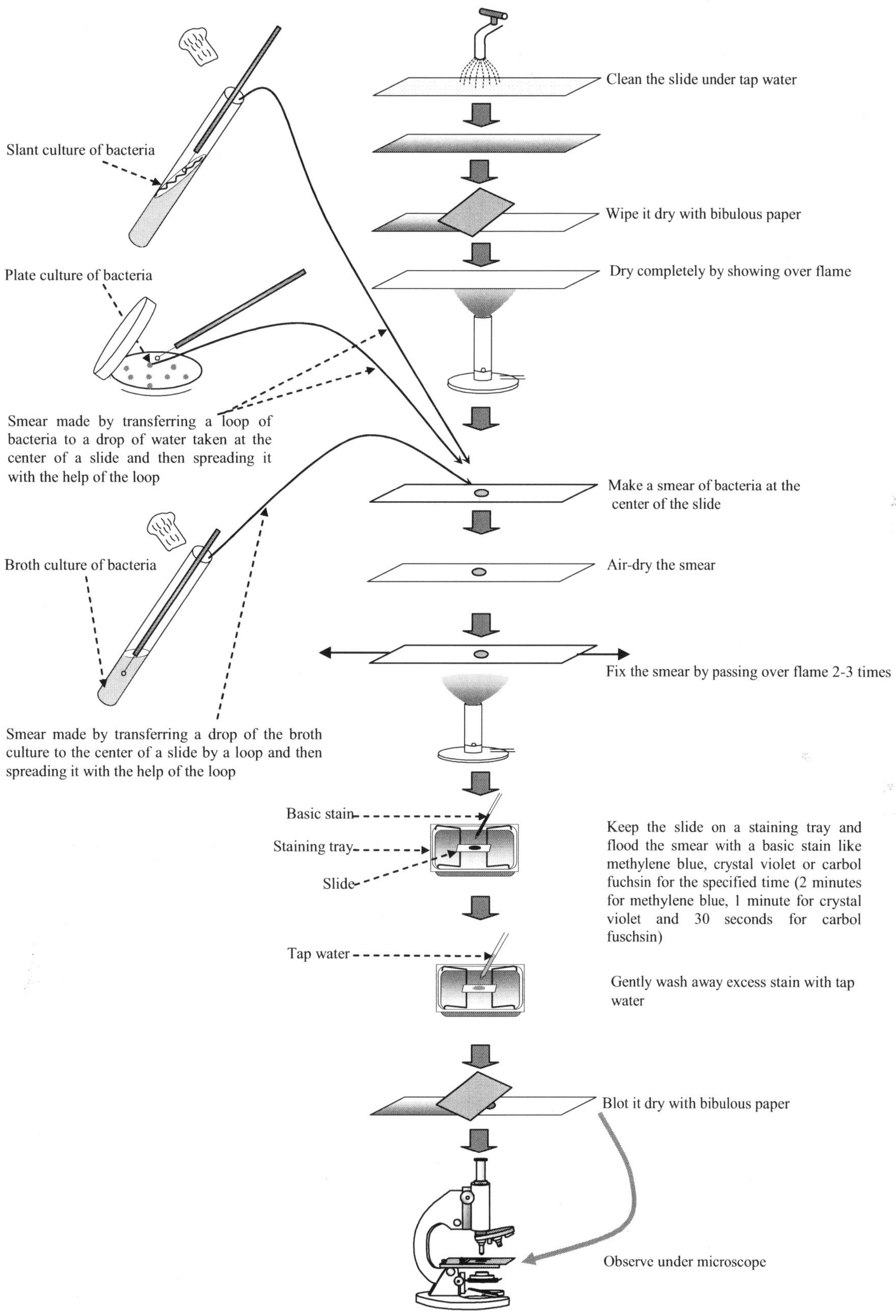

Figure 5.8: Simple basic staining

3. *Arrangement of bacteria*: Pairs (diplobacillus/diplococcus)
In fours (tetrads)
In chains (streptococcus/streptobacillus)
Grape-like clusters (staphylococcus)
Cuboidal (sarcinae or octet)

4. *Size of bacteria*: By eye estimation, make drawing of the field under oil-immersion objective.

Experiment 18

(*ii*) Simple Acidic Staining

***Aim*: To perform simple basic staining of a bacteria, to observe its shape, size and arrangement.**

Purpose

It is not possible to observe the natural shape, size and arrangement of bacteria by basic staining, as these characteristics are distorted by heat-fixation. Besides, some bacteria (*e.g.* spirilli) are difficult to be stained. Thus, negative staining is performed for two reasons as follows.

(*a*) To observe the natural shape, size and arrangement of bacteria, as no heat-fixation is done here.

(*b*) To observe those bacteria, which are difficult to be stained.

Principle

Bacteria cells carry negative charge on their surface, due to which they are surrounded by cations, such as Na^+ and K^+ (Figure 5.9). In acidic staining, an acidic stain is used, which ionises into an anionic chromogen (negatively charged dye ion) and a cation. The negatively charged chromogens are repelled by the surface negative charges on the bacteria cells, due to which the dye cannot penetrate the cell. Now, the unstained cells are easily discernible against the coloured background.

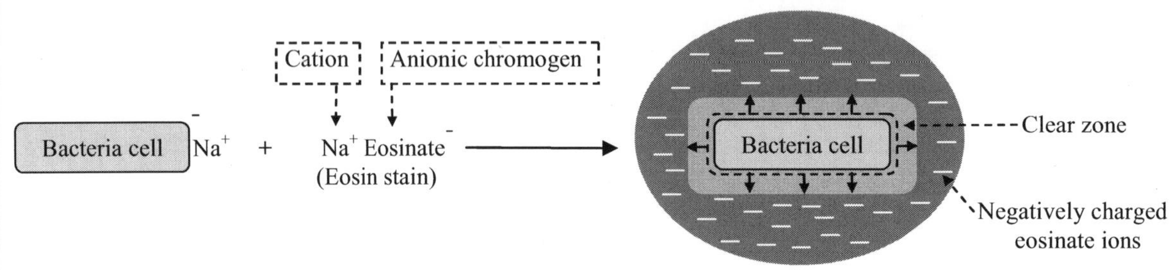

Figure 5.9: Principle of simple acidic staining (Negative staining)

Materials Required

Slides, loop, acidic stain (eosin/nigrosin) (*See* Appendix II at page 251), broth/plate/slant culture of bacteria, microscope, immersion oil.

Procedure

1. A slide is cleaned properly under tap water, such that water does not remain as drops on its surface (Figure 5.10).
2. The adhering water is wiped out with bibulous paper and the slide is air-dried.
3. A small drop of the acidic stain (nigrosin/eosin) is placed close to one end of the slide.
4. A loop is sterilised over flame and cooled. Aseptically, a loop of bacteria from agar plate or slant or a loop of bacteria suspension from a liquid broth is transferred to the drop of stain. A suspension of bacteria in the stain is made by gently mixing the loop of bacteria in the drop of stain, in such a way that, the drop does not spread.

5. Another clean slide is held at an angle of 30° to the first slide, in such a way that, one narrow edge of the former touches the surface of the later towards the end without the stain drop.
6. In that inclined position, the second slide is pulled forward towards the stain drop, till its edge just touches the drop and the drop gets spread along its edge.
7. In that inclined position, the second slide is pushed backward to form a thin smear of bacteria.
8. The smear is air-dried. Heat-fixation is not done here.
9. The slide is clipped to the stage of the microscope and the smear observed under low power and high dry objectives.
10. A drop of immersion oil is put on the smear.
11. The smear is observed under oil-immersion objective (*See* point 13 at page 78).

Observations (Under Oil-immersion Objective)

1. *Shape of bacteria*:	Spherical (coccus)
	Rod-shaped (bacilli)
	Comma-like (vibrio)
	Spiral (spirochetes)
2. *Arrangement of bacteria*:	Pairs (diplobacillus/diplococcus)
	In fours (tetrads)
	In chains (streptococcus/streptobacillus)
	Grape-like clusters (staphylococcus)
	Cuboidal (sarcinae or octet)
3. *Size of bacteria*:	By eye estimation, make drawing of the field under oil-immersion objective.

Experiment 19

(iii) Gram Staining

***Aim*: To perform gram staining of a bacteria, to find out whether it is gram-positive or gram-negative.**

Purpose

The most important differential staining used in microbiology is gram staining. It is named after Dr. Christian Gram who categorised bacteria, based on the differences in the composition of their cell wall, into two groups as follows (For details of the differences in chemical composition of gram-positive and gram-negative bacteria, *see* pages 10–13).

(1) Gram-positive Bacteria

After staining a bacteria with crystal violet, if its cell wall resists decolourisation[2] by washing with a decolourising agent (ethanol or acetone), it is a gram-positive bacteria. Examples: *Bacillus, Staphylococcus*.

(2) Gram-negative Bacteria

After staining a bacteria with crystal violet, if its cell wall allows to undergo decolourisation by washing with a decolourising agent (ethanol or acetone), it is a gram-negative bacteria. Examples: *Escherichia, Salmonella, Vibrio.*

Differentiation of bacteria into gram-positive and gram-negative groups provides the most important clue for proceeding further in proper direction for identification of unknown bacteria. It is also useful for simple differentiation of bacteria into gram-positive and gram-negative groups. It also gives an idea about the shape and arrangement of the bacteria cells.

---

2 *Decolourisation*: Making 'colourless' by removal of the colour. It is different from 'discolouration', which means change of original desirable colour to some undesirable colour. For example, in brown discolouration of red meat, the original red colour changes to undesirable brown colour.

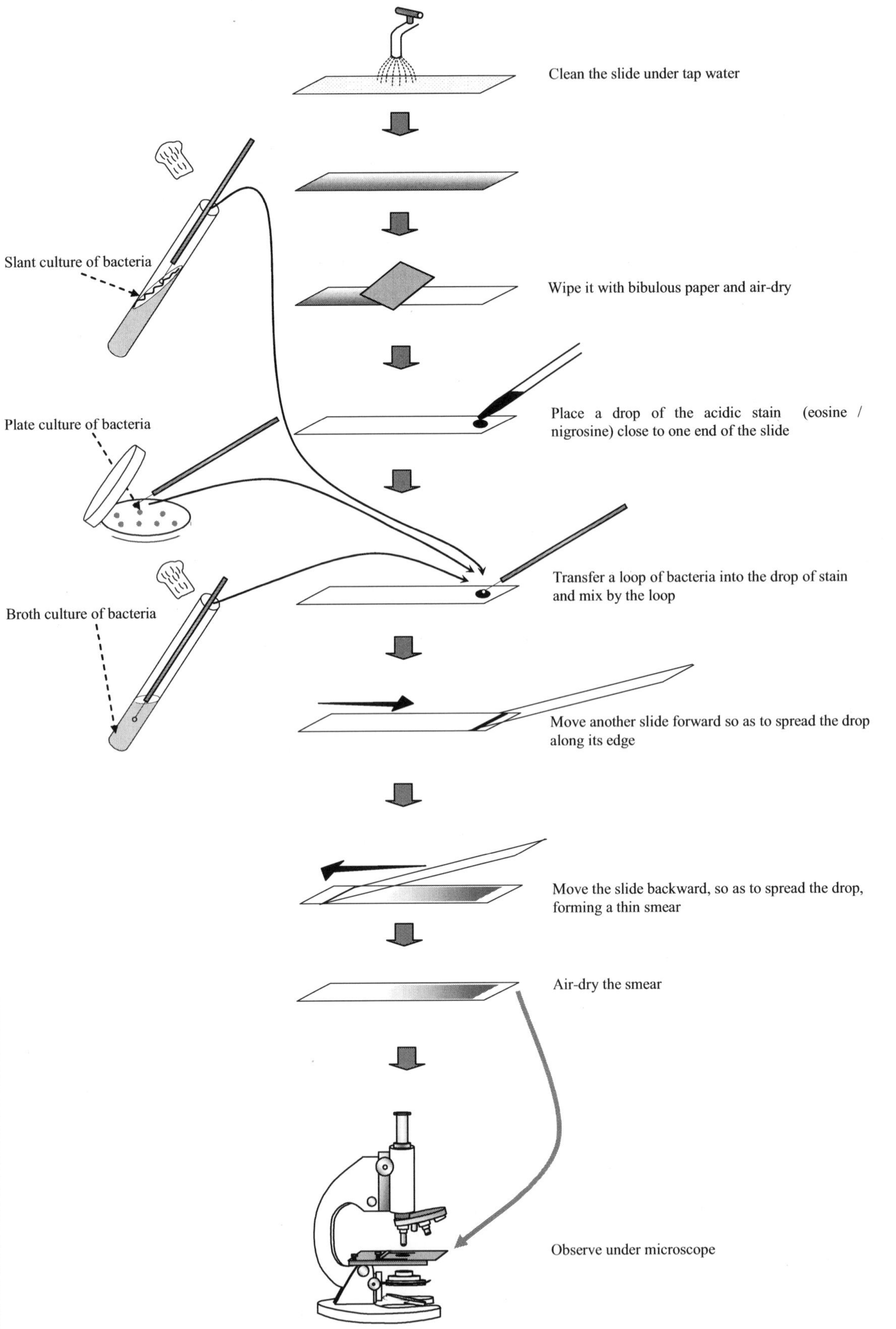

Figure 5.10: Simple acidic staining (Negative staining)

Principle

In gram staining, the bacteria cells are first stained with a primary stain, crystal violet that enters into the cells and stain them purple-blue. Then, the cells are treated with a mordant, gram's iodine, which enters into the cells and binds to the primary stain forming an insoluble dye-mordant complex (crystal violet-iodine complex), thus making the escape of the stain difficult. Then, the cells are treated with a decolourising agent, such as ethanol or acetone. It acts as a lipid solvent and as a protein-dehydrating agent. In gram-positive cells, the decolourising agent acts initially as a lipid solvent, dissolving out the little quantity of lipid present in the cell wall, thereby forming minute pores in it. Subsequently, it dehydrates the cell wall proteins (peptides), which close the pores. Now, the stain-mordant complex is difficult to be removed by the decolourising agent and the cells retain the purple-blue colour of the primary stain. When counter-stained by a pink-red coloured stain, safranin, it cannot enter into the cells, as the pores have been closed. The cells finally retain the purple-blue colour of the primary stain. On the other hand, the gram-negative cell wall contains large quantity of lipid (LPS), which is dissolved out by the decolourising agent, resulting in the formation of large pores. These pores do not close appreciably on dehydration of cell wall proteins. That is why, the stain-mordant complex escapes through the pores, when washed by the decolourising agent and the cells appear colourless. When counter-stained by safranin, it enters into the cells through the pores and finally the cells take the pink-red colour of the counter-stain.

Materials Required

Slide, loop, primary stain (crystal violet), mordant (gram's iodine), decolourising agent (95% ethanol), counter-stain (safranin) (*See* Appendix II at page 251), broth/slant/plate culture of bacteria, microscope, immersion oil.

Procedure

1. A slide is cleaned properly under tap water, such that water does not remain as drops on its surface (Figure 5.11).
2. The adhering water is wiped out with bibulous paper and the slide is air-dried.
3. A smear of bacteria is prepared at the center of the slide in two methods as follows.
   (*a*) If bacteria grown on agar plate or agar slant is to be observed, a drop of water is put at the center of the slide and a loop of bacteria from the plate or slant is transferred to it by a loop sterilised over flame. Then, by slow rotation of the loop in the drop, a bacteria suspension is made and it is spread till a smear is obtained.
   (*b*) If bacteria grown in liquid broth is to be observed, a drop of the bacteria suspension is directly placed at the center of the slide by a flame-sterilised loop and a smear is made by spreading.
4. The smear is air-dried.
5. The smear is fixed by heating. Heating results in coagulation of the cellular proteins, due to which the cells stick to the slide surface and do not get washed away during staining, Heat-fixation is done by quickly passing the slide high above a flame 2-3 times, with the smear surface facing upward, so that the smear does not get heated up.
6. The slide is kept on a staining tray and flooded with the primary stain, crystal violet, for 1 minute.
7. Excess stain is washed away from the smear under gently-flowing tap water, in such a way that, water does not fall directly on the smear.
8. The smear is flooded with the mordant, gram's iodine, for 1 minute.
9. Excess mordant is washed away from the smear under gently-flowing tap water, in such a way that, water does not fall directly on the smear.

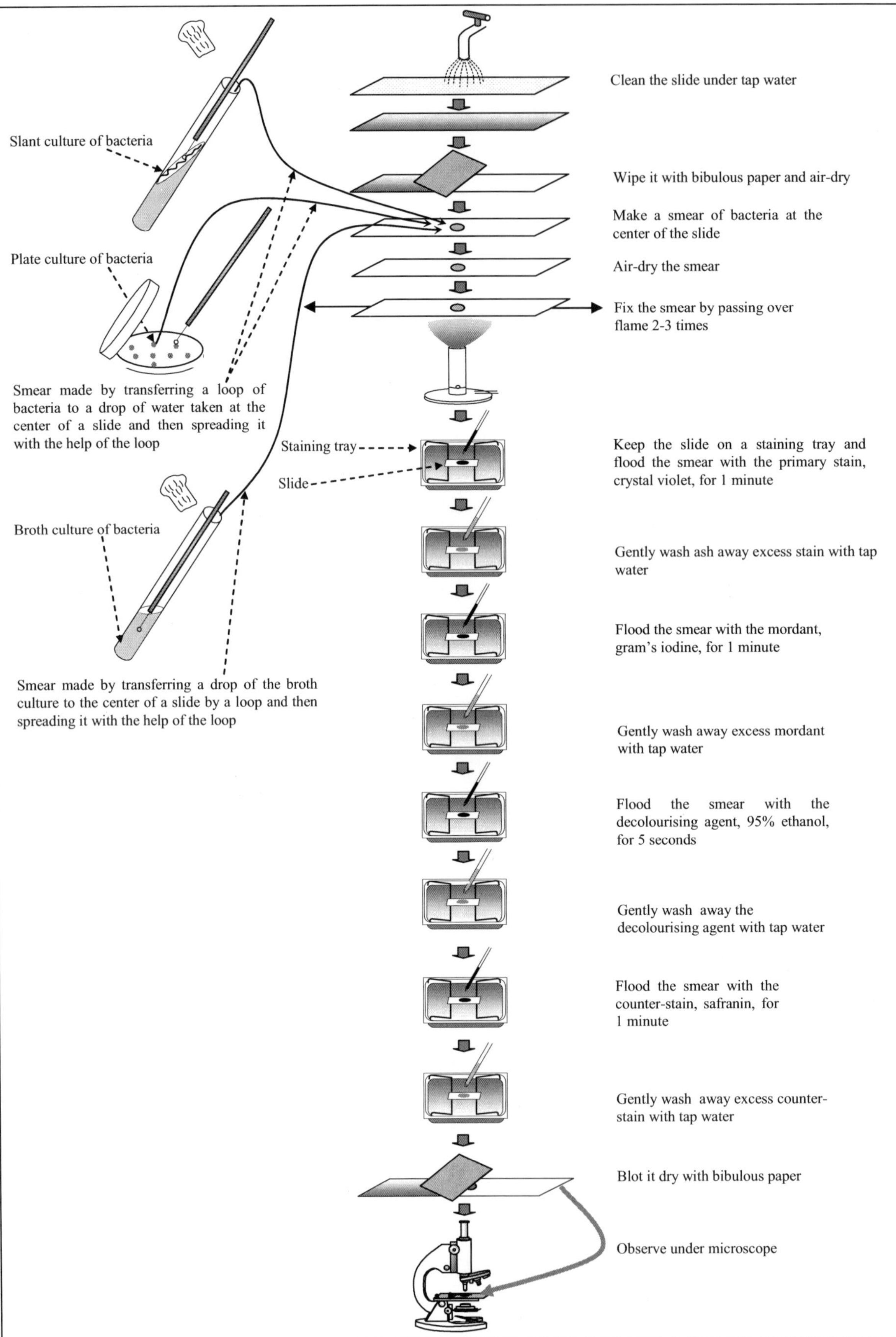

Figure 5.11: Gram staining of bacteria

10. The smear is flooded with the decolourising agent, 95% ethanol, for 5 seconds, taking care, so that the smear is not over-decolourised.
11. The ethanol is quickly washed away from the smear under gently-flowing tap water, so as to prevent over-decolourisation. Care is taken, so that, water does not fall directly on the smear.
12. The smear is flooded with the counter-stain, safranin, for 1 minute.
13. Excess counter-stain is washed away from the smear under gently-flowing tap water, in such a way that, water does not fall directly on the smear.
14. The slide is blotted dry with bibulous paper.
15. The slide is clipped to the stage of the microscope and the smear observed under low power and high dry objectives.
16. A drop of immersion oil is put on the smear.
17. The smear is observed under oil-immersion objective (*See* point 13 at page 78).

Observations (Under Oil-immersion Objective)

1. *Colour of the cells*:	Purple-blue: Gram-positive bacteria
	Pink–red: Gram-negative bacteria
2. *Shape of bacteria*:	Spherical (coccus)
	Rod-shaped (bacilli)
	Comma-like (vibrio)
	Spiral (spirochetes)
3. *Arrangement of bacteria*:	Pairs (diplobacillus/diplococcus)
	In fours (tetrads)
	In chains (streptococcus/streptobacillus)
	Grape-like clusters (staphylococcus)
	Cuboidal (sarcinae or octet)
4. *Size of bacteria*:	By eye estimation, make drawing of the field under oil-immersion objective.

Gram-variable Reaction

In some cases, the gram-positive cells appear as gram-negative cells. This is called gram-variable reaction. The reasons are as follows.

(*a*) Over-decolourisation may occur, due to which the gram-positive cells also lose their violet colour.

(*b*) Over-fixation may occur, due to which the gram-positive cells lose their ability to resist decolourisation

(*c*) If old culture of bacteria is used, the components of the cell wall may change with the age of the cells allowing decolourisation.

Experiment 20

(*iv*) Acid-fast Staining (Ziel-Neelsen Method)

***Aim*: To perform acid-fast staining of a bacteria, to find out whether it is acid-fast or non-acid-fast.**

Purpose

Most of the bacteria can be stained, either by simple basic staining or by gram staining, as their cells take up stains easily. However, some bacteria possess a thick waxy cell wall made of lipid materials. Such bacteria are extremely difficult to be stained, as ordinary aqueous stains cannot enter into their cells easily, but once stained, it is equally difficult to remove the stain out of their cells, even with vigorous use of acid-alcohol as decolourising agent. These bacteria are stained by acid-fast staining. Thus, acid-fast staining, similar to gram staining, is a differential staining method, which differentiates bacteria, based on the nature of their cell wall, into two groups as follows.

(1) Acid-fast Bacteria

A bacteria, which is extremely difficult to be stained, but once stained, it is equally difficult to remove the stain out of its cells, even with vigorous use of acid-alcohol as decolourising agent, is an acid-fast bacteria (acid-loving bacteria). Examples: *Mycobacterium* spp. [*M. tuberculosis* (TB bacteria), *M. leprae* (leprosy bacteria), *M. smegmatis* (natural bacteria of smegma) and *M. marinum* (TB bacteria of marine fishes). They possess a thick waxy cell wall made of lipid materials.

(2) Non-acid-fast Bacteria

A bacteria, which is easy to be stained and is also easy to be decolourised by acid-alcohol as decolourising agent, is a non-acid-fast bacteria (non-acid-loving bacteria). Examples: All bacteria except *Mycobacterium* spp. In these bacteria, the cell wall is not thick and waxy.

Acid-fast staining is useful in differentiating acid-fast and non-acid-fast bacteria and also in the identification of bacteria belonging to the genus *Mycobacterium.*

Principle

The acid-fast bacteria are different from the non-acid-fast bacteria in that, they possess a thick waxy cell wall made of lipid materials. Ordinary aqueous stains, such as methylene blue or crystal violet cannot enter into their cells through this waxy cell wall. However, the red coloured phenolic primary stain carbol fuchsin (carbolic acid or phenol + basic fuchsin), which is soluble in the lipid materials of the cell wall, can enter into their cells through the cell wall and can be retained inside the cells imparting red colour to them. Penetration is further augmented by application of heat, which drives carbol fuchsin through the lipoidal wall into the cytoplasm. (A slight modification of this Ziel-Neelsen method describes the addition of a wetting agent, Turgitol, to the stain, which reduces the surface tension between the cell wall and the stain, thereby requiring no heating). The cells are allowed to cool, so as to harden the waxy cell wall. When the cells are exposed to the decolourising agent, acid-alcohol, they resist decolourisation, as the primary stain is more soluble in the cellular waxes than in the decolourising agent. Subsequently, when counter-stained with methylene blue, it cannot enter into the cells through the waxy cell wall. Thus, finally the acid-fast bacteria retain the red colour of the primary stain and appear red. On the other hand, the non-acid-fast bacteria take up the primary stain easily and undergo decolourisation easily. When counter-stained with methylene blue, these colourless cells also take up the counter-stain easily and appear blue, unlike the acid-fast bacteria, which appear red.

Materials Required

Slide, loop, primary stain (carbol fuchsin), decolourising agent (acid-alcohol), counter stain (methylene blue) (*See* Appendix II at page 251), hot plate, broth/slant/plate culture of bacteria, microscope, immersion oil.

Procedure

1. A slide is cleaned properly under tap water, such that water does not remain as drops on its surface (Figure 5.12).
2. The adhering water is wiped out with bibulous paper and the slide is air-dried.
3. A smear of bacteria is prepared at the center of the slide in two methods as follows.
   (*a*) If the bacteria grown on agar plate or agar slant is to be observed, a drop of water is put at the center of the slide and a loop of bacteria from the plate or slant is transferred to it by a loop sterilised over flame. Then, by slow rotation of the loop in the drop, a bacteria suspension is made and it is spread till a smear is obtained.

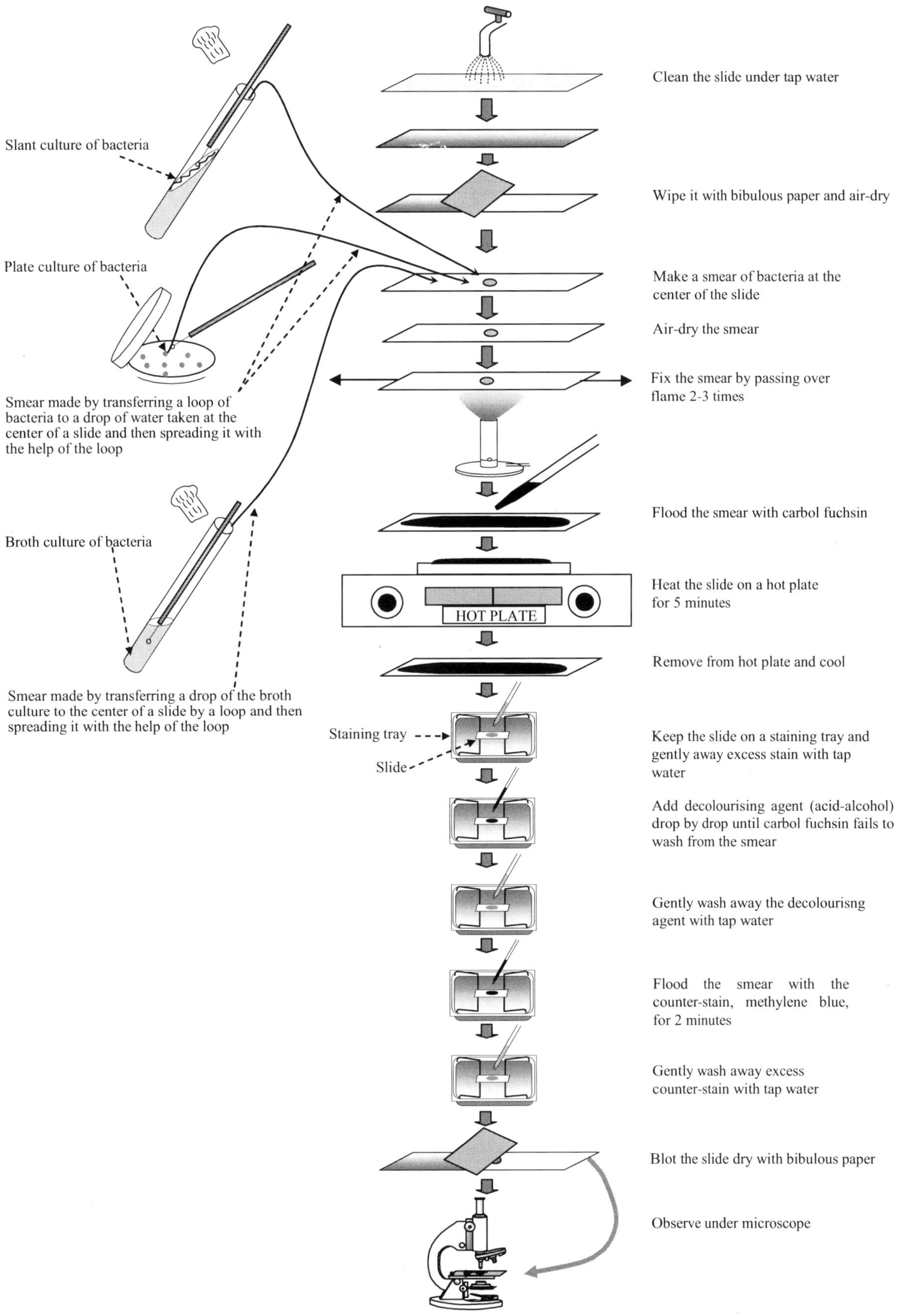

Figure 5.12: Acid-fast staining of bacteria (Ziel-Neelsen method)

   (b) If bacteria grown in liquid broth is to be observed, a drop of the bacteria suspension is directly placed at the center of the slide by a flame-sterilised loop and a smear is made by spreading.

4. The smear is air-dried.
5. The smear is fixed by heating. Heating results in the coagulation of the cellular proteins, due to which the cells stick to the slide surface and do not get washed away during staining. Heat-fixation is done by quickly passing the slide high above a flame 2-3 times, with the smear surface facing upward, so that the smear does not get heated up.
6. The smear is flooded with carbol fuchsin
7. The slide is placed on a warm hot plate, allowing the preparation to steam for 5 minutes. The temperature of the hot plate is so adjusted that, the preparation does not boil and get evaporated quickly. The evaporation loss is replenished, so that the smear does not dry up. (For heatless method, the smear is flooded for 3-5 minutes with carbol fuchsin containing Turgitol).
8. The slide is removed from the hot plate and cooled.
9. Excess stain is washed away from the smear under gently-flowing tap water, in such a way that, water does not fall directly on the smear.
10. The decolourising agent, acid-alcohol, is added on the smear drop by drop, until carbol fuchsin fails to wash from the smear.
11. The acid-alcohol is washed away from the smear under gently-flowing tap water, in such a way that, water does not fall directly on the smear.
12. The smear is flooded with the counter-stain, methylene blue, for 2 minutes.
13. Excess counter-stain is washed away from the smear under gently-flowing tap water, in such a way that, water does not fall directly on the smear.
14. The slide is blotted dry with bibulous paper.
15. The slide is clipped to the stage of the microscope and the smear observed under low power and high dry objectives.
16. A drop of immersion oil is put on the smear.
17. The smear is observed under oil-immersion objective (*See* point 13 at page 78).

Observations (Under Oil-immersion Objective)

1. *Colour of the cells*: Red: Acid-fast
   Blue: Non-acid-fast
2. *Shape of bacteria*: Spherical (coccus)
   Rod-shaped (bacilli)
   Comma-like (vibrio)
   Spiral (spirochetes)
3. *Arrangement of bacteria*: Pairs (diplobacillus/diplococcus)
   In fours (tetrads)
   In chains (streptococcus/streptobacillus)
   Grape-like clusters (staphylococcus)
   Cuboidal (sarcinae or octet).
4. *Size of bacteria*: By eye estimation, make drawing of the field under oil-immersion objective.

Experiment 21

(*v*) Spore Staining (Schaeffer-Fulton Method)

***Aim*: To perform spore staining of a bacteria, for differentiation between bacterial spore and vegetative cell forms.**

Purpose

All bacteria remain in their 'vegetative forms', if the environmental conditions are favourable for their normal metabolic activities. In this form, they take up nutrients, grow and reproduce. On the other hand, most of them die, when the environmental conditions become adverse, such as, severe cold, extreme heat, ageing, lack of nutrients, exposure to radiation and toxic chemicals. However, few species of bacteria, can survive under such adverse conditions by changing themselves to highly resistant, metabolically inactive forms called 'spores' (*See* page 18-21). In adverse conditions, a spore is produced within a vegetative cell by dehydration and contraction of its cell contents. This spore, formed inside the bacteria cell, is called 'endospore' (Figure 2.14). If adverse conditions worsen, the cell ruptures, releasing the endospore, which now becomes an independent dormant cell called 'spore'. The process of spore formation is called 'sporogenesis'. The spore has thick, relatively impervious layers, such as spore cortex and spore coat, which protect the cell from any physical damage. The spore gains its resistance by several mechanisms, which have not yet been clearly explained. When the conditions become favourable, the layers covering the spore rupture and the spore gives rise to a metabolically active vegetative cell. This process is called 'germination' (*See* page 18-21). Thus, based on the ability to form spores, bacteria can be divided into two groups as follows.

(1) Spore-forming Bacteria (Spore-formers)

A bacteria, which can produce a spore to survive under adverse environmental conditions is a spore-forming bacteria (spore-former). Mostly, the following three genera of rod-shaped bacteria can produce spores under adverse environmental conditions.

A. Aerobic rod-shaped bacteria

1. *Bacillus* spp.

B. Anaerobic rod-shaped bacteria

2. *Clostridium* spp.
3. *Desulfotomaculum* spp.

(2) Non-spore-forming Bacteria (Non-spore-formers)

A bacteria, which cannot produce a spore and therefore, dies in its vegetative form under adverse environmental conditions, is a non-spore-forming bacteria (non-spore-former).

The purpose of spore staining is to differentiate the spores and vegetative cells of a spore-former and to differentiate spore-formers from non-spore-formers. Spore staining is also helpful in identification of the bacteria belonging to the genera *Bacillus, Clostridium* and *Desulfotomaculum.*

Principle

The spores are different from the vegetative cells in that they possess thick, relatively impervious layers around them (Figure 2.14). The primary stain, malachite green, cannot penetrate into the spores through these layers. Therefore, penetration of the primary stain is augmented by the application of heat, which drives it through the covering layers into the spore protoplast. Now, the spores appear green. When the spores are treated with the decolourising agent, tap water, they do not undergo decolourisation, as they exclude water (*See* page 21). The tap water removes only the excess primary stain present in the surrounding of the spores. Thus, the spores retain the green colour. Subsequently, when counter-stained with safranin, the safranin molecules cannot enter into the spores through the covering layers. Thus, finally the spores retain the green colour of the primary stain and appear green.

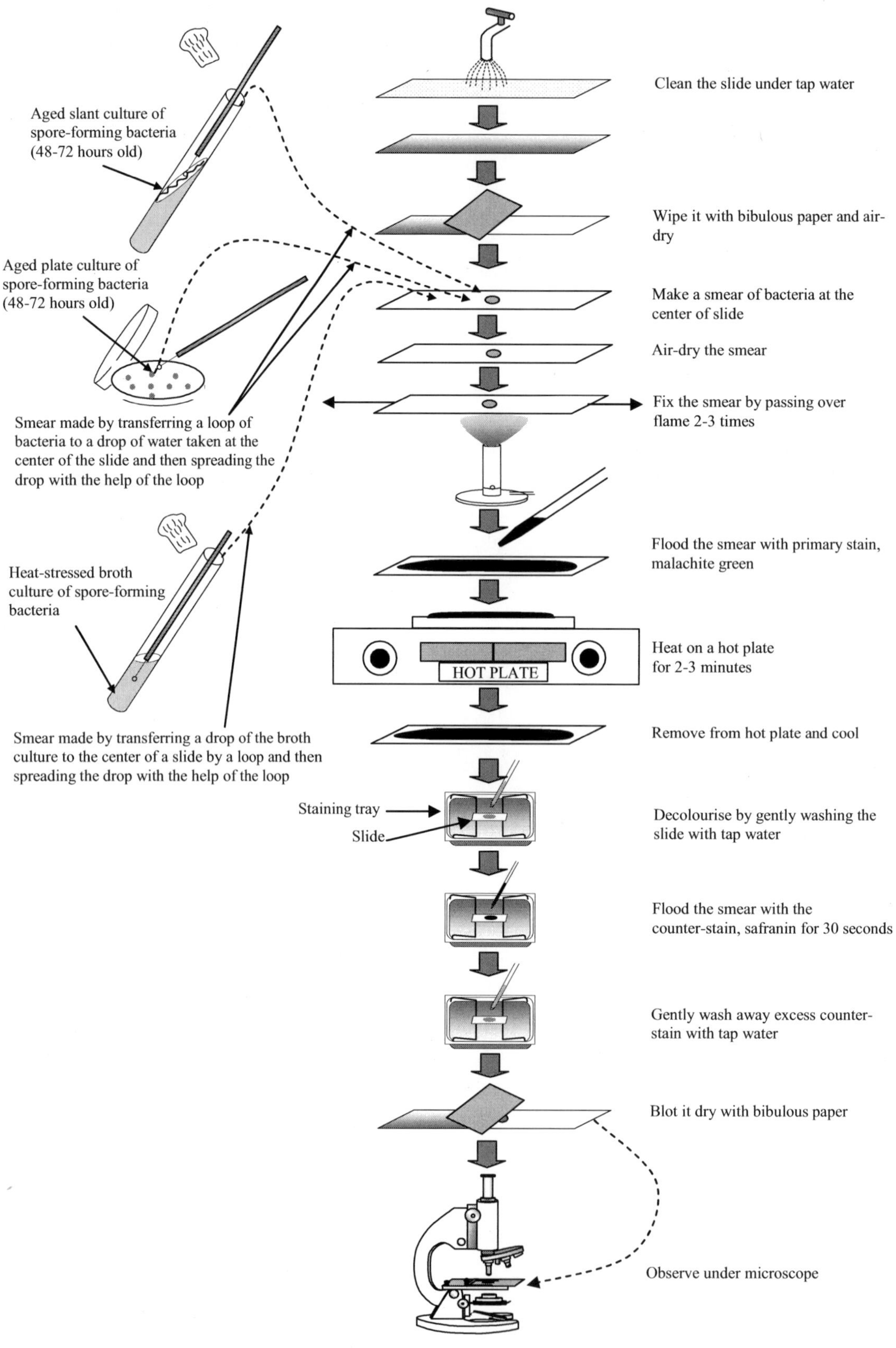

Figure 5.13: Spore staining of bacteria (Schaeffer-Fulton method)

On the other hand, the vegetative bacteria cells take up the primary stain, malachite green, easily, but the stain does not have strong affinity for vegetative cell components, due to which it is washed away, when decolourised under tap water. Now, the vegetative cells appear colourless. When counter-stained with safranin, the colourless vegetative cells take up the stain and appear red unlike the spores, which appear green.

Materials Required

Slide, loop, malachite green, safranin (*See* Appendix II at page 251), spore-forming bacteria, hot plate, microscope, immersion oil.

Procedure

1. A slide is cleaned properly under tap water, such that water does not remain as drops on its surface (Figure 2.14).
2. The adhering water is wiped out with bibulous paper and the slide is air-dried.
3. A smear of spore-forming bacteria is made at the center of a slide in two methods as given below.
   (*a*) If spore-former grown on agar plate or agar slant is to be observed, a drop of water is placed at the center of the slide. A loop is sterilised over flame and a *Clostridium* loop of bacteria from an aged plate or slant culture (48-72 hours old) of spore-former, such as *Clostridium sporogenes* or *Bacillus subtilis* is transferred to the water drop. Then, by gentle rotation of the loop in the water drop, a bacteria suspension is made and the drop is spread till a smear is obtained. As the age of spore-forming bacteria on plate or slant cultures increases, they form spores.
   (*b*) If spore-former grown in liquid broth is to be observed, the broth culture, containing only vegetative cells, is subjected to heat stress, by heating on a water bath for 15 minutes, so that some of the vegetative cells form spores to overcome the heat stress. A drop of the mixed spore-vegetative cell suspension from the broth culture is directly placed at the center of the slide by a sterile loop and a smear is made by spreading.
4. The smear is air-dried.
5. The smear is fixed by heating. Heating results in coagulation of the cellular proteins, due to which the cells stick to the slide surface and do not get washed away during staining, Heat-fixation is done by quickly passing the slide high above a flame 2-3 times, with the smear surface facing upward, so that the smear does not get heated up.
6. The smear is flooded with the primary stain, malachite green.
7. The slide is kept on a warm hot plate and the preparation allowed to steam for 2-3 minutes. The temperature of the hot plate is so adjusted that, the preparation does not boil and get evaporated quickly. The evaporation loss is replenished, so that the smear does not get dried up.
8. The slide is removed from the hot plate and cooled.
9. The smear is decolourised by washing under gently-flowing tap water, in such a way that, water does not fall directly on the smear.
10. The smear is flooded with the counter-stain, safranin, for 30 seconds.
11. Excess counter-stain is completely washed away from the smear under gently-flowing tap water, in such a way that, water does not fall directly on the smear.
12. The slide is blotted dry with bibulous paper.
13. The slide is clipped to the stage of the microscope and the smear observed under low power and high dry objectives.

14. A drop of immersion oil is put on the smear.
15. The smear is observed under oil-immersion objective (*See* point 13 at page 78).

Observations (Under oil-immersion objective):

1. *Colour of the cells*: Green: Spore (Notice the location of the spore)
   Red: Vegetative cell
2. *Shape of bacteria*: Spherical (coccus)
   Rod-shaped (bacilli)
   Comma-like (vibrio)
   Spiral (spirochetes)
3. *Arrangement of bacteria*: Pairs (diplobacillus/diplococcus)
   In fours (tetrads)
   In chains (streptococcus/streptobacillus)
   Grape-like clusters (staphylococcus)
   Cuboidal (sarcinae or octet)
4. *Size of bacteria*: By eye estimation, make drawing of the field under oil-immersion objective.

Experiment 22

(*vi*) Capsule Staining

***Aim*: To perform capsule staining of a bacteria, to observe bacterial capsule.**

Purpose

In some bacteria, the cell wall is surrounded by a viscous cell envelope called 'capsule' (*See* page 8-9). It is made of polysaccharide, glycoprotein or polypeptide. When the capsule is too thin to be observed under light microscope, it is called 'microcapsule' and when it is so thick that many cells are embedded in the capsular matrix, it is called 'slime' (Figure 2.8). Based on presence or absence of capsule, bacteria are of two types as follows.

(1) Capsulated Bacteria

A bacteria, which possesses capsule is a capsulated bacteria.

(2) Non-capsulated Bacteria

A bacteria, which does not possess capsule is a non-capsulated bacteria

The purpose of capsule staining is to observe bacterial capsule by distinguishing capsular material from the bacteria cell.

Principle

In capsule staining, a smear of bacteria is made at the center of a slide. It is not heat-fixed, as the cell shrinkage caused by heating may create a clear zone around the cell, which may be mistaken as capsule. Moreover, as the capsular material is water-soluble and may be washed away with vigorous washing, only two reagents are used in staining without any in-between water-washing. One of the two reagents is the primary stain, crystal violet. It imparts dark purple-blue colour to both, the cell as well as the capsule. However, it is 'absorbed' into the cell due to the ionic nature of the cellular components, whereas it simply 'adheres' to the capsule, because of the non-ionic nature of the capsular material. To prevent dislodging of the capsular material, the smear is not water-washed. The second reagent, copper sulphate acts both as a decolourising agent and a counter-stain. It decolourises by removing excess crystal violet from around the cells as well as the crystal violet adhering to the capsule. It also counter-stains the capsule and imparts a light blue colour to it. The capsule now appears light blue, whereas the cell appears deep purple-blue.

Materials Required

Slide, loop, immersion oil, microscope, crystal violet stain, copper sulphate solution (20%) (*See* Appendix II at page 251).

Procedure

1. The slide is cleaned properly under tap water, such that water does not remain as drops on its surface (Figure 5.14).
2. The adhering water is wiped out with bibulous paper and the slide is air-dried.
3. A smear of bacteria is prepared at the center of the slide in two methods as follows.
   (*a*) If bacteria grown on agar plate or agar slant is to be observed, a drop of water is put at the center of the slide and a loop of bacteria from the plate or slant is transferred to it by a loop sterilised over flame. Then, by slow rotation of the loop in the drop, a bacteria suspension is made and it is spread till a smear is obtained.
   (*b*) If bacteria grown in liquid broth is to be observed, a drop of the bacteria suspension is directly placed at the center of the slide by a flame-sterilised loop and a smear is made by spreading.
4. The smear is air-dried. No heat-fixation is done as the resultant cell shrinkage may create a clear zone around the bacteria, which may be mistaken as capsule.
5. The smear is flooded with the primary stain, crystal violet, for 5–7 minutes.
6. The smear is washed with 20% copper sulphate solution. To prevent dislodging of the capsular material, the smear is not water-washed.
7. The slide is blotted dry with bibulous paper.
8. The slide is clipped to the stage of the microscope and the smear observed under low power and high dry objectives.
9. A drop of immersion oil is put on the smear.
10. The smear is observed under oil-immersion objective (*See* point 13 at page 78).

Observations

1. *Colour of the area surrounding the cells*:	Light blue: Capsule present (capsulated bacteria) Dark purple-blue: Capsule absent (non-capsulated bacteria)
2. *Colour of the cells*:	Dark purple-blue
3. *If capsulated, size of the capsules*:	Small, moderate or large.
4. *Relative size of cells and capsules*:	By eye estimation, make drawing of the field under the oil-immersion objective, indicating the relative size of the cells and the capsules.

Experiment 23

(4) Micrometry

***Aim*: To measure the size of microorganisms under microscope.**

Purpose

Micrometry (*micro*: microscopic, *metry*: measurement) is the measurement of the dimensions of microscopic objects[3] in terms of length, breadth, diameter and thickness. Microorganisms are microscopic

3 Besides measuring the dimensions of microbes, micrometry also has other applications such as measurement of the dimensions of microscopic plant and animal cells as well as their sub-cellular components. Micrometry is also useful in the measurement of the dimensions of non-living objects like the diameter of different fibers (synthetic and natural), thickness of the thin-coatings over metals surfaces etc.

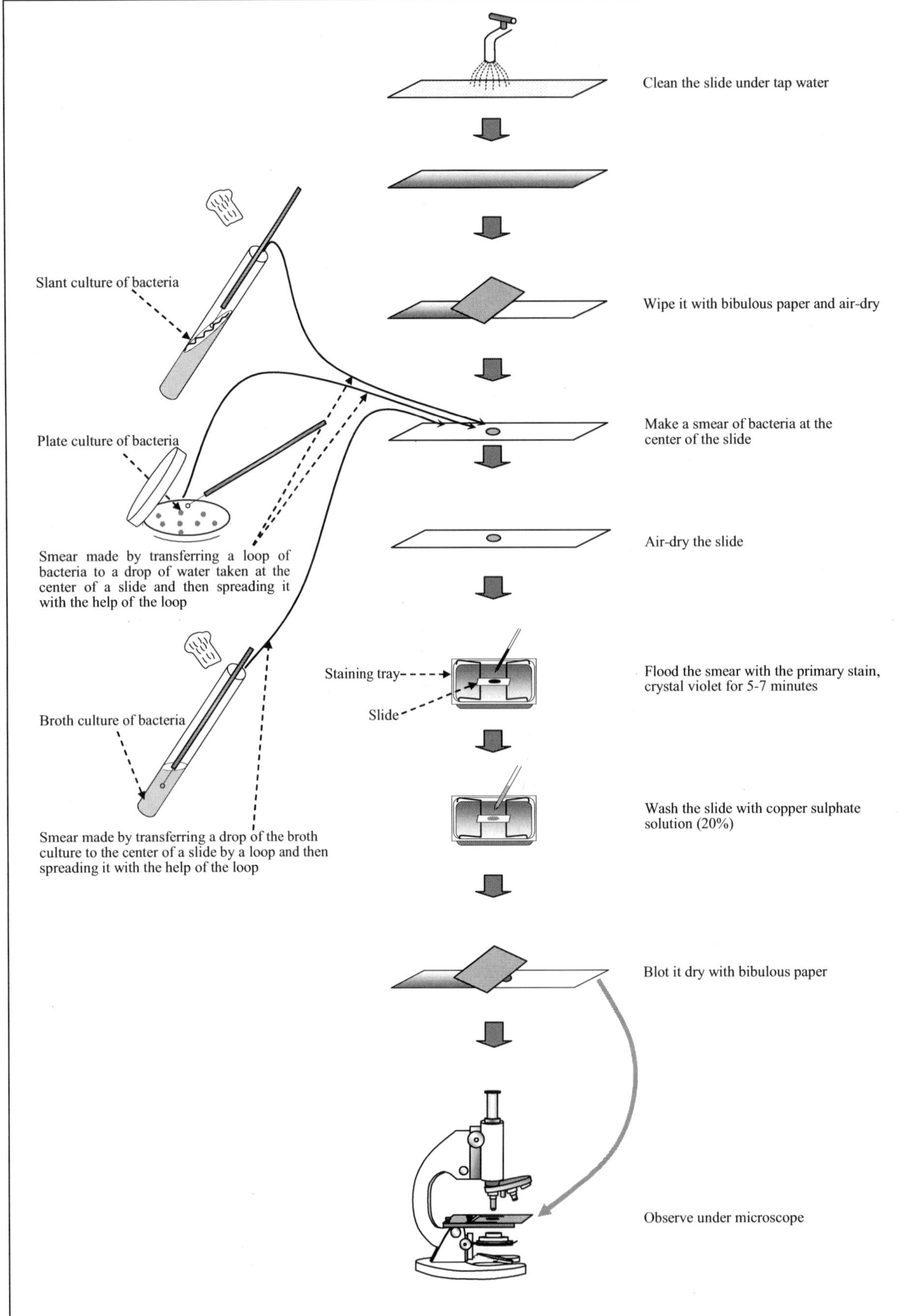

Figure 5.14: Capsule staining of bacteria

objects, as they are not visible to naked eye and can only be observed under microscope. Very often, it is required to measure their dimensions in terms of length, breadth and diameter. Because of their minute size, measurement of their dimensions has to be done under microscope. Thus, the purpose of micrometry is to measure the dimensions of microorganisms under microscope.

Principle

Measurement of the dimensions of microorganisms is done under microscope with the help of two micro-scales called 'micrometers'. Both the micrometers have microscopic graduations etched on their surfaces. One of them, the 'ocular micrometer' is a circular glass disc, which fits into the circular shelf inside the eyepiece. It has arbitrary graduations etched on its surface. However, the distance between the etched graduations is constant for a particular ocular micrometer. The other micrometer, called 'stage micrometer', is a special glass slide, which is clipped to the stage of the microscope. It has standard graduations etched on its surface, which are 10 μ apart.

Calibration

Using the required objective, the graduations on the ocular micrometer are calibrated against the standard graduations on the stage micrometer. Calibration is required, because the distance between ocular graduations varies depending on the objective being used, which determines the size of the field. For calibration, both the micrometer etchings are superimposed by rotating the eyepiece. The number of ocular divisions (O.D.) coinciding with the number of stage divisions (S.D.) is found out. From this, the calibration factor for one ocular division (O.D.) is calculated as follows.

If 10 O.D. coincide with 2 S.D., then

$$10 \text{ O.D.} = 2 \text{ S.D.} = 2 \times 10\ \mu = 20\ \mu \quad (\because 1 \text{ S.D.} = 10\ \mu)$$

$$1 \text{ O.D.} = \frac{20}{10}\ \mu = 2\ \mu$$

Thus, the distance between two adjacent ocular etchings is 2 μ (*i.e.* calibration factor is 2 μ).

Measurement

After calibration, the stage micrometer is removed and the microbe, whose dimensions are to be measured is placed on the stage on a slide and focused. Now, the number of ocular divisions occupied by the microorganism is counted. Then, by multiplying this number of divisions with the calibration factor, the size of the microbe is determined as follows.

If the microbe occupies 6 O.D. in length, then

length of microbe = 6 x calibration factor = 6 x 2 = 12 μ.

It is possible to measure the size of microbes by directly observing them on a stage micrometer. This would avoid calibration and calculations. But the stage micrometer is a standard scale, which is costly because of the micro etchings on it. If used frequently for direct observation, its etchings get worn away. Moreover, the etchings on the stage micrometer are more widely spaced (about 10 times) than those on the ocular micrometer. Thus, the dimensions cannot be precisely determined with a stage micrometer. That is why, it is never used for direct measurement.

Materials Required

Ocular micrometer, stage micrometer, slide, microscope, microbe.

Procedure

1. The eyepiece is removed from the microscope, and its top lid is unscrewed. The lid is removed. Carefully, the eye lens (Figure 4.9 and Figure 5.15) is removed. The ocular micrometer (a circular etched glass piece, which slips into the eye piece) is placed carefully into the eyepiece. The eye

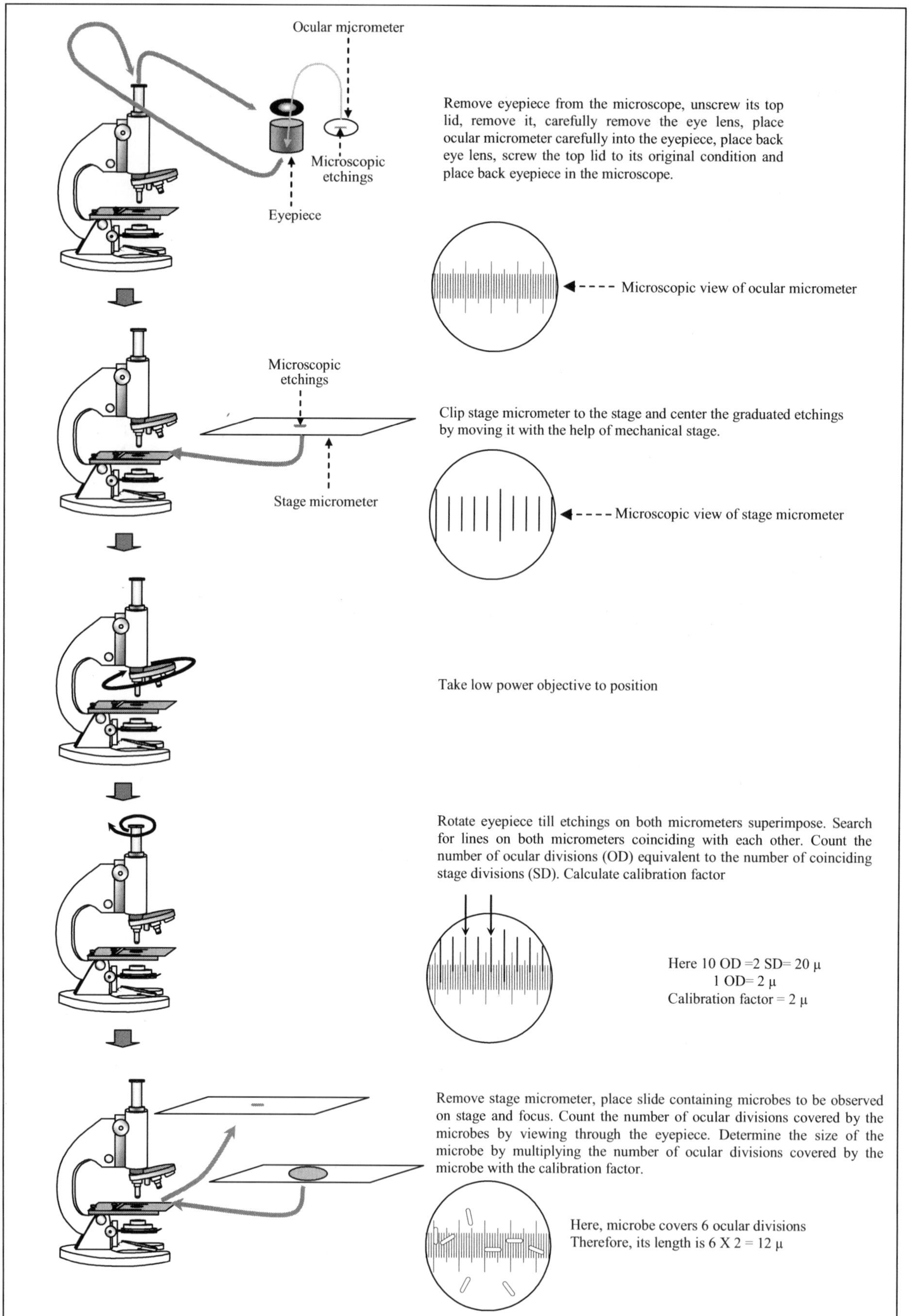

Figure 5.15: Measurement of the size of microbes by micrometry

lens is placed back and the top lid is screwed to its original condition. The eyepiece is placed back in the microscope.

2. The stage micrometer is clipped to the stage and the etchings centered by moving the mechanical stage.
3. The low power objective is taken to position.
4. The eyepiece is rotated till the etchings on both the micrometers superimpose.
5. The required objective is taken to position. The required objective is that, using which the whole microorganism can be viewed and it covers the microscopic field to the maximum possible extent.
6. With the required objective in position (for oil-immersion objective, a drop of oil is put on the stage micrometer) the mechanical stage is moved, so that a line on the stage micrometer coincides with a line on the ocular micrometer. Then, another line is searched on the ocular micrometer, which coincides with another line on the stage micrometer. The number of divisions between the coinciding lines is counted for both the micrometers.
7. The calibration factor for the objective used is calculated.
8. In a similar way, calibration factors are calculated for the other objectives.
9. The stage micrometer is removed.
10. The slide containing the microbe to be observed is placed on the stage and focused.
11. The number of ocular divisions covered by the microbe is counted by viewing through the eyepiece.
12. The size of the microorganism is determined by multiplying the number of ocular divisions covered by the microbe with the calibration factor.

Observations

	Calibration			*Measurement*	
1. Low power objective					
Organism	Number of ocular divisions between the lines of coincidence (X_1)	Number of stage divisions between the lines of coincidence (Y_1)	Calibration factor $F_1 = 10 \times \frac{Y_1}{X_1}\ \mu$	Number of ocular divisions covered by the microbe (N_1)	Size of the microbe $N_1 \times F_1$ (μ)
Bacteria					
Protozoa					
Algae					
Yeast					
2. High power objective					
Bacteria					
Protozoa					
Algae					
Yeast					
3. Oil-immersion objective					
Bacteria					
Protozoa					
Algae	10	2	2	6	6 X 2 = 12 μ
Yeast					

6

Cultivation of Bacteria

Bacteria are present universally almost everywhere; in soil, air, water and even inside mouth and intestine of all animals. 'Cultivation of bacteria' or 'bacteria culture' means growing these minute invisible bacteria in nutritionally rich substances and suitable environmental conditions, which support their rapid growth and multiplication. This results in their manifestation as large population visible to naked eye (as colonies or turbid suspension). Thus, there are two basic requirements for the cultivation of bacteria, such as (*I*) Abundant nutrients and (*II*) Optimum environmental conditions.

(*I*) Abundant Nutrients

In nature, bacteria take up the complex nutrients available around them after degrading them into simpler forms by the enzymes secreted by them. But in laboratory, rapid growth is augmented by growing them in substances containing nutrients in simpler forms. These substances containing adequate quantity of nutrients in simpler forms for rapid growth and multiplication of bacteria are called 'culture media'. There are a number of culture media now available containing different ingredients (*See* page 59-61 and Appendix I). Culture media are obtained in the following three 'physical forms'.

1. Liquid Media or Broth

These are clear liquids containing water and nutrients in simpler forms for growth of bacteria, which have been sterilised in autoclave. When bacteria is inoculated into them and incubated in conditions suitable for their growth, they grow profusely into thick suspensions of bacteria cells, due to which the media become turbid.

2. Solid Media

These are solidified substances, in which liquid broths have been supplemented with a solidifying agent called 'agar', at a level more than 1%. Agar is a powder (sometimes called agar agar) extracted from seaweeds and is a complex carbohydrate composed mainly of galactose. It is important to note that, agar is a solidifying agent and has no nutritional value for bacteria. It serves as an excellent solidifying agent, as in aqueous solution it liquefies at 100°C and solidifies at 40°C. Most of the pathogenic bacteria of human are grown at 37°C (normal human body temperature). Agar does not melt at this temperature and provides a hard surface. On this nutritionally rich hard surface, each single bacterium grows, multiplies and gives rise to an isolated colony of that bacteria. Such isolation is not possible in liquid media, where bacteria grow in suspension. Solid agar media can be prepared in the following forms.

(*a*) Agar Plates

Agar powder, at a level of more than 1%, is dissolved completely in liquid broth by warming. Then, it is sterilised in an autoclave. It remains liquid in hot condition and solidifies as it cools. In the warm liquid state, it is poured into sterilised petri dishes (20 ml in each petri dish) and allowed to cool, so that it forms a thick layer at the bottom of the petri dishes. These petri dishes containing a thick layer of solidified agar media are called 'agar plates' or simply 'plates'. Bacteria are grown as isolated colonies on these plates for their enumeration and isolation. The characteristics of these colonies also help in the identification of bacteria. Petri dishes are available in different sizes to meet different experimental conditions. For routine purposes, however, petri dishes of 15 cm diameter are used.

(*b*) Agar Slants

To prepare 'agar slants' or simply 'slants', agar powder, at a level of more than 1%, is dissolved completely in liquid broth by warming. In the warm liquid state, it is distributed into test tubes (20 ml in each test tube), cotton-plugged and sterilised in autoclave. The sterilised medium in test tubes is allowed to solidify in slanting position, so as to get the slants. The slants are used for maintenance of pure stock cultures of bacteria obtained by isolating on agar plates. These are also used for maintenance of standard reference stock cultures obtained from international standard laboratories. Pure cultures and standard cultures are maintained by periodically (usually 15 days to 1 month) transferring to fresh slants aseptically. The growth characteristics on slants also help in identification of bacteria.

(*c*) Agar Deep Tubes

Agar deep tubes are prepared following the same procedure as followed in the preparation of agar slants except that, here the media, after sterilisation, are allowed to solidify in up right position. These are primarily used for study of gaseous requirements of bacteria.

3. Semi Solid Media

They contain agar at a level less than 1%, so that they remain in a semisolid state. They are used for specific studies.

(*II*) Optimum Environmental Conditions

Several environmental conditions influence the growth of bacteria. To cultivate a bacteria, it should be provided with a set of optimum environmental conditions. The most important environmental conditions to be provided during cultivation of bacteria are given below.

1. pH of the Media

Each species of bacteria can grow within a specific pH range. For most bacteria this range is between 4 and 9. However, the maximum growth of each species of bacteria occurs within a very narrow pH range. This optimum pH range for most bacteria is 6.5-7.5 and that for most of the fungi, molds and yeasts is 4-6, as they prefer acidic environments. For maximum growth to occur, the pH of the culture media has to be adjusted to this pH during its preparation. Chemical substances that act as buffers (*e.g.* KH_2PO_4, K_2HPO_4) are also added to the media to prevent any shift in pH that may occur due to accumulation of acidic or basic metabolic end products produced by the bacteria during their growth.

2. Temperature of Incubation

Mesophiles are incubated at 37°C, thermophiles at 55°C and psychrophiles at 4°C

Experiment 24

A. Cultivation of Bacteria

***Aim*: To cultivate bacteria from solid, liquid and swab samples.**

Purpose

The main purposes of cultivation of bacteria are as follows.

1. Increasing the number of bacteria, so as to get them in visible forms, as colonies or suspensions.
2. Isolation of bacteria.
3. Maintenance of pure stock culture and standard cultures.
4. Enumeration of bacteria in samples.
5. Detection of particular bacteria of interest in a sample and its enumeration.
6. Identification of bacteria from colony characteristics, growth characteristics on slants and biochemical activities in different media.

However, the purpose of this experiment is only to cultivates bacteria from liquid, solid and surface samples in solid and liquid media, so as to get them in visible forms as colonies or suspension respectively.

Principle

Bacteria are cultured in sterilised, nutritionally rich liquid or solid media. The liquid media, called broth, is contained in test tubes to form 'broth tubes', while the solid media, called agar media, is contained in petri dishes to form 'agar plates' or simply 'plates'. Cultivation of bacteria needs some material, which is suspected to contain bacteria. Most of the things we see contain bacteria. They are present in teeth scrape, food, soil, water, fecal mater and even in the unsterilised microbiological media itself. A definite amount of the homogenous suspension of any of the bacteria-containing material is inoculated into the sterilised media aseptically and incubated in an incubator at 37°C for 24 hours. In liquid broth, the bacteria grow as suspension and make it turbid. On solid agar plates, they grow as colonies; each colony growing from a single bacterium. Cultivation of bacteria is done in the following five steps.

1. Preparation of media
2. Sterilisation of media and glasswares
3. Inoculation
4. Incubation
5. Observation

1. Preparation of Media

Usually, in preparation of liquid broth and semisolid media, the ingredients are weighed in the prescribed proportions and dissolved in the required amount of water. At present, ready-made media powders containing the ingredients in required proportions are available. In preparation of liquid broth media, the prescribed quantity of powder (as mentioned on the label of the pack) is weighed and dissolved in the required amount of water in a conical flask. The ingredients are dissolved by warming, poured into test tubes and sterilised in autoclave. But in preparation of solid plates, slants and deep tubes, the prescribed quantity of powder (as mentioned on the label of the pack) is weighed and dissolved in required amount of water in a conical flask. This prepared medium is first sterilised in autoclave and then allowed to cool for sometime. While still warm, before it solidifies, it is poured into sterilised petri dishes or test tubes and allowed to solidify upon cooling to room temperature. Media, in very hot condition should never be poured into containers, as it leads to condensation of water on the wall of the containers, which drop on the surface of the media and may lead to its contamination.

2. Sterilisation

Glasswares are sterilised in hot air oven at 180°C for 3 hours and media in autoclave at 121°C (15 psi pressure) for 15 minutes. Glasswares can also be sterilised in autoclave, but media should never be sterilised in the oven, as water escapes from the media and they dehydrate.

3. Inoculation

Liquid samples are assumed to be homogenous suspensions of bacteria. Therefore, for cultivation in broth, a definite volume of the sample is pipetted into the broth aseptically. For cultivation on agar plates, a definite volume of the sample is pipetted onto the solid agar plate and spread on the surface of the medium aseptically.

For solid samples, a sample of definite weight is homogenised aseptically in a definite volume of normal physiological saline (0.85% sodium chloride) using a sterilised pestle and mortar or a blender. Most of the human pathogens are isotonic to human body (0.85% sodium chloride). Usually the ratio of sample to saline is 1: 9 (1g + 9 ml; 10g + 90 ml; 25g + 225 ml or 50g + 450 ml). A definite volume of this homogenised liquid, which is assumed to be a homogenous suspension of bacteria, is pipetted aseptically to the sterilised broth in test tubes for broth culture. For culture on agar plates, the liquid suspension is pipetted onto the surface of the plates and spread aseptically.

For surface samples taken to study the microbiology of solid surfaces (table tops, body surfaces or wounds), the surface is rubbed with a sterilised swab. The swab is touched to the surface of a sterilised agar plate. From the point of touch, streaks are made by sterilised loop aseptically, so as to isolate the bacteria.

4. *Incubation*

The inoculated broth tubes and plates are incubated at 37°C for 24 hours in an incubator.

5. *Observation*

Turbidity in liquid broth and colonies on agar plates indicate growth of bacteria.

Material Required

Petri dishes (6 nos.), 2-ml pipettes (5 nos.), test tubes (5 nos.), conical flasks (100 ml, 250ml and 500ml–1 each), 250 ml beaker (2 nos.), glass spreader, stainless steel pipette case, craft paper, thread (or rubber band), non-absorbent cotton, small sticks, loop, ethyl alcohol, sodium chloride (NaCl), 0.1N hydrochloric acid (HCl), 0.1N sodium hydroxide (NaOH), distilled water, nutrient broth (*See* Appendix I at page 247), nutrient agar (*See* Appendix I at page 247), liquid sample (*e.g.* pond water), solid sample (*e.g.* soil), surface sample(*e.g.* table top, body surface, wound), pH paper (or pH meter), pestle and mortar (or homogeniser), bunsen burner, hot air oven, autoclave, incubator, laminar flow chamber.

Procedure

1. Five pipettes (in a stainless steel pipette case), six petri dishes and a pair of pestle and mortar (or one homogeniser cup) are sterilised at 180°C for 3 hours in a hot air oven. Alternatively, they can be covered with craft paper, tied with thread or rubber band and sterilised in autoclave along with the media (Figure 6.1).
2. 0.85 g of NaCl is dissolved in 100 ml of distilled water in a 250 ml beaker and 90 ml of this saline solution is poured into a 100 ml conical flask. The mouth is cotton-plugged, covered with craft paper and tied with thread or rubber band.
3. The ingredients of nutrient broth medium (*See* Appendix I at page 247) required for 100 ml of the broth are weighed. Alternatively, prescribed amount of ready-made nutrient broth powder (ingredient mixture) is weighed.
4. The ingredients (or the ready-made powder) are dissolved in 100 ml of distilled water in a 250 ml conical flask by shaking and swirling. Its pH is determined using a pH paper or pH meter. The pH is adjusted to 7.0 using 0.1N HCl if it is more or using 0.1N NaOH if it is less. The flask is heated, if required, to dissolve the ingredients completely.
5. The broth is distributed into 5 test tubes (approximately 10 ml each), their mouths cotton-plugged, covered with craft paper and tied with thread or rubber band.
6. The ingredients of nutrient agar medium (*See* Appendix I at page 247) or its ready-made powder required for 200 ml of the medium is weighed and dissolved in 200 ml of distilled water in a 500 ml conical flask by shaking and swirling. Its pH is determined using a pH paper or pH

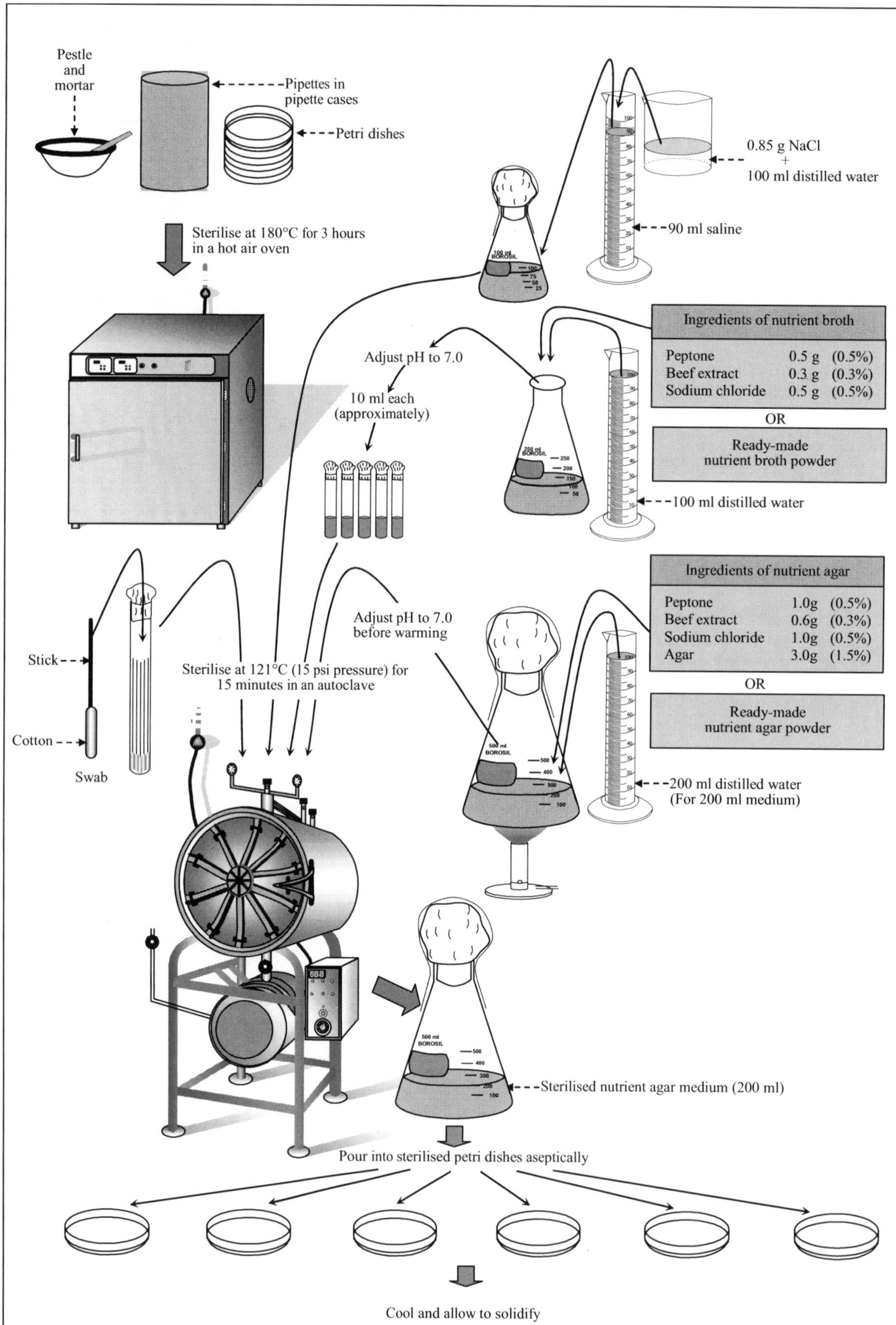

Figure 6.1: Cultivation of bacteria: Preparation and sterilisation of media

meter and adjusted to 7.0 using 0.1N HCl if it is more or using 0.1N NaOH if it is less. The flask is heated to dissolve the agar in the medium completely. Then, it is cotton-plugged, covered with craft paper and tied with thread or rubber band.

7. Swabs are made by twisting cotton around the tips of small sticks. Few such swabs are kept in a test tube with the cotton tips downward. The test tube is cotton-plugged, covered with craft paper and tied with thread or rubber band.
8. The 100 ml conical flask with 90 ml saline, the 5 test tubes with nutrient broth, the 500 ml conical flask containing 200 ml nutrient agar medium and the test tube containing the swabs are sterilised at 121°C (15 psi pressure) for 15 minutes in an autoclave.
9. After sterilisation, the sterilised materials are removed from the autoclave and allowed to cool for sometime, without allowing the medium to solidify. Cooling of the medium prevents condensation and accumulation of water droplets inside the plates. If the medium has already been prepared and solidified during storage, it has to be liquefied by heating carefully till it melts completely.
10. [1]To prepare nutrient agar plates, before the sterilised nutrient agar medium cools and solidifies, in warm molten condition, it is poured aseptically, into the 6 sterilised petri dishes (approximately 20 ml each), so that the molten medium covers the bottom of the petri dishes completely. Then, the plates are covered with their lids and allowed to cool, so as to solidify the medium in them. Water vapour that may condense on the inner surface of the plates and lids is evaporated by keeping the plates and lids in inverted position in an incubator at 37°C for about 1 hour.
11. The liquid sample (suspected to contain bacteria, *e.g.* pond water) is taken. One ml each of the sample is aseptically pipetted into 2 broth tubes (Figure 6.2). The tubes are swirled. The liquid sample is also pipetted aseptically onto 2 agar plates, 0.1 ml each, and spread on the surface of the agar medium using a flame-sterilised glass spreader. Before each spreading by the glass spreader, it is dipped in alcohol and flamed over a bunsen burner. The inoculated broth tubes and plates are incubated at 37°C for 24 hours in an incubator. The plates are incubated in inverted position, top down.
12. For the solid sample (*e.g.* soil), 10g of the sample is aseptically weighed and homogenised in the sterilised pestle and mortar or homogeniser cup after adding 90 ml of the sterilised saline from the 100 ml conical flask. This homogenous bacteria suspension is aseptically pipetted into 2 broth tubes and 2 agar plates as in step 11 and incubated at 37°C for 24 hours in the incubator (Figure 6.2). The plates are incubated in inverted position, top down.
13. For surface sampling, the surface suspected to contain bacteria (table top, body surface, wound) is marked for a unit area (*e.g.* 1 cm^2), which is rubbed by a sterilised swab. The swab is touched onto the surface of the two left out agar plates. Streaking is done aseptically by a flame-sterilised loop. For streaking, almost parallel lines are drawn by the loop from the swab-touch point. These form the primary streaks. After flame-sterilisation of the loop, secondary streaks are

---

1 Steps 10 to 13 should be performed following 'aseptic technique', preferably in a laminar flow chamber. Before use, the platform of the laminar flow chamber is cleaned and disinfected with lysol. Bunsen burner is connected and then, the glass door is closed. The UV light is switched on for 10 minutes to sterilise the environment inside the chamber and then, switched off. The glass door should never be opened, when the UV light is on, because UV light has detrimental effect on skin and vision. The blower is switched on and then, the glass door is opened. Now, the bunsen burner is lighted and media transfer or inoculation is carried out in the chamber aseptically. The mouths of the containers containing sterilised media or samples should be shown over flame of bunsen burner after removing the cotton plugs and before putting them back. Loops or needles, before use have to be sterilised over flame by heating to red hot and then cooling for 30 seconds to cool to room temperature. They should never be used, when very hot, as they kill the microbes when touch them. For aseptic use of glass spreader, before use, its portion to come in contact with samples or cultures is dipped in ethyl alcohol taken in a 250 ml beaker and then shown over bunsen flame to catch fire and burn off the alcohol. After cooling to room temperature, it is used.

drawn almost diagonally to the primary streaks. In similar manner, tertiary and quaternary streaks are made aseptically.

14. Then, the plates are incubated in inverted position, top down, at 37°C for 24 hour in the incubator (Figure 6.2).
15. One uninoculated agar plate and one uninoculated broth tube are incubated as control to ensure proper sterilisation as indicated by no growth in them. This step is optional.

Observations (Cultural Characteristics)

1. ***Broth Culture***

(*i*) *Turbidity Observed*: Growth has taken place. It is observed for growth characteristics as follows (Figure 6.3).

(*a*) *Uniform Fine Turbidity*: Finely dispersed growth throughout.

(*b*) *Flocculant*: Flaky aggregates dispersed throughout.

(*c*) *Pellicle*: Thick pad-like growth on surface.

(*d*) *Sediment*: Concentration of growth at the bottom of broth culture; may be granular, flaky or flocculant.

(*ii*) *No Turbidity*: No growth has taken place. The sample used is bacteria-free.

2. ***Spread Plate Culture***

(*i*) *Colonies Observed*: Growth has taken place. It is observed for colony characteristics as follows (Figure 6.3).

1. *Size*: Pinpoint, small, moderate or large.
2. *Pigmentation*: Colour of colony.
3. *Form*: The shape of the colony is described as follows.

(*a*) *Circular*: Unbroken peripheral edge.

(*b*) *Irregular*: Indented peripheral edge.

(*c*) *Rhizoid*: Root-like spreading growth.

4. *Margin*: The appearance of the outer edge of the colony is described as follows.

(*a*) *Entire*: Sharply defined, even.

(*b*) *Lobate*: Marked indentations.

(*c*) *Undulate*: Wavy indentations.

(*d*) *Serrate*: Tooth-like appearance.

(*e*) *Filamentous*: Thread-like spreading edge.

5. *Elevation*: The degree, to which colony is raised is described as follows

(*a*) *Flat*: Elevation not discernible.

(*b*) *Raised*: Slightly elevated.

(*c*) *Convex*: Dome-shaped elevation.

(*d*) *Umbonate*: Raised with elevated convex central region.

(*ii*) *No Colony*: No growth has taken place on the plate. The sample used is bacteria-free.

3. ***Streak Plate Culture***

(*i*) *Colonies Observed*: Growth has taken place. It is observed for colony characteristics as described above.

(ii) *No Colony*: No growth has taken place: The surface sample used is bacteria-free.

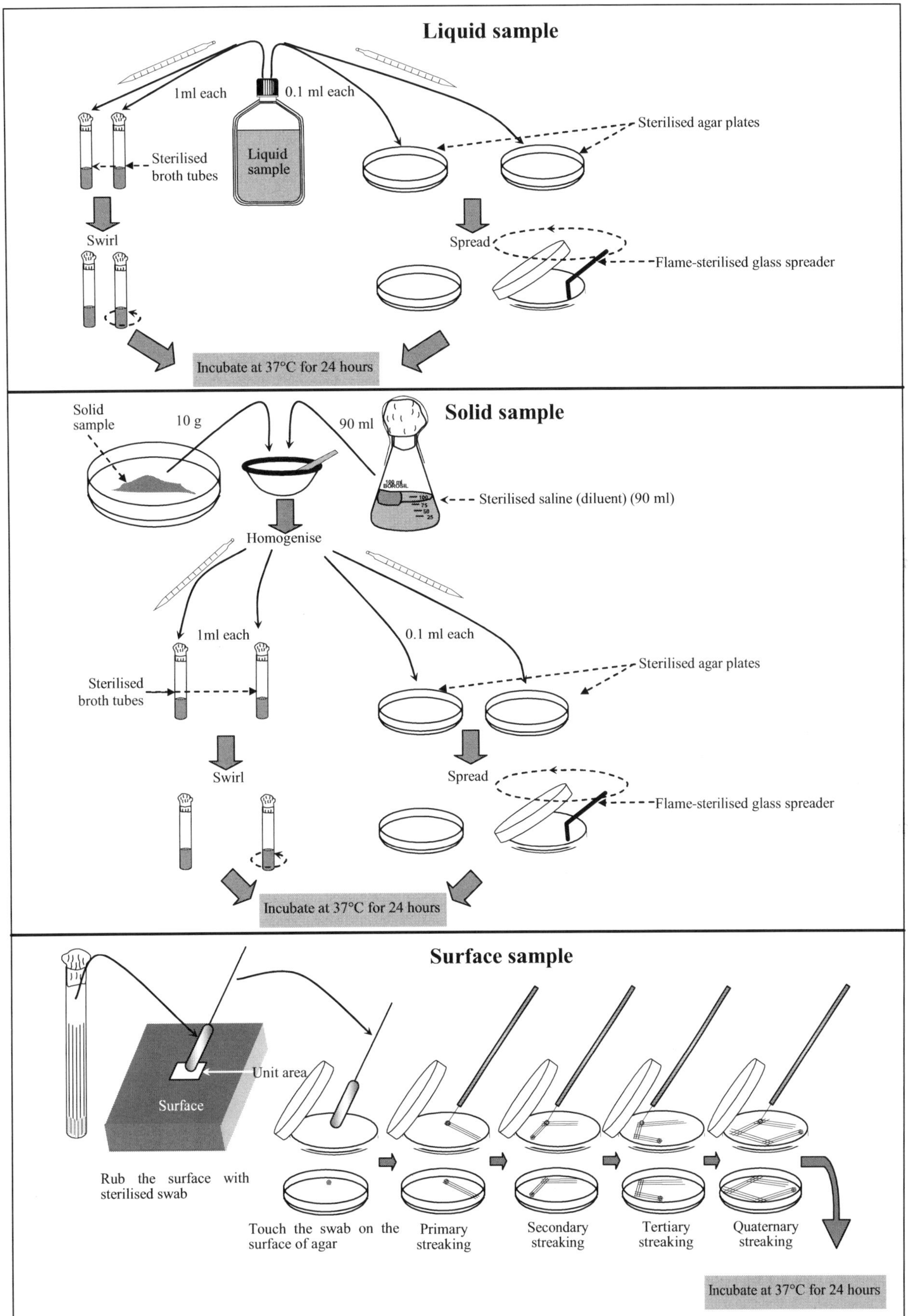

Figure 6.2: Cultivation of bacteria: Inoculation of bacteria and incubation

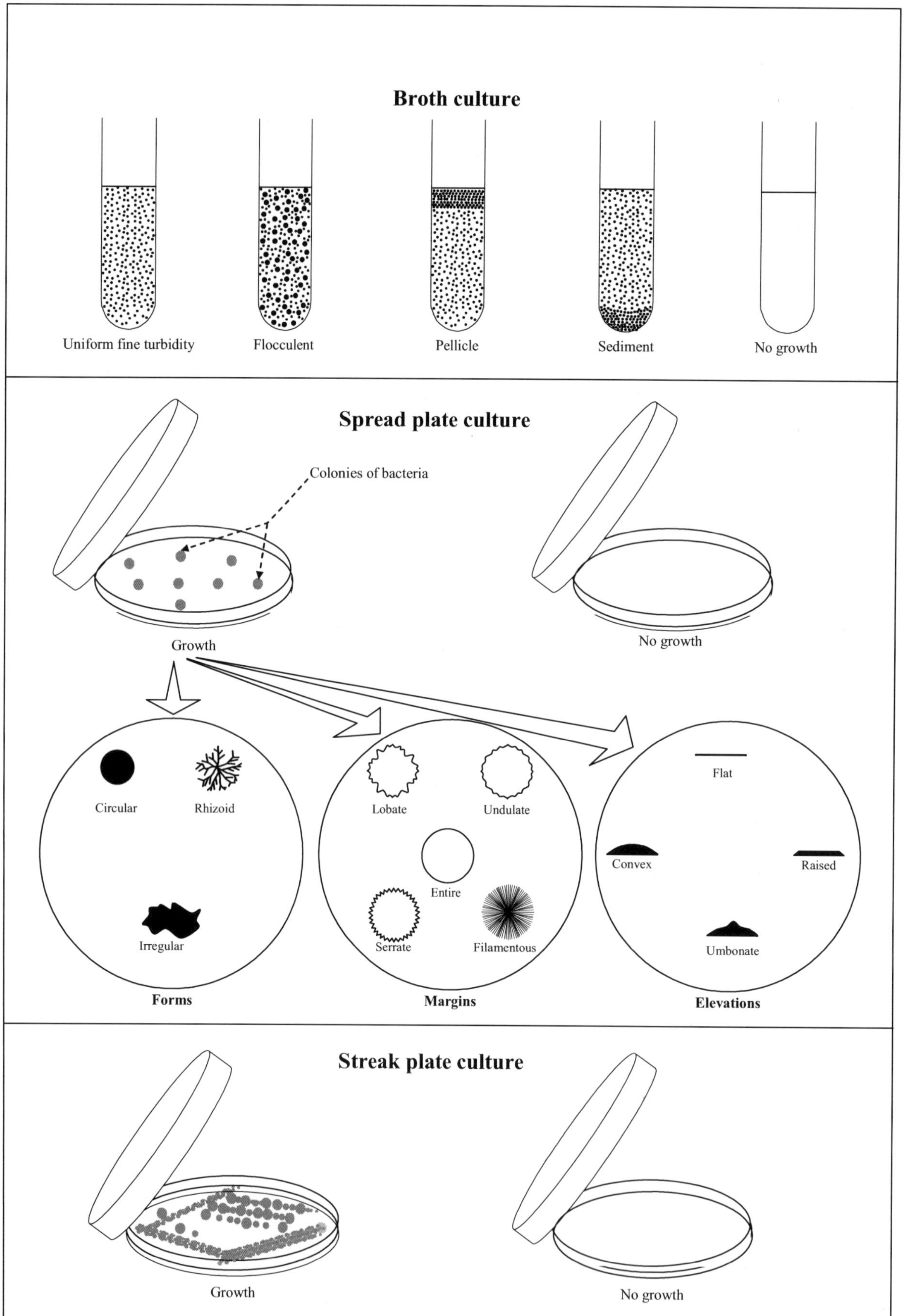

Figure 6.3: Cultivation of bacteria: Observation of growth (Cultural characteristics)

Experiment 25

B. Isolation of Bacteria and Maintenance of Pure Culture

***Aim*: To isolate different bacteria present in a given sample and maintain their pure cultures.**

Purpose

Bacteria found in nature, do not occur as segregated species, rather they occur as mixed populations of different species. Therefore, to study the individual species of bacteria, it is first required to segregate them from the mixed population. This process is called 'isolation of bacteria'. It is accomplished by growing the mixed population of bacteria on the surface of a solid medium into discrete colonies. 'Colonies' are individual, macroscopically visible masses of bacteria grown on the surface of solid medium, each representing the multiplication of a single bacterium. As each colony comes from the growth and repeated multiplication of a single bacterium, all the bacteria present in the colony belong to the same species. Thus, each colony represents a very large population of a single species of bacteria. These colonies are transferred aseptically to separate nutrient agar slants and allowed to grow there. The isolated species of bacteria, grown separately on agar slants are called 'pure cultures'. In every 15 to 30 days, they are transferred to fresh slants, so that they do not lose their original characteristics due to over-crowding, lack of nutrients and accumulation of metabolites. In this way, pure cultures of bacteria are maintained in the laboratory by repeated transfer to fresh slants at regular intervals. This process is known as 'maintenance of pure culture'. Pure cultures are maintained in the laboratory for their subsequent identification by various staining, biochemical, serological and molecular techniques as well as for their future use. 'Stock cultures' are standard pure cultures, whose identification has been established internationally to genus, species, sub-species, type, or sub-type level. They are maintained in internationally recognised microbiology laboratories. Other laboratories can obtain them from these laboratories and maintain in their own laboratories as their stock cultures, by repeated transfer to fresh slants at regular intervals. They are used for confirmed identification of pure cultures obtained in these laboratories by comparison of their characteristics with those of the standard stock cultures (*See* page 37).

Principle

The mixed population of bacteria present in a given material (solid, liquid or surface) is grown on nutrient agar plates by spread plate or streak plate method as described previously under 'Cultivation of bacteria'. Each isolated colony found on an agar plate consists of one species of bacteria, as each colony grows from a single bacterium. Thus, bacteria are isolated on agar plates by two techniques as follows.

(*a*) Spread plate technique

(*b*) Streak plate technique

Representative colonies (colonies having dissimilar characteristics) are selected and aseptically inoculated to separate agar slants to get the pure cultures. After each 15 to 30 days, they are transferred to fresh slants for maintenance of these pure cultures.

Materials Required

Test tubes (5 nos.), 250 ml conical flask (1 no), 0.1N NaOH, 0.1N HCl, distilled water, nutrient agar (*See* Appendix I at page 247), non-absorbent cotton, loop, craft paper, thread (or rubber band), pH paper (or pH meter), bunsen burner, autoclave, laminar flow chamber, incubator, plates containing isolated colonies of bacteria (spread plate or streak plate).

Procedure

1. The ingredients of nutrient agar medium (*See* Appendix I at page 247) or its ready-made powder required for 100 ml of the medium is weighed and dissolved in 100 ml of distilled water in a 250 ml conical flask by shaking and swirling (Figure 6.4).

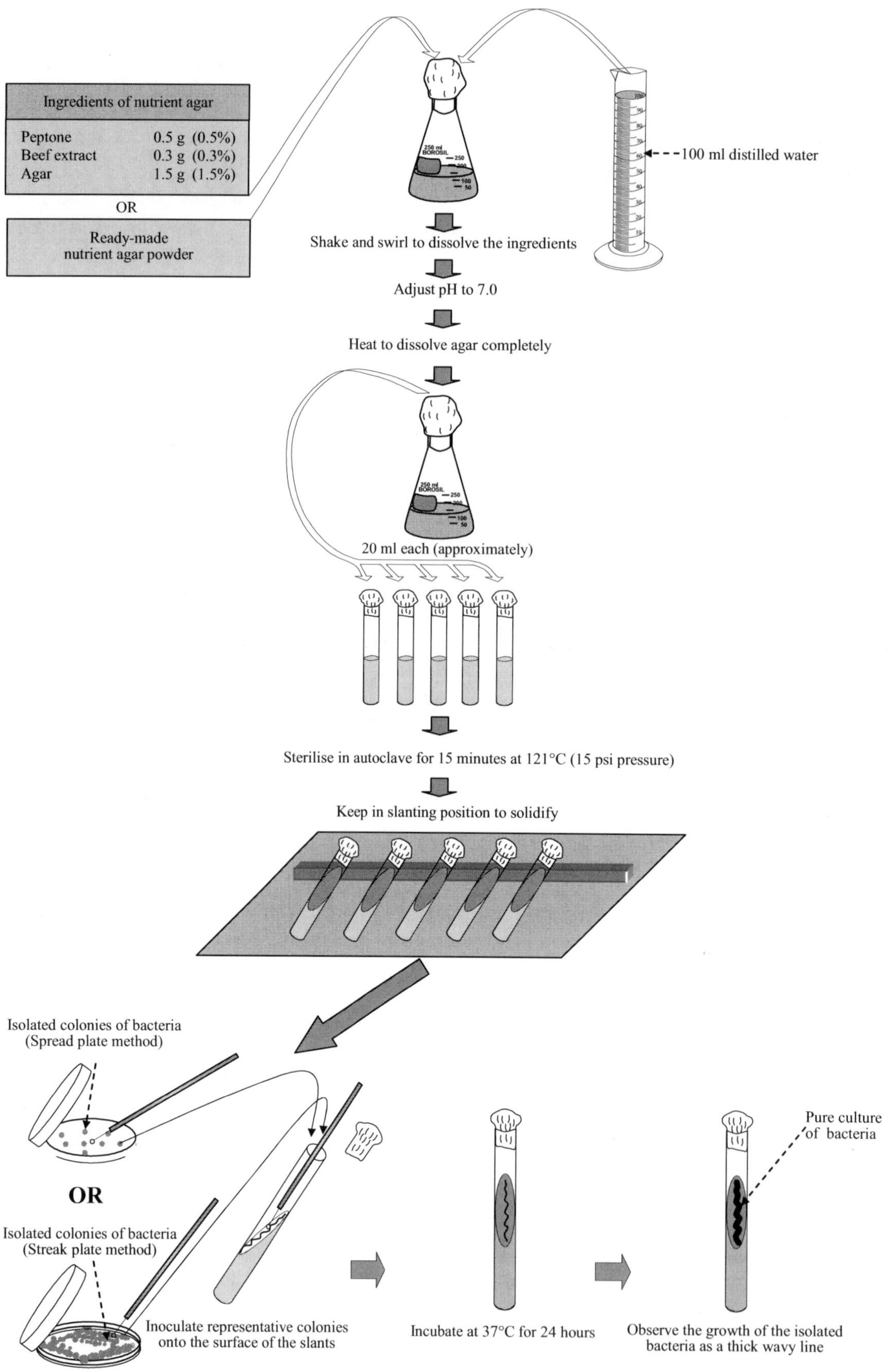

Figure 6.4: Isolation of bacteria and maintenance of pure culture

2. Its pH is determined using a pH paper or pH meter and adjusted to 7.0 using 0.1N HCl if it is more or using 0.1N NaOH if it is less.
3. The flask is heated to dissolve the agar in the medium completely.
4. Before it solidifies, the medium in warm molten condition, is distributed into 5 test tubes (approximately 20 ml each).
5. The test tubes are cotton-plugged, covered with craft paper and tied with thread or rubber band.
6. They are sterilised at 121°C (15 psi pressure) for 15 minutes in an autoclave.
7. After sterilisation, they are removed from the autoclave and kept in a slanting position to cool and solidify the medium. These test tubes containing solidified nutrient agar medium in slanting condition are called 'nutrient agar slants'.
8. Steps 10 and 11 should be performed following aseptic technique preferably in a laminar flow chamber. The mouth of the containers containing sterilised media or cultures should be shown over flame of bunsen burner after removing the cotton plug and before putting it back. Loops, before use have to be sterilised over flame by heating to red hot and then cooling for 30 seconds to cool to room temperature. They should never be used when very hot, as they kill the microbes when touch them.
9. In the previous experiment, if isolated colonies could be observed on the spread plate or streak plate, five colonies with dissimilar characteristics are selected as representative colonies.
10. A loop is sterilised over flame and a loop of bacteria from each of the representative colonies is taken aseptically. The loop is introduced into the agar slant, so that the loop of bacteria goes to the end of the slant. The loop is moved outward in a wavy manner touching the surface of the slant, so that a wavy line is formed.
11. The loop is flame-sterilised and in similar manner the rest of the four representative colonies are inoculated separately into the left over four slants. The loop is sterilised after each inoculation.
12. The five inoculated slants are incubated at 37°C for 24 hours in an incubator.

Observations (Cultural Characteristics)

*(i) **A Wavy Line with Growth Along its Length Observed:*** Growth has taken place

The slant is observed for slant characteristics as follows (Figure 6.5).

1. *Abundance of Growth*: The amount of growth is designated as none, slight, moderate or large.
2. *Pigmentation*: Chromogenic microorganisms may produce intracellular pigments that are responsible for the colouration of the organism as seen in surface colonies. Other organisms produce extracellular soluble pigments that are excreted into the medium and also produce a colour. Most organisms, however, are non-chromogenic and will appear white to gray.
3. *Optical Characteristics*: Optical characteristics may be evaluated on the basis of the amount of light transmitted through the growth. These characteristics are described as
   (*a*) *Opaque*: No light transmission.
   (*b*) *Translucent*: Partial light transmission.
   (*c*) *Transparent*: Full light transmission.
4. *Form*: The appearance of the single line streak of growth on the agar surface is designated as follows.
   (*a*) *Filiform*: Continuous, threadlike growth with smooth edges.
   (*b*) *Echinulate*: Continuous, threadlike growth with irregular edges.
   (*c*) *Beaded*: Non-confluent to semi-confluent colonies.

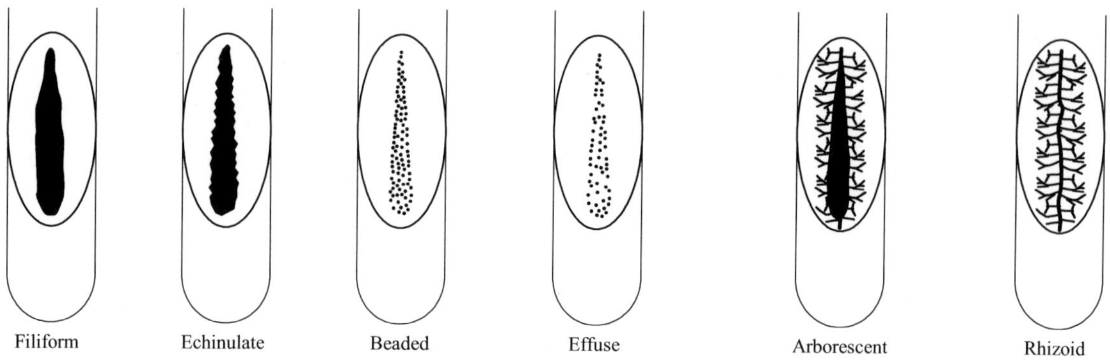

Figure 6.5: Cultural characteristics of bacteria on nutrient agar slants

(*d*) *Effuse*: Thin, spreading growth.

(*e*) *Arborescent*: Tree-like growth.

(*f*) *Rhizoid*: Root-like growth.

(ii) No Growth Along the Line of Inoculation: Faulty technique of inoculation. Inoculation is repeated

C. Enumeration of Bacteria

The extent of bacterial activity in a given sample in a definite set of conditions mainly depends on the total number of bacteria present in it irrespective of their species. Therefore, it is very often required to find out the total number of bacteria present in samples of food, water, soil, air and tissue during their microbiological analysis. Estimating the number of bacteria in a given sample is called 'enumeration of bacteria'. There are various methods of enumeration of bacteria as given below. All of these methods need bacteria to be present in a homogenous suspension. That is why, liquid samples are assumed to be homogenous suspensions of bacteria and are directly used, while solid samples are homogenised in sterile saline solutions, so as to get homogenous suspensions of bacteria.

(*I*) Direct Methods

(*a*) Direct microscopic count

(*b*) Electronic cell counter

(*II*) Indirect Methods

(*c*) Chemical methods

(*d*) Turbidimetric method

(*e*) Membrane filter count

} *Not used commonly* [(a)–(e)]

(*f*) Serial dilution-agar plating method or Total Plate Count method (TPC method) } *Most widely used*

(*a*) Direct Microscopic Count

In this method, the number of bacteria present in an aliquot of the homogenous suspension of bacteria is counted directly under a microscope and the total number of bacteria in the sample is determined mathematically. The advantage of this method is that, it is very rapid. The disadvantages are that, both living (viable) and dead cells are counted and the method is not sensitive to populations of fewer than one million bacteria per milliliter. Counting can be done in two methods as follows.

(i) Petroff-Hauser Chamber

It is a specialised counting chamber, in which an aliquot of the homogenous suspension of bacteria is put for counting directly under a microscope.

(ii) Breed Smear

Bacteria cells are directly counted under microscope using stained smears confined to an area of 1 mm^2 on the slide. It is mainly used for the enumeration of bacteria in milk.

(*b*) Electronic Cell Counter

An electronic cell counter such as 'Coulter counter' is used to directly count the number of bacteria cells. A homogenous suspension of bacteria cells prepared in a conducting fluid is allowed to pass through a minute orifice, across which an electric current flows. The resistance at the orifice is electronically recorded. When a cell passes through the orifice, being non-conductor, it increases the resistance momentarily. The number of times resistance increases momentarily is recorded electronically, which indicates the number of bacteria present in the suspension. The advantage of this method is that, it is extremely rapid. The disadvantages are that, both living (viable) and dead cells are counted and the instrument cannot distinguish between bacteria cells and inert particulate matter.

(*c*) Chemical Methods

These methods estimate the quantity of those substances, mainly chemicals, which increases with the increase in bacterial population. The main parameters estimated are as follows.

(*i*) Protein concentration
(*ii*) DNA concentration
(*iii*) Dry weight
(*iv*) Carbon dioxide production
(*v*) Oxygen uptake
(*vi*) Lactic acid production

(*d*) Turbidimetric Method

When bacteria are grown in liquid nutrient-rich media (*e.g.* nutrient broth), their profuse growth makes the media turbid, as the bacteria cells mostly remain suspended in them. The turbidity increases with increase in the number of cells in the media. As turbidity increases, the 'absorbance' or 'optical density (OD)' of the media increases. The OD of the suspension of bacteria cells in the media is measured using a spectrophotometer at 600 nm. The number of bacteria cells in the suspension is found out by comparing the OD with a standard curve prepared by plotting the OD values for different known concentrations of bacteria. The method is rapid, but limited to bacterial suspensions of more than 10 million cells.

(*e*) Membrane Filter Count

This method is used, when the number of bacteria in a liquid sample is very less. To increase the concentration of bacteria, first the liquid sample is filtered aseptically through a sterilised membrane filter apparatus using a sterile membrane filter. The membrane filter containing the trapped bacteria is aseptically transferred to a sterile petri dish containing an absorbent pad saturated with a selective differential liquid medium. The medium oozes onto the surface of the filter. After incubation, the number of colonies formed on the filter is counted using a simple microscope.

(*f*) Serial Dilution-Agar Plating Method or TPC Method

It is the most versatile and widely used method for enumeration of bacteria (*See* Expiment 26).

Experiment 26

Total Plate Count (TPC)

Aim: **To enumerate bacteria present in a sample by serial dilution-agar plating method or total plate count (TPC) method.**

Purpose

The extent of bacterial activity in a given sample in a definite set of conditions mainly depends on the total number of bacteria present in it irrespective of their species. Therefore, it is very often required to find out the total number of bacteria present in samples of food, water, soil, air and tissue during their microbiological analysis. This total number of bacteria includes both living and dead bacteria. Dead bacteria cannot grow and reproduce. It is only the living bacteria (viable bacteria), which can grow and multiply resulting in specific bacterial activity. Therefore, it is very often required to enumerate the viable bacteria cells in different samples. However, most of the enumeration methods like direct microscopic count, electronic cell count, chemical methods and spectrophotometric method count both living as well as dead cells. These methods cannot discriminate between living and dead cells. Therefore, serial dilution-agar plating method, which enumerates only the viable bacteria cells, is the universally used method for counting living viable cells in different samples.

Principle

A definite weight of solid sample is homogenised aseptically in nine volumes of sterile saline to get a homogenous suspension of bacteria. The liquid sample is directly used as homogenous suspension of bacteria. The suspensions of bacteria so obtained are diluted serially (10 times, 100 times, 1000 times etc.). Here 10^{-1}, 10^{-2}, 10^{-3} etc. are called dilutions. Their reciprocals (10^1,10^2,10^3 etc.) are called dilution factors. A definite volume of the suspension of bacteria from each dilution is inoculated onto agar plates and spread properly, so as to space the individual bacteria cells wide apart and isolate them from each other. The inoculation of bacteria for its enumeration is done in two techniques as follows.

1. **Pour plate technique**
2. **Spread plate technique**

1. *Pour Plate Technique*

In this technique, 1 ml of the bacteria suspension is dropped onto a sterilised petri dish and then liquefied nutrient agar medium is poured over it. The petri dish is swirled gently, so as to allow the suspension to mix with the medium uniformly. It is allowed to cool and solidify.

2. *Spread Plate Technique*

In this technique 0.1 ml of the bacteria suspension is dropped onto a prepared agar plate. Then, the drop of suspension is spread uniformly on the agar plate by a sterilised glass spreader.

To minimise error, each diluted suspension is plated onto 2-5 replicate plates. The inoculated plates are incubated at 37°C for 24 hours. During this period, each isolated individual bacteria cell on the agar plate grows and multiplies rapidly to produce a macroscopic visible mass of bacteria cells called a 'colony'. Thus, the number of colonies on the plate represents the number of bacteria in the sample. However, very often, during spreading, some cells may not get separated properly and few such unseparated cells may give rise to a single colony. Moreover, few cells have tendency to remain in pairs, chains or clusters. Here, each pair, chain or cluster produces a colony. Thus, each colony, in strict sense, does not represent a single bacterium. That is why, instead of expressing the counts of bacteria as 'No. of bacteria/gm or ml of sample', it is very often expressed as number of colony forming units per gm or ml (CFU/gm or ml). The total plate count (TPC) in the original sample is calculated by multiplying the number of CFUs with the respective dilution factors. The 'rules of enumeration' (*See* pages 129–130) are followed, while calculating the number of bacteria in the original sample.

Materials Required

Petri dishes (15 nos.), 2-ml pipettes (10 nos.), 10-ml pipette (1 no.), test tubes (10 nos.), conical flasks (500 ml and 1 liter–1 no. each), 500 ml beaker (2 nos.), glass spreader, stainless steel pipette case, craft paper, thread (or rubber band), non-absorbent cotton, ethyl alcohol, sodium chloride (NaCl), 0.1N hydrochloric acid (HCl), 0.1N sodium hydroxide (NaOH), distilled water, nutrient agar (*See* Appendix I at page 247), liquid sample (*e.g.* pond water/sewage water), solid sample (*e.g.* soil/fish meat/oyster meat/processed food), pH paper (or pH meter), pestle and mortar (or homogeniser), bunsen burner, hot air oven, autoclave, incubator, laminar flow chamber, Quebec colony counter.

Procedure

1. Ten pipettes (in a stainless steel pipette case), 15 petri dishes and a pair of pestle and mortar (or one homogeniser cup) are sterilised in hot air oven at 180° C for 3 hours. Alternatively, they can be covered with craft paper, tied with thread or rubber band and sterilised in autoclave along with the medium (Figure 6.6). The number of petri dishes and accordingly the amount of medium to be used is calculated depending on the number of replications and dilutions required. Here, the glasswares and the medium have been taken for single replication and dilution upto 10^{-6}. The number of glasswares and the amount of medium taken for sterilisation is slightly more to avoid any incidental error, because sterilisation is a lengthy process.
2. 4.25 g of NaCl is dissolved in 500 ml of distilled water to get physiological saline (0.85%). 225 ml of this saline solution is poured into a 500 ml conical flask. Its mouth is cotton-plugged, covered with craft paper and tied with thread or rubber band. It is used as the first diluent to dilute the solid sample.
3. 9.0 ml of the left over saline is also pipetted into each of the 10 test tubes. Their mouths are cotton-plugged, covered with craft paper and tied with thread or rubber band. These are used as diluents for serial dilution.
4. The ingredients of nutrient agar medium (*See* Appendix I at page 247) or its ready-made powder required for 500 ml of the medium is weighed and dissolved in 500 ml of distilled water in a 1 liter conical flask by shaking and swirling. Its pH is determined using a pH paper or pH meter and adjusted to 7.0 using 0.1N HCl if it is more or using 0.1N NaOH if it is less. The flask is heated to dissolve the agar in the medium completely. Then, it is cotton-plugged, covered with craft paper and tied with thread or rubber band.
5. The 500 ml conical flask containing 225 ml of saline, the 10 test tubes containing 9 ml of saline each and the 1 liter conical flask containing 500 ml of nutrient agar medium are sterilised at 121°C (15 psi pressure) for 15 minutes in an autoclave.
6. After sterilisation, the sterilised materials are removed from the autoclave and allowed to cool for sometime, without allowing the medium to solidify. Cooling of the medium prevents condensation and accumulation of water droplets inside the plates. If the medium has already been prepared and solidified during storage, it has to be liquefied by heating carefully till it melts completely.
7. [2]To prepare agar plates, before the sterilised nutrient agar medium cools and solidifies, in warm molten condition, it is poured aseptically into the 6 sterilised petri dishes (approximately

2 Steps 7 to 12 should be performed following 'aseptic technique', preferably in a laminar flow chamber. Before use, the platform of the laminar flow chamber is cleaned and disinfected with lysol. Bunsen burner is connected and then, the glass door is closed. The UV light is switched on for 10 minutes to sterilise the environment inside the chamber and then, switched off. The glass door should never be opened, when the UV light is on, because UV light has detrimental effect on skin and vision. The blower is switched on and then the glass door is opened. Now, the bunsen burner is lighted and media transfer or inoculation is carried out in the chamber aseptically (*See* page 115). The mouths of the containers containing sterilised media or samples should be shown over flame of bunsen burner after removing the cotton plugs and before putting them back. For aseptic use of glass spreader, before use, its portion to come in contact with samples or cultures is dipped in ethyl alcohol taken in a 250 ml beaker and then shown over bunsen flame to catch fire and burn off the alcohol. After cooling to room temperature, it is used.

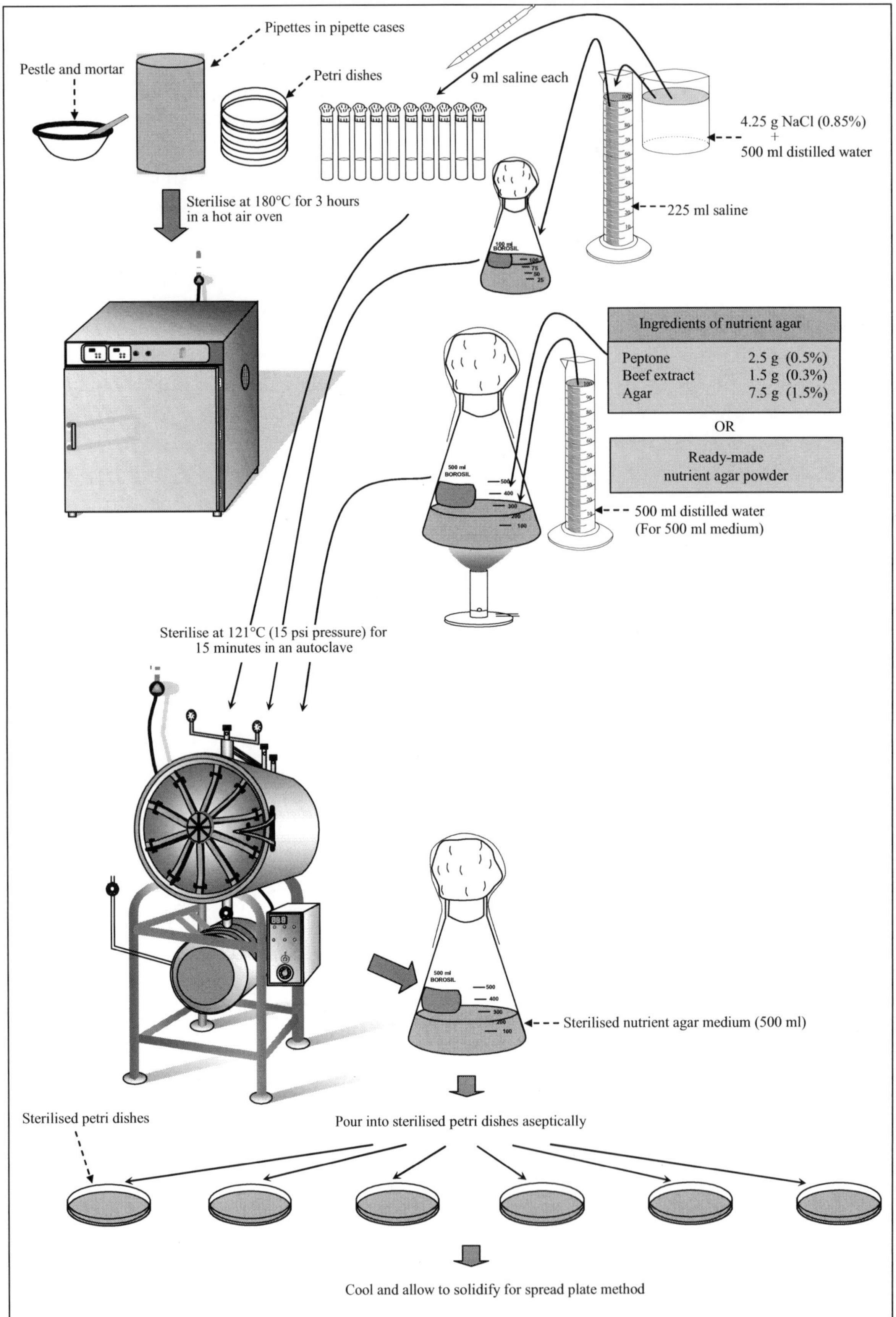

Figure 6.6: Enumeration of bacteria: Preparation and sterilisation of medium

20 ml each), so that the molten medium covers the bottom of the petri dishes completely. Then, the plates are covered with their lids and allowed to cool, so as to solidify the medium in them. Water vapour that may condense on the inner surface of the plates and lids is evaporated by keeping the plates and lids in inverted position in an incubator at 37°C for about 1 hour.

8. 25 g of the solid sample (*e.g.* fish meat/oyster meat/processed food) is weight and homogenised in 225 ml sterilised saline (diluent) aseptically (Figure 6.7). This gives a 10 times dilution (dilution = 10^{-1}). For the liquid sample, 1ml of sample is pipetted aseptically into a 9 ml sterilised saline tube. This also gives a 10 times dilution (dilution = 10^{-1}).
9. 1 ml of the 10^{-1} dilution is transferred to 9 ml sterilised saline in another test tube. This gives 100 times dilution (dilution =10^{-2}). From the 10^{-2} dilution, 1 ml is dropped into a sterilised petri dish and 0.1 ml onto an agar plate, from the same pipette. For each dilution a separate sterilised pipette is used. After use it is dipped in the dispose jar.
10. 1 ml of the 10^{-2} dilution is transferred to 9 ml sterilised saline in another test tube. This gives 1000 times dilution (dilution =10^{-3}). From the 10^{-3} dilution, 1 ml is dropped into a sterilised petri dish and 0.1 ml onto an agar plate, from the same pipette. In a similar way, dilution is continued upto 10^{-6} serially, each time transferring 1ml to a sterilised petri dish and 0.1 ml to an agar plate from the same pipette.
11. Then, the drops of suspension on the agar plates are spread aseptically by a sterilised glass spreader. After spreading in each plate, it is flame-sterilised by dipping in alcohol and showing over a flame. This is the 'spread plate technique'.
12. The petri dishes containing 1ml of bacteria suspension each are taken and sterilised liquefied nutrient agar is poured into them. They are swirled gently, so as to allow the suspension to mix with the medium uniformly. The plates are allowed to cool till the medium solidifies. This is 'pour plate technique'.
13. Then, the plates are incubated in inverted position, top down, at 37°C for 24 hours in an incubator (Figure 6.7).
14. An uninoculated agar plate is incubated as control to ensure proper sterilisation as shown by no growth on it.

Observations

The number of colonies of bacteria on the plates is counted directly or with the help of a Quebec colony counter. From this, the number of bacteria present per gram or ml of the original sample is calculated. This is called enumeration. This is done using the 'rules of enumeration' as described at the end of this chapter and tabulating the values as given below.

Sample	*Technique*	*Replications*	*Dilutions*						*Total Plate Count (TPC)*
			10^{-1}	10^{-2}	10^{-3}	10^{-4}	10^{-5}	10^{-6}	
Gut of fish	Pour plate technique	R_1							No. x 10^{c}/gm or ml
		R_2							
		R_3							
		R_4							
		R_5							
	Spread plate technique	R_1							No. x 10^{c+1}/gm or ml
		R_2							
		R_3							
		R_4							
		R_5							

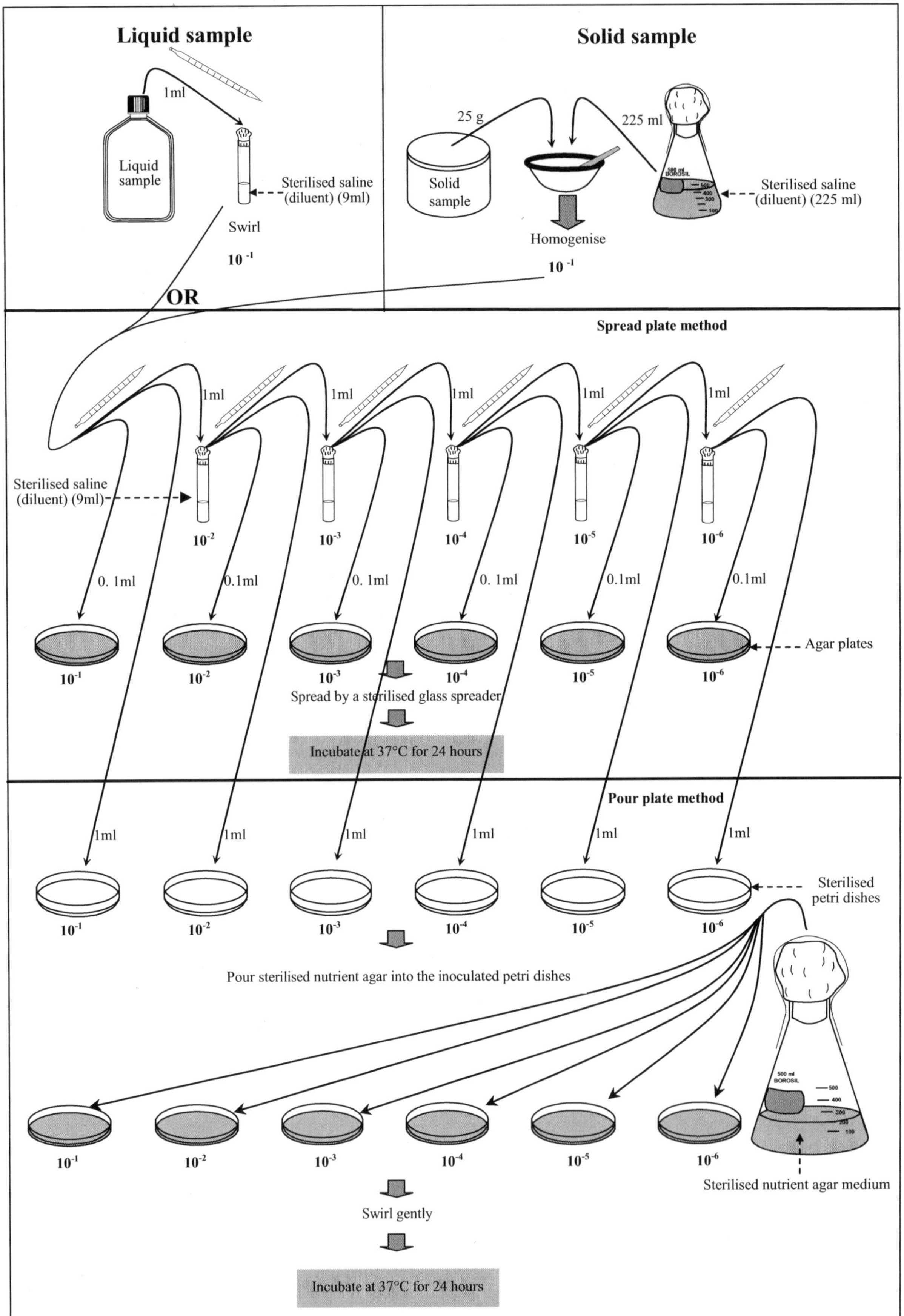

Figure 6.7: Enumeration of bacteria: Inoculation of bacteria and incubation

Rules of Enumeration

1. Petri dishes with 30 to 300 colonies should be considered.

10^{-1}	10^{-2}	10^{-3}	10^{-4}	10^{-5}	10^{-6}
>300	>300	>300	✓ 288	✓ 32	<30

2. Average numbers of duplicates and triplicates (R_1, R_2, R_3 ...) are considered only if one count is not more than double of the other. If one is more than double of the other lower value is taken.

10^{-1}	10^{-2}	10^{-3}	10^{-4}	10^{-5}	10^{-6}	
>300	>300	>300	✓ 282	✓ 32	<30	R_1
>300	>300	>300	✓ 296	68	<30	R_2
---	---	---	$\frac{286+296}{2}$ =289	32	---	

68 is more than double of 32 (32X2=64), whereas 296 is not more than double of 282 (282X2=564).

3. For pour plate technique, bacterial count is No.X 10^c/gm, where c = dilution factor. For spread plate technique, bacterial count is No. X10^{c+1}/gm, where c = dilution factor. The number is converted to two decimal places in the form of (x.yz X 10^m). For example, 288 X 10^4 is expressed as 2.88 X 10^6.

10^{-1}	10^{-2}	10^{-3}	10^{-4}	10^{-5}	10^{-6}
>300	>300	>300	✓ 288	<30	<30

For pour plate technique, the number of CFU/ g or ml = 288 X 10^4 = <u>2.88 X 10^6 CFU/g or ml</u>

10^{-1}	10^{-2}	10^{-3}	10^{-4}	10^{-5}	10^{-6}
>300	>300	✓ 282	<30	<30	<30

For spread plate technique, the number of CFU/ g or ml = 282 X 10^{3+1} = 282 X 10^4 = <u>2.82X10^6 CFU/g or ml</u>

4. If, in all dilutions, colony number is more than 300, count for the highest dilution and if in all dilutions, it is less than 30, count for the lowest dilution is considered. In both cases count is

represented as: Estimated No. X 10^c/gm or ml for pour plate technique and Estimated No. X 10^{c+1}/gm or ml for spread plate technique.

10^{-1}	10^{-2}	10^{-3}	10^{-4}	10^{-5}	10^{-6}
>300	>300	>300	>300	>300	✓ 346

The number of CFU/ g or ml = Est. 346 X 10^6 = Est. 3.46 X 10^8 CFU/g or ml (For pour plate)

The number of CFU/ g or ml = Est. 346 X 10^{6+1} = Est. 3.46 X 10^9 CFU/g or ml (For spread plate)

10^{-1}	10^{-2}	10^{-3}	10^{-4}	10^{-5}	10^{-6}
✓ 28	8	1	Nil	Nil	Nil

The number of CFU/ g or ml = Est. 28 X 10^2 = Est.2.80 X 10^3 CFU/g or ml (For pour plate)

The number of CFU/ g or ml = Est. 28 X 10^{2+1} = Est. 2.80 X 10^4 CFU/g or ml (For spread plate)

5. If no colony is observed in any dilution taken, it is represented as: Estimated <1 x lowest dilution.

10^{-1}	10^{-2}	10^{-3}	10^{-4}	10^{-5}	10^{-6}
Nil	Nil	Nil	Nil	Nil	Nil

The number of CFU/ g or ml = Est.<1X 10^1 CFU/g or ml (For pour plate)

10^{-1}	10^{-2}	10^{-3}	10^{-4}	10^{-5}	10^{-6}
Nil	Nil	Nil	Nil	Nil	Nil

The number of CFU/ g or ml = Est.<1X 10^{1+1} = Est.<1X 10^2 CFU/g or ml (For spread plate)

6. As the serial dilution takes place in terms of 10 times, mathematically it is obvious that no two dilutions can have colonies between 30 and 300. For example, if 10^{-3} has 50 colonies, 10^{-2} should have 500 (*i.e.*>300) and 10^{-4} should have 5 (*i.e.*<30) colonies. However, this does not occur in reality, as bacteria do not occur as a homogenous solution, rather occur as a suspension in the diluent. If there are two dilutions having countable colonies (between 30 and 300) first calculate the number of colony forming units/gm or ml using each dilution. If one value is more than double of the other, report the lower value. If not, take the average of the two values and report that value.

10^{-1}	10^{-2}	10^{-3}	10^{-4}	10^{-5}	10^{-6}	
>300	>300	>300	282	32	<30	**R_1**
>300	>300	>300	296	60	<30	**R_2**
---	---	---	$\frac{282+296}{2}$ =289	$\frac{32+60}{2}$ = 46	---	

No of CFU /g or ml = 289 X 10^4 =2.89 X 10^6 (For pour plate method) (Using 289 colonies found)
No of CFU /g or ml = 46 X 10^5 =4.60 X 10^6 (For pour plate method) (Using 46 colonies found)
4.60 X 10^6 is not more than double of 2.89 X 10^6 .
Therefore average is taken *i.e.* $\frac{2.89+4.60}{2}$ X10^6 =3.74 X 10^6.

If the average number of colonies in the same two dilutions were 289 and 66 (instead of 46), then the No of CFU /g or ml would have been 2.89 X 10^6 and 6.60 X 10^6. Here 6.60 X 10^6 is more than double of 2.89 X 10^6 (double of 2.89 X 10^6 is 5.78 X 10^6). Therefore, the value to be reported is the lower value *i.e.* 2.89 X 10^6.

7

Biochemical Tests of Bacteria

A. What are Biochemical Tests ?

Biochemical tests are the tests used for the identification of bacteria species based on the differences in the biochemical activities of different bacteria. Bacterial physiology differs from one species to the other. These differences in carbohydrate metabolism, protein metabolism, fat metabolism, production of certain enzymes, ability to utilise a particular compound etc. help them to be identified by the biochemical tests.

B. Importance of Biochemical Tests

The identification of higher plants and animals involves the observations of the structural differences, both internal and external, which exist among them. Most of these structural differences are visible to naked eye. Even the identification of microscopic plants and animals involves the observations of their structural differences under a microscope. Such identification based on structural differences is not possible in case of bacteria, because structural differences, which may differentiate one species of bacteria from the other are not discernible even under a microscope. The structural differences with respect to shape, size and arrangement of bacteria only help in the process of identification, because there are many species of bacteria having similar shape, size and arrangement. Therefore, ultimately, the identification of bacteria is mostly based on the differences in their biochemical activities. A list of some of the most commonly used biochemical tests performed for the identification of bacteria has been given in Figure 7.1.

Each species of bacteria has a well-defined set of metabolic activities different from all other species. These biochemical fingerprints are properties controlled by the bacterial enzymes (Figure 7.2). The bacterial enzymes can be grouped into two categories as follows.

1. Intracellular Enzymes (Endoenzymes)

These enzymes function inside the bacteria cells. They are mainly responsible for the synthesis of new protoplasmic substances and production of cellular energy from simple substances permeating into the cells through the cell membrane. There are many intracellular enzymes, which help in the utilisation of these simple substances. It is necessary for cellular survival and function and is the basis of cellular metabolism. As a result of these metabolic processes, metabolic products are formed and excreted by the cells into the environment. Assay of these end products aids in the identification of bacteria.

2. Extracellular Enzymes (Exoenzymes)

These are the enzymes secreted by the bacteria cells to the surrounding to hydrolyse high molecular weight or complex substances, such as proteins, polysaccharides and fats, which cannot permeate the

BIOCHEMICAL TESTS

Intracellular enzyme activity

1. Indole test
2. Methyl red test
3. Voges-Proskauer test
4. Citrate utilisation test

(Tests 1–4: **IMViC test**)

5. Triple sugar iron (TSI) test

(Tests 1–5: Special tests for separation of enteric bacteria)

6. Carbohydrate fermentation test
7. Oxidation-fermentation test (O/F test)
8. Nitrate reduction test
9. Amino acid decarboxylase test
10. Litmus milk test
11. Hydrogen sulphide test
12. Urease test
13. O-Nitrophenyl galactoside test (ONPG test)
14. Phenylalanine deaminase test
15. Catalase test
16. Oxidase test

Extracellular enzyme activity

17. Gelatinase test
18. Starch hydrolysis test
19. Lipid hydrolysis test
20. Deoxyribonuclease test (DNase test)
21. Coagulase test

Figure 7.1: Some common biochemical tests performed for the identification of bacteria

bacterial cell membrane, because of their large size (proteins and polysaccharides) or because of their complex nature (fats). The extracellular enzymes hydrolyse them into their respective simple building blocks. Proteins are hydrolysed to amino acids, polysaccharides like starch to glucose and fats like triglycerides to glycerol and fatty acids. The low molecular weight simple substances, so produced, can permeate through the cell membrane into the bacteria cells, where they are utilised with the help of the intracellular enzymes with the liberation of metabolic wastes. The ability of a bacteria to produce these extracellular enzymes is species specific and therefore, is used for the identification of bacteria.

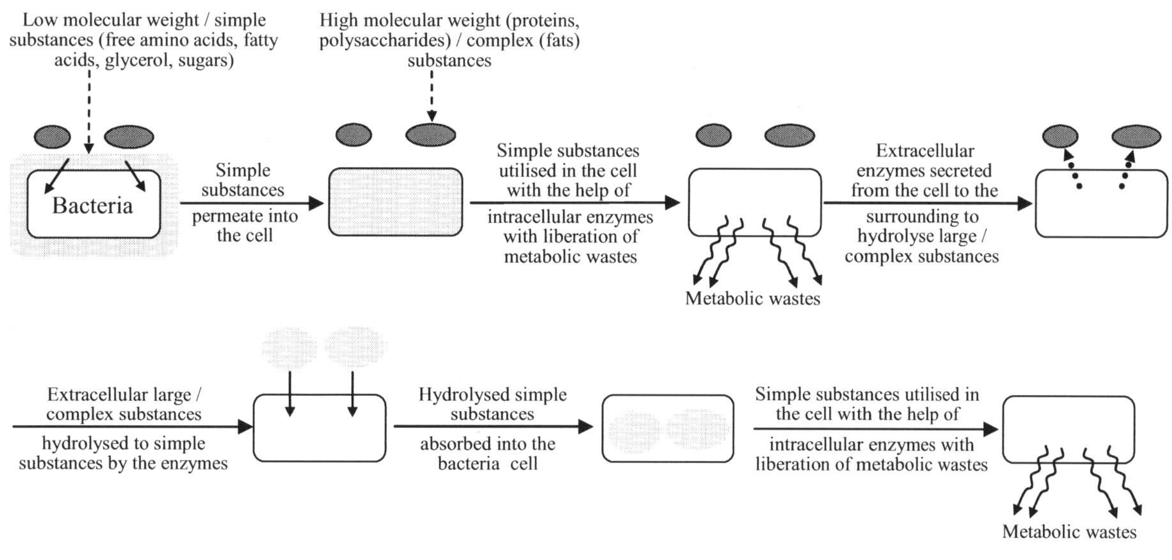

Figure 7.2: Activities of intracellular and extracellular enzymes in bacteria

C. Common Biochemical Tests

Some of the common biochemical tests used for the identification of bacteria are given below.

Experiment 27

(1) Indole Test[1]

Aim: **To perform indole test, to find out the ability of a bacteria to hydrolyse the amino acid tryptophan to indole.**

Principle

Some bacteria have the ability to hydrolyse the amino acid tryptophan to indole, as they can produce the enzyme 'tryptophanase'. Tryptophan is hydrolysed with the production of indole, pyruvic acid and ammonia. Indole is detected by the colour reagent, paradimethylaminobenzaldehyde (p-DMAB, *i.e.* Kovac's reagent), which produces a pink ring. Indole reacts with p-DMAB to produce the compound 'quinoidal red violet compound (rosindole dye)', which is pink in colour. The ring is produced at the surface, as the reagent is prepared in amyl alcohol.

In the indole test, the test bacteria is grown in a broth medium containing tryptophan. If the bacteria has the ability to hydrolyse tryptophan to indole, a pink ring is formed at the surface of the broth culture upon addition of p-DMAB.

Materials Required

Test tubes, conical flask, cotton plugs, inoculating loop, autoclave, bunsen burner, laminar flow chamber, dispose jar, incubator, tryptone broth (*See* Appendix I at page 247), Kovac's reagent (para-dimethylaminobenzaldehyde) (*See* Appendix II at page 251), isolated colonies or pure cultures of bacteria.

---

1 The four biochemical tests, namely 1) Indole test, 2) Methyl red test, 3) Voges-Proskauer test and 4) Citrate utilisation test, which are performed for the differentiation of the principal groups of bacteria belonging the family Enterobacteriaceae, are collectively called 'IMViC test'. The family Enterobacteriaceae includes the groups of bacteria that can be found in the intestinal tract of humans and lower mammals. They are short, gram-negative, non-spore-forming bacilli. This family includes the following groups.

1) 'Pathogens' such as members of the genera *Salmonella* and *Shigella*.

2) 'Occasional pathogens' such as members of the genera *Proteus* and *Klebsiella*.

3) 'Normal intestinal flora' such as members of the genera *Escherichia* and *Enterobacter*, which are saprophytic inhabitants of the intestinal tract.

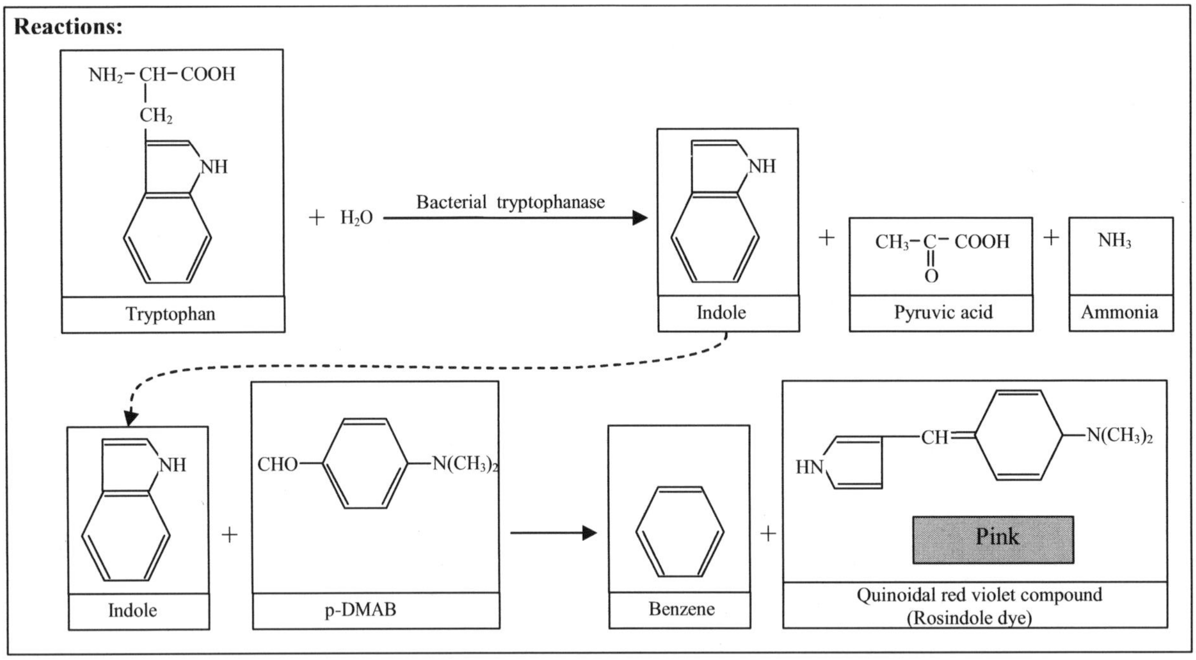

Procedure

1. The ingredients of tryptone broth medium (*See* Appendix I at page 247) or its ready-made powder required for 100 ml of the broth is weighed and dissolved in 100 ml of distilled water in a 250 ml conical flask by shaking and swirling. Tryptone acts as a source of tryptophan. Therefore, addition of tryptophan to the broth is optional (Figure 7.3).
2. Its pH is determined using a pH paper or pH meter and adjusted to 7.5 using 0.1N HCl if it is more or using 0.1N NaOH if it is less. The flask is heated, if required, to dissolve the ingredients completely.
3. The broth is distributed into five test tubes (approximately 5 ml each), cotton-plugged, covered with craft paper and tied with thread or rubber band.
4. The broth tubes are sterilised at 121°C (15 psi pressure) for 15 minutes in an autoclave.
5. The broth tubes are allowed to cool to room temperature.
6. The test bacteria is inoculated aseptically, preferably in a laminar flow chamber, into the broth with the help of an inoculating loop sterilised over bunsen flame. The loop is sterilised after each inoculation.
7. The inoculated broth tubes are incubated at 37°C for 48 hours in an incubator.
8. The colour reagent, para-dimethylaminobenzaldehyde (p-DMAB), (*i.e.* Kovac's reagent) (*See* Appendix II at page 251) is dropped into the broth tubes (0.5 ml each) and observed after 1 minute.

Alternatively

7. Paper strips soaked in oxalic acid are put at the mouth of the inoculated broth tubes, so that about half of the paper strips remain inside the tubes without touching the broth and the other half remain to outside. For this, filiter paper is cut into strips of approximately 35 mm long and 5 mm wide. The strips are soaked in hot saturated aqueous solution of oxalic acid and dried before use.
8. The inoculated broth tubes are incubated at 37°C for 48 hours in an incubator.

Observations

1. *Pink ring produced*: Indole positive (*i.e.* the bacteria can convert tryptophan to indole).
2. *Pink ring not produced*: Indole negative (*i.e.* the bacteria cannot convert tryptophan to indole).

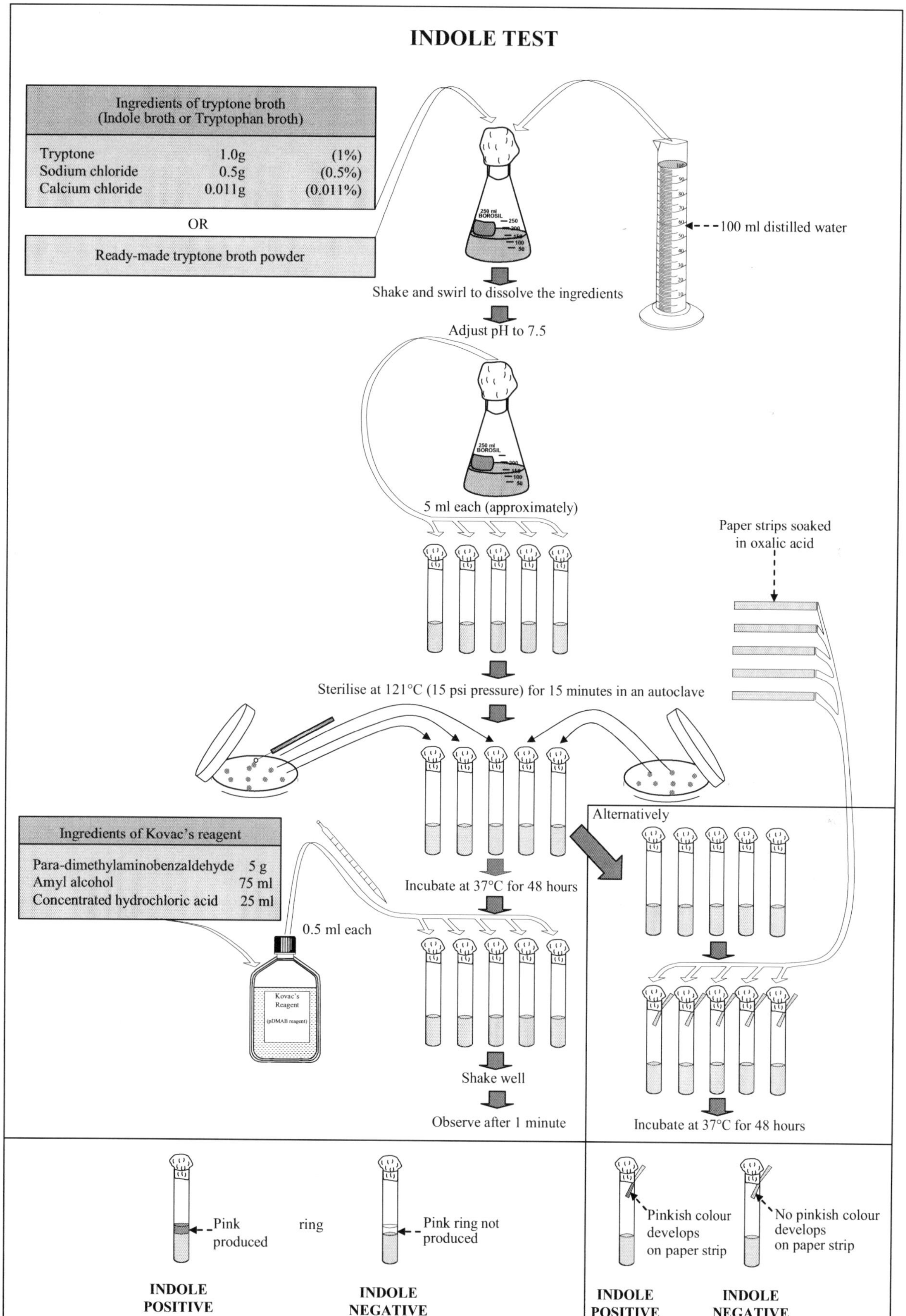

Figure 7.3: Indole test

Alternatively

1. *Pink colour produced on paper strip*: Indole positive (*i.e.* the bacteria can convert tryptophan to indole).
2. *Pink colour not produced on paper strip*: Indole negative (*i.e.* the bacteria cannot convert tryptophan to indole).

Experiment 28

(2) Methyl Red Test (MR Test)[2]

Aim: **To perform methyl red test (MR test), to find out the ability of a bacteria to utilise glucose with the production of a stable acid as the end product.**

Principle

Some bacteria have the ability to utilise glucose and convert it to a stable acid like lactic acid, acetic acid or formic acid as the end product. These bacteria initially metabolise glucose to pyruvic acid, which is further metabolised through the 'mixed acid pathway'[3] to produce the stable acid. The type of acid produced differs from species to species and depends on the specific enzymatic pathways present in the bacteria. The acid so produced decreases the pH to 4.5 or below, which is indicated by a change in the colour of methyl red from yellow to red.

In the methyl red test (MR test), the test bacteria is grown in a broth medium containing glucose. If the bacteria has the ability to utilise glucose with production of a stable acid, the colour of the methyl red changes from yellow to red, when added into the broth culture.

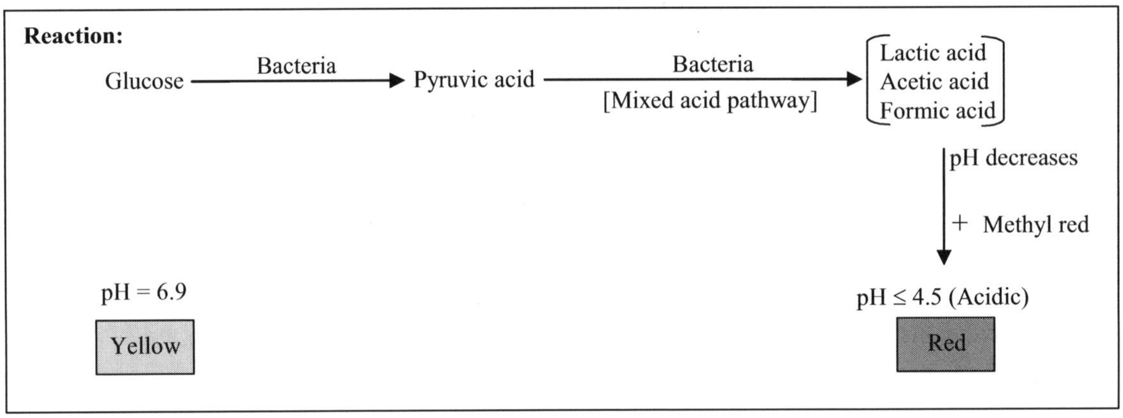

Materials Required

Test tubes, conical flask, cotton plugs, inoculating loop, autoclave, bunsen burner, laminar flow chamber, dispose jar, incubator, MR-VP broth (methyl red-Voges Proskauer broth or glucose phosphate broth) (*See* Appendix I at page 247), methyl red solution (*See* Appendix II at page 251), isolated colonies or pure cultures of bacteria.

Procedure

1. The ingredients of MR-VP broth[4] medium (*See* Appendix I at page 247) (containing glucose as the main component) or its ready-made powder required for 100 ml of the broth is weighed

---

2 Methyl red test is a part of the IMViC test performed for differentiation of the groups of bacteria belonging to the family Enterobacteriaceae (*See* page 133).

3 All the bacteria, which can utilise glucose, initially hydrolyse it to pyruvic acid. The subsequent metabolism of pyruvic acid can take place in either of the two pathways such as (1) 'Mixed acid pathway' to produce lactic acid, acetic acid or formic acid, as done by the methyl red positive bacteria (MR positive bacteria) or (2) 'Butylene glycol pathway' to produce the neutral end product, acetylmethylcarbinol (acetoin) as done by the Voges-Proskauer positive bacteria (VP positive bacteria).

4 As the same medium is used for methyl red test (MR test) as well as for Voges-Proskauer test (VP test), it is called MR-VP broth. When both the tests are performed simultaneously, it is called MR-VP test.

and dissolved in 100 ml of distilled water in a 250 ml conical flask by shaking and swirling. MR-VP broth is also called glucose phosphate broth (Figure 7.4).

2. Its pH is determined using a pH paper or pH meter and adjusted to 6.9 using 0.1N HCl if it is more or using 0.1N NaOH if it is less. The flask is heated, if required, to dissolve the ingredients completely.
3. The broth is distributed into five test tubes (approximately 10 ml each), cotton-plugged, covered with craft paper and tied with thread or rubber band.
4. The broth tubes are sterilised at 121°C (15 psi pressure) for 15 minutes in an autoclave.
5. The broth tubes are allowed to cool to room temperature.
6. The test bacteria is inoculated aseptically, preferably in a laminar flow chamber, into the broth with the help of an inoculating loop sterilised over bunsen flame. The loop is sterilised after each inoculation.
7. The inoculated broth tubes are incubated at 37°C for 24 to 48 hours in an incubator.
8. Alcoholic solution of methyl red (*See* Appendix II at page 251) (3-4 drops) is dropped into each test tube.

Observations

1. *Red colour produced*: MR positive (*i.e.* The bacteria has converted glucose to a stable acid, as indicated by conversion of methyl red from yellow to red colour. It indicates mixed acid fermentation).
2. *Red colour not produced*: MR negative (*i.e.* The glucose in the medium has not been converted to a stable acid. This indicates butylene glycol fermentation).

Experiment 29

(3) Voges-Proskauer Test (VP Test)[5]

Aim: **To perform Voges-Proskauer test (VP test), to find out the ability of a bacteria to utilise glucose with the production of acetylmethylcarbinol (acetoin) as the neutral end product.**

Principle

Some bacteria have the ability to utilise glucose and convert it to acetylmethylcarbinol (acetoin), which is a neutral end product. These bacteria initially metabolise glucose to pyruvic acid, which is further metabolised through the metabolic intermediate acetic acid to acetylmethylcarbinol (acetoin) and CO_2 via the 'butylene glycol pathway' (*See* page 136). Acetylmethylcarbinol is oxidised to diacetyl in presence of α-naphthol under alkaline condition (40 per cent KOH). Diacetyl reacts with the guanidine group of creatine (from peptone used in the culture medium) to produce rose pink colour.

In the Voges-Proskauer test (VP test), the test bacteria is grown in a broth medium containing glucose. If the bacteria has the ability to utilise glucose with production of acetylmethylcarbinol (acetoin) as the neutral end product, the broth acquires a rose pink colour upon addition of α-naphthol solution followed by 40% KOH.

Materials Required

Test tubes, conical flask, cotton plugs, inoculating loop, autoclave, bunsen burner, laminar flow chamber, dispose jar, incubator, MR-VP broth (or glucose phosphate broth) (*See* Appendix I at page 247), VP solution I (Barritt's reagent solution A) and VP solution II (Barritt's reagent solution B) (*See* Appendix II at page 251), isolated colonies or pure cultures of bacteria.

5 The Voges-Proskauer test is a part of the IMViC test performed for differentiation of the groups of bacteria belonging to the family Enterobacteriaceae (*See* page 133).

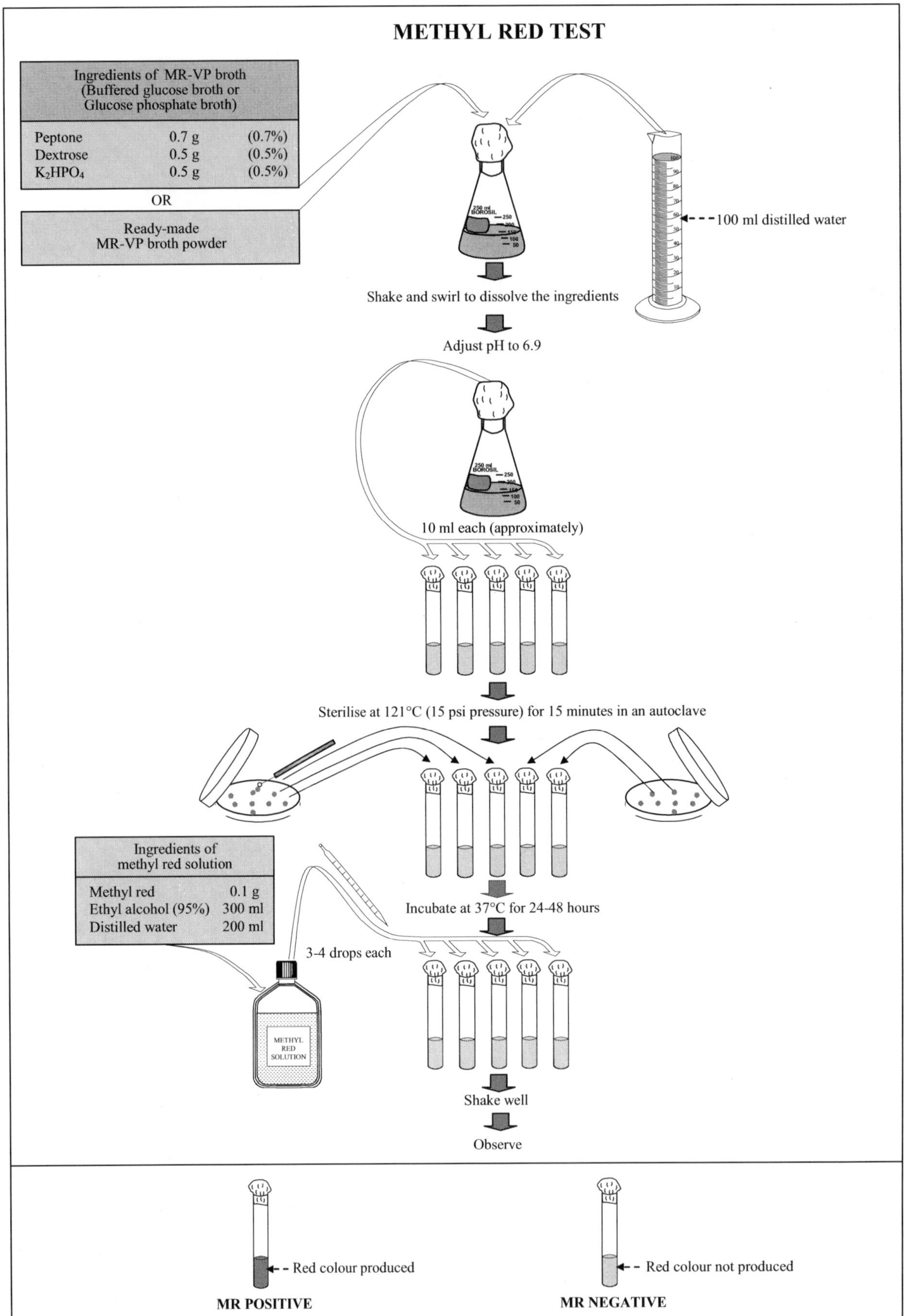

Figure 7.4: Methyl red test (MR test)

Reactions:

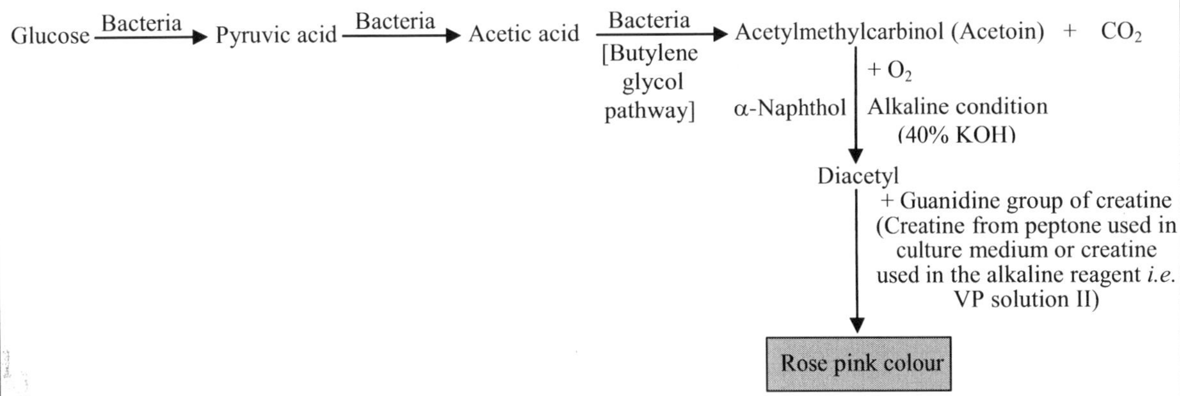

Procedure

1. The ingredients of MR-VP broth medium (*See* Appendix I at page 247) (containing glucose as the main component) or its ready-made powder required for 100 ml of the broth is weighed and dissolved in 100 ml of distilled water in a 250 ml conical flask by shaking and swirling (Figure 7.5). The broth used for methyl red test can also be used here. Usually the same broth is used for both the tests (MR and VP) at the same time.
2. Its pH is determined using a pH paper or pH meter and adjusted to 6.9 using 0.1N HCl if it is more or using 0.1N NaOH if it is less. The flask is heated, if required, to dissolve the ingredients completely.
3. The broth is distributed into five test tubes (approximately 10 ml each), cotton-plugged, covered with craft paper and tied with thread or rubber band.
4. The broth tubes are sterilised at 121°C (15 psi pressure) for 15 minutes in an autoclave.
5. The broth tubes are allowed to cool to room temperature.
6. The test bacteria is inoculated aseptically, preferably in a laminar flow chamber, into the broth with the help of an inoculating loop sterilised over bunsen flame. The loop is sterilised after each inoculation.
7. The inoculated broth tubes are incubated at 37°C for 48 to 72 hours in an incubator.
8. VP solution I (containing α-naphthol) (*See* Appendix II at page 251) is dropped into the broth tubes (0.2 ml each) and mixed thoroughly.
9. VP solution II (containing KOH) (*See* Appendix II at page 251) is dropped into the broth tubes (0.6 ml each), mixed thoroughly and allowed to stand for 30 minutes to 2 hours.

Observations

1. *Rose pink colour produced*: VP positive.
2. *Rose pink colour not produced*: VP negative.

Experiment 30

(4) Citrate Utilisation Test[6]

Aim: **To perform citrate utilisation test, to find out the ability of a bacteria to utilise citrate as the sole source of carbon.**

Principle

Some bacteria have the ability to grow in media without organic C and N. They can utilise sodium citrate as the sole source of C and ammonium dihydrogen phosphate ($NH_4H_2PO_4$) as the sole source of

6 The citrate utilisation test is a part of the IMViC test performed for differentiation of the groups of bacteria belonging to the family Enterobacteriaceae (*See* page 133).

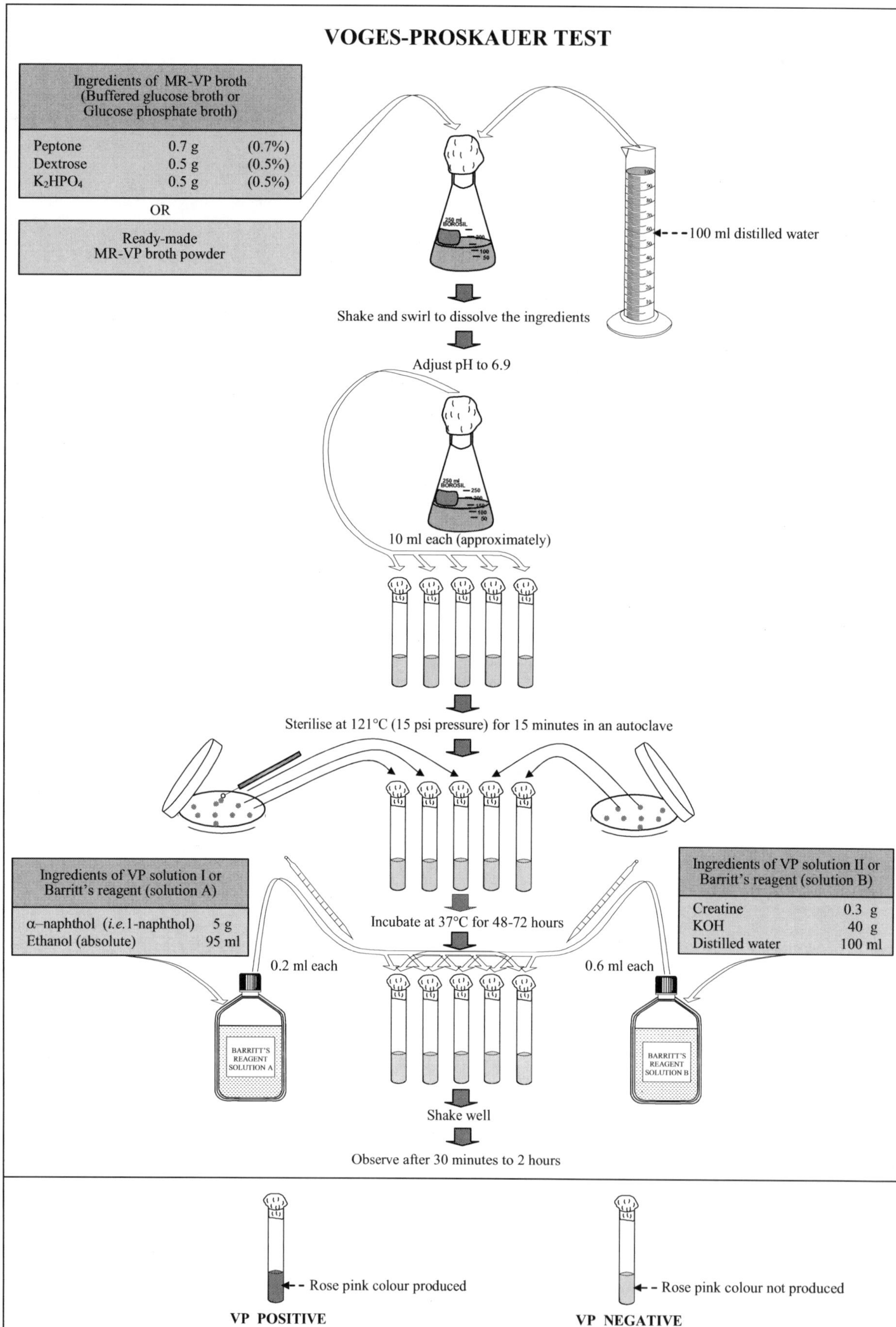

Figure 7.5: Voges-Proskauer test (VP test)

N. They utilise $NH_4H_2PO_4$ to get N with production of NH_3, which increases the pH resulting in a change in the colour of bromothymol blue from green (pH = 6.9) to blue (pH above 7.6).

In the citrate utilisation test, the test bacteria is grown on agar slants containing no organic C or N, rather containing sodium citrate, $NH_4H_2PO_4$ and bromothymol blue. If the bacteria has the ability to utilise citrate as the sole source of C, it shows growth on the slants. It also utilises $NH_4H_2PO_4$ as the sole source of N resulting in a change in the colour of the slants from green to blue.

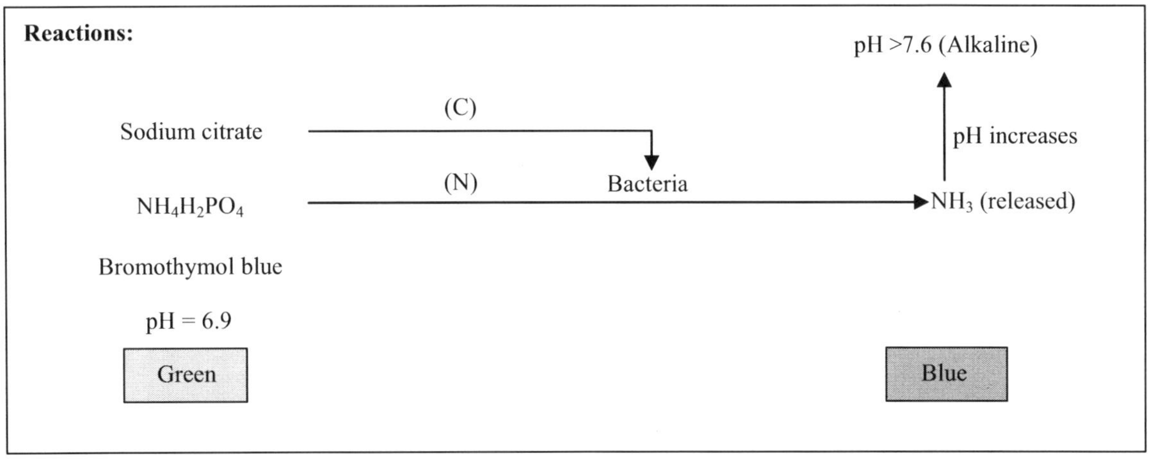

Materials Required

Test tubes, conical flask, cotton plugs, inoculating needle, autoclave, bunsen burner, laminar flow chamber, dispose jar, incubator, Simmons citrate agar (*See* Appendix I at page 247), isolated colonies or pure cultures of bacteria.

Procedure

1. The ingredients of Simmons citrate agar medium (*See* Appendix I at page 247) (containing sodium citrate, $NH_4H_2PO_4$ and bromothymol blue as the main ingredients) or its ready-made powder required for 100 ml of the medium is weighed and dissolved in 100 ml of distilled water in a 250 ml conical flask by shaking and swirling (Figure 7.6).
2. Its pH is determined using a pH paper or pH meter and adjusted to 6.9 using 0.1N HCl if it is more or using 0.1N NaOH if it is less.
3. The flask is heated to dissolve the agar in the medium completely.
4. Before it solidifies, the medium in warm molten condition, is distributed into 5 test tubes (approximately 20 ml each).
5. The test tubes are cotton-plugged, covered with craft paper and tied with thread or rubber band.
6. They are sterilised at 121°C (15 psi pressure) for 15 minutes in an autoclave.
7. After sterilisation, they are removed from the autoclave and kept in a slanting position to cool and solidify the medium, so as to get citrate agar slants.
8. The test bacteria is inoculated aseptically, preferably in a laminar flow chamber, into the slants by stabbing into the butt and streaking on the surface of the slants with the help of a flame-sterilised needle. The needle is sterilised after each inoculation.
9. The inoculated slants are incubated at 37°C for 24 to 48 hours in an incubator.

Observations

1. *Growth on slant and colour changes from green to blue*: Citrate utilisation positive.
2. *No growth and colour remains green*: Citrate utilisation negative.

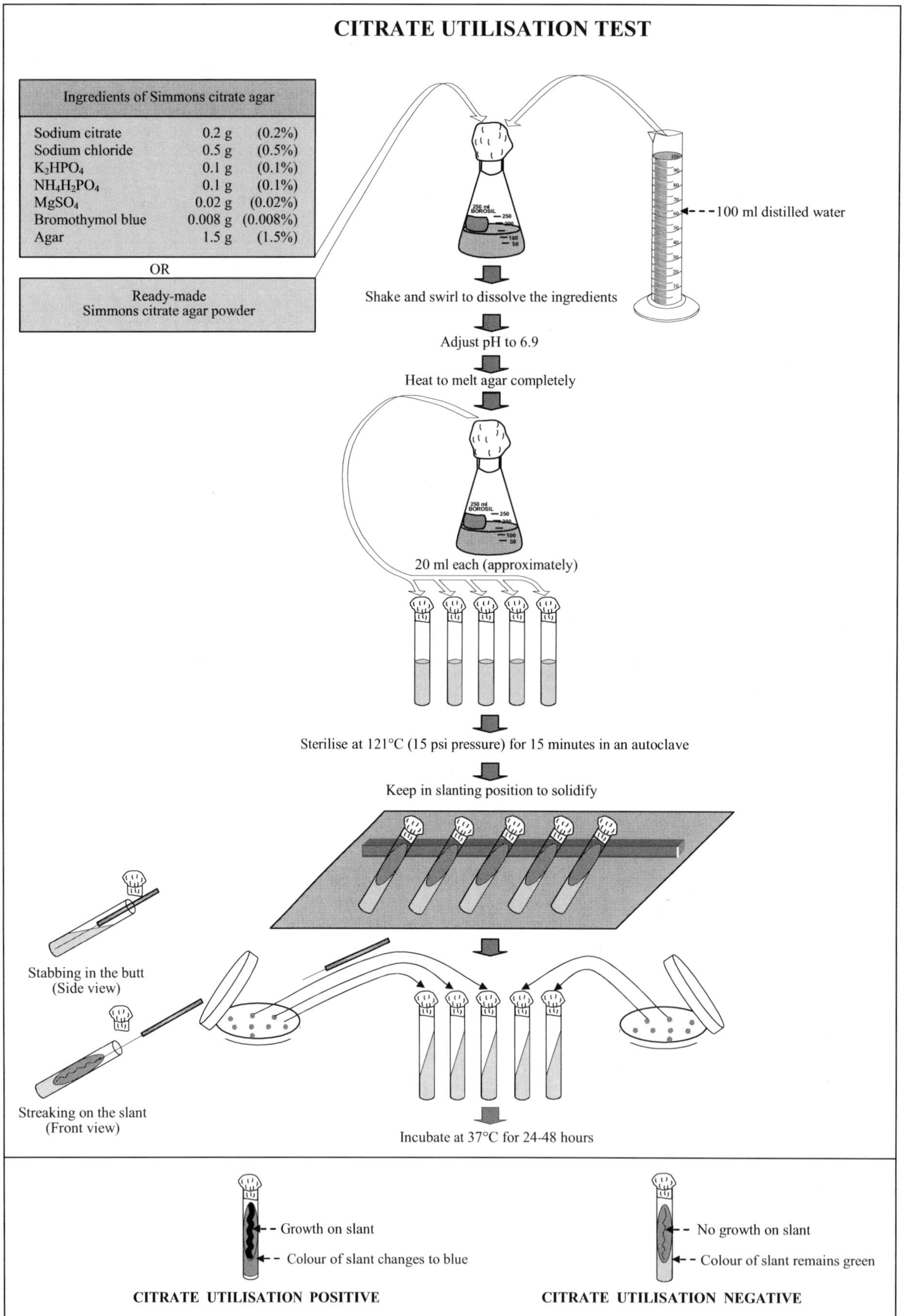

Figure 7.6: Citrate utilisation test

Experiment 31

(5) Triple Sugar Iron Test (TSI Test)

***Aim*: To perform triple sugar iron test (TSI test), to find out the ability of a bacteria to utilise any one or more of the three sugars, such as glucose, sucrose and lactose as well as its ability to produce hydrogen sulphide (H_2S), which reduces iron.**

Principle

Some bacteria have the ability to utilise one or more of the three sugars such as glucose, sucrose and lactose. If any one or more of the three sugars (triple sugars) are utilised, acid is produced, which reduces the pH changing the colour of phenol red from red to yellow. Moreover, some bacteria have the ability to produce hydrogen sulphide (H_2S) by utilising sulphur compounds. The H_2S so produced combines with the iron compound, ferrous sulphate, to form black precipitates of ferrous sulphide.

In the triple sugar iron test (TSI test), the test bacteria is grown on agar slants containing glucose, sucrose, lactose, phenol red, sodium thiosulphate and ferrous sulphate. While the medium contains glucose (*i.e.* D-glucose or dextrose) at a low concentration of 0.1%, the concentration of sucrose and lactose is kept high at 1%. If the bacteria has the ability to utilise any one or more of the three sugars, colour of the medium changes from red to yellow. If the bacteria has the ability to produce H_2S, the medium acquires a black colour. As three sugars and an iron compound are used in the medium, the test is called triple sugar iron test.

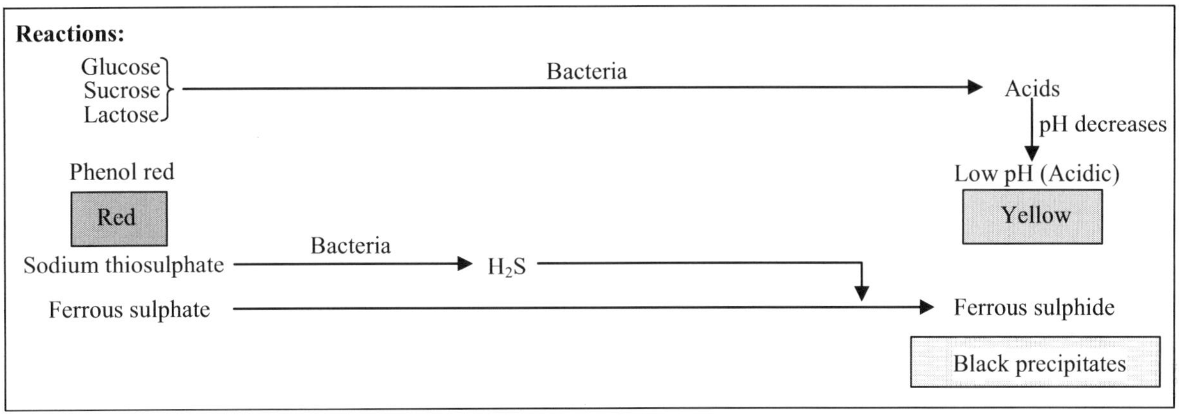

Materials Required

Test tubes, conical flask, cotton plugs, inoculating needle, autoclave, bunsen burner, laminar flow chamber, dispose jar, incubator, triple sugar iron (TSI) agar (*See* Appendix I at page 247), isolated colonies or pure cultures of bacteria.

Procedure

1. The ingredients of TSI agar medium (*See* Appendix I at page 247) (containing the 3 sugars and iron as the main components) or its ready-made powder required for 100 ml of the medium is weighed and dissolved in 100 ml of distilled water in a 250 ml conical flask by shaking and swirling (Figure 7.7).
2. Its pH is determined using a pH paper or pH meter and adjusted to 7.4 using 0.1N HCl if it is more or using 0.1N NaOH if it is less.
3. The flask is heated to dissolve the agar in the medium completely.
4. Before it solidifies, the medium in warm molten condition, is distributed into 5 test tubes (approximately 20 ml each).
5. The test tubes are cotton-plugged, covered with craft paper and tied with thread or rubber band.
6. They are sterilised at 121°C (15 psi pressure) for 15 minutes in an autoclave.

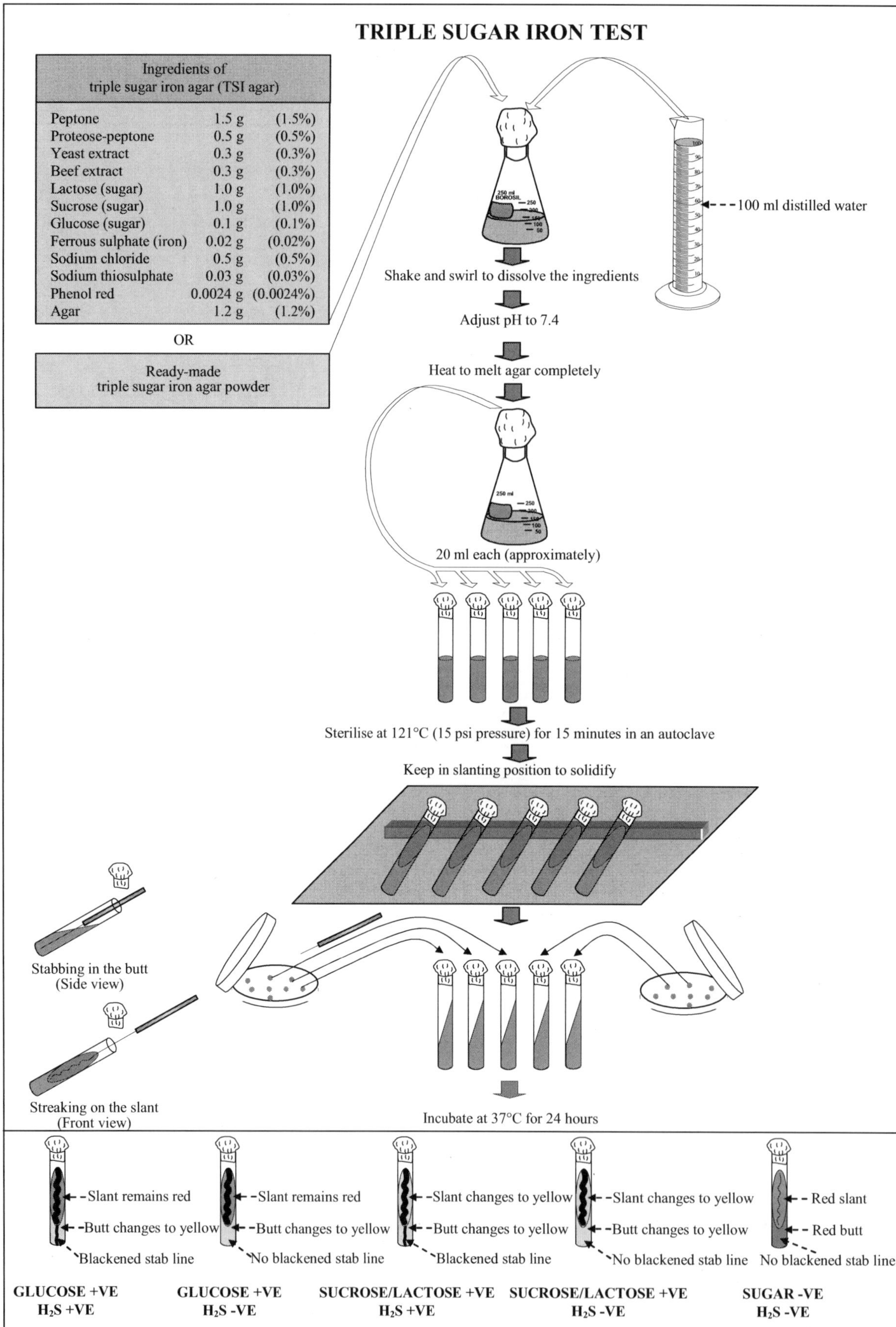

Figure 7.7: Triple sugar iron test (TSI test)

7. After sterilisation, they are removed from the autoclave and kept in a slanting position to cool and solidify the medium, so as to get TSI agar slants.
8. The test bacteria is inoculated aseptically, preferably in a laminar flow chamber, into the slants by stabbing into the butt and streaking on the surface of the slants with the help of a flame-sterilised needle. The needle is sterilised after each inoculation.
9. The inoculated slants are incubated at 37°C for 24 hours in an incubator.

Observations

1. *Yellow butt and red slant with or without gas production (breaks in the agar butt)*: Acid butt and alkaline slant has been formed. Here only glucose has been used anaerobically (fermentatively) making the butt acidic (yellow). No other sugar has been utilised. Since concentration of glucose is less (0.1%), the small amount of acid produced on the slant surface is oxidised rapidly making it alkaline (red). Further, oxidative deamination of peptone present in the medium produces NH_3, which makes the slant alkaline (red). However, in the butt, the acid condition is maintained due to reduced availability of oxygen and slower growth of the bacteria. Thus, the bacteria is glucose positive.
2. *Yellow butt and yellow slant with or without gas production*: Acid butt and acid slant has been formed. Here, lactose and/or sucrose have been fermented. Since their concentration in the medium is high, they produce large quantity of acids resulting in acidic slant and acidic butt and maintain the acidic condition. Thus, the bacteria is sucrose/lactose positive.
3. *Red butt and red slant*: None of the three sugars has been fermented. Instead, peptones have been catabolised under anaerobic and/or aerobic conditions, resulting in an alkaline condition due to production of ammonia. If only aerobic degradation of peptones occurs, only the slant surface becomes alkaline (red). If there is aerobic and anaerobic degradation of peptone, both the slant as well as the butt becomes alkaline (red). Thus, the bacteria is sugar negative.
4. *Blackening of the butt*: In addition to any one of the above conditions, if blackening of butt occurs, it indicates that, the bacteria is capable of producing H_2S utilising the inorganic sulphur (sodium thiosulphate) present in the medium. The H_2S combines with the ferrous sulphate in the medium to form black precipitates of ferrous sulphide resulting in a change in the colour of the medium to black. Thus, the bacteria is H_2S positive.
5. *No blackening of butt*: The bacteria is not capable of producing H_2S utilising the inorganic sulphur (sodium thiosulphate) present in the medium. Thus, the bacteria is H_2S negative.

Experiment 32

(6) Carbohydrate Fermentation Test

Aim: **To perform carbohydrate fermentation test, to find out the ability of a bacteria to ferment carbohydrates (sugars) with the production of an acid or acid and gas.**

Principle

Some bacteria have the ability to ferment carbohydrates, particularly sugars. Among them, each bacteria can ferment only some of the sugars, while it cannot ferment the others. Thus, the sugars, which a bacteria can ferment and the sugars, which it cannot is the characteristic of the bacteria. The carbohydrate fermentation test is performed to test, separately, the ability of a bacteria to ferment the sugars like glucose, sucrose, lactose, maltose and xylose as well as their alcoholic derivatives like aesculin, salicin, adonitol, dulcitol and sorbitol. If the bacteria can ferment a sugar or sugar derivative, acid is produced, which reduces the pH changing the colour of bromocresol purple from purple to yellow. Moreover, if it is an 'aerogenic bacteria', both acid and gas (CO_2) are produced, while if it is an 'anaerogenic bacteria', only acid is produced without any gas. Production of gas is indicated by its accumulation as a bubble in an inverted Durham tube (a miniature test tube).

In the carbohydrate fermentation test, the test bacteria is grown in a broth medium containing one of the sugars or sugar derivatives and bromocresol purple. An inverted Durham tube is kept submerged in it. If the bacteria has the ability to ferment the sugar or sugar derivative, the colour of the broth changes from purple to yellow. If gas accumulation is seen as a bubble in the Durham tube, it is an aerogenic bacteria, while if no gas accumulation is seen, it is an anaerogenic bacteria.

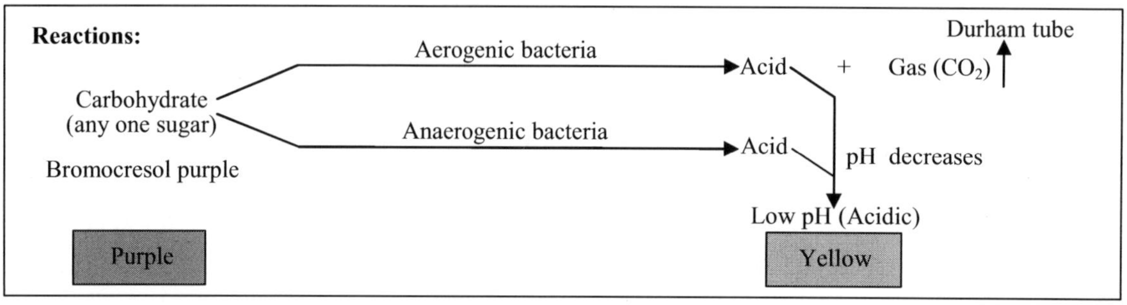

Materials Required

Test tubes, Durham tubes, conical flask, cotton plugs, inoculating loop, autoclave, bunsen burner, laminar flow chamber, dispose jar, incubator, carbohydrate broth (*See* Appendix I at page 247) (broth containing the specific sugar or sugar derivatives like glucose, sucrose, lactose, maltose, xylose, aesculin, salicin, adonitol, dulcitol, sorbitol etc.), isolated colonies or pure cultures of bacteria.

Procedure

1. The ingredients of carbohydrate broth medium (*See* Appendix I at page 247) (containing the required carbohydrate and bromocresol purple as the main components) or its ready-made powder required for 100 ml of the broth is weighed and dissolved in 100 ml of distilled water in a 250 ml conical flask by shaking and swirling (Figure 7.8).
2. Its pH is determined using a pH paper or pH meter and adjusted to 6.8 using 0.1N HCl if it is more or using 0.1N NaOH if it is less. The flask is heated, if required, to dissolve the ingredients completely.
3. The broth is distributed into five test tubes (approximately 10 ml each).
4. One Durham tube is put in inverted condition into the broth in each test tube. The Durham tubes contain air in them and float. During sterilisation, hot steam displaces this air, due to which they immerse in the broth. Thus, there is no need to remove air from within the Durham tubes by filling them with the broth before sterilisation to keep them immersed in the broth.
5. The test tubes are cotton-plugged, covered with craft paper and tied with thread or rubber band.
6. The broth tubes are sterilised at 121°C (15 psi pressure) for 15 minutes in an autoclave. Alternatively, 90 ml of the basal medium (medium without the carbohydrate) is sterilised in the autoclave and to this, after cooling, 10 ml of the carbohydrate solution (10%) sterilised by membrane filtration is added. This is particularly essential for heat-sensitive carbohydrates, which undergo degradation during heat sterilisation.
7. The broth tubes are allowed to cool to room temperature.
8. The test bacteria is inoculated aseptically, preferably in a laminar flow chamber, into the broth with the help of an inoculating loop sterilised over bunsen flame. The loop is sterilised after each inoculation.
9. The inoculated broth tubes are incubated at 37°C for 24 hours in an incubator.

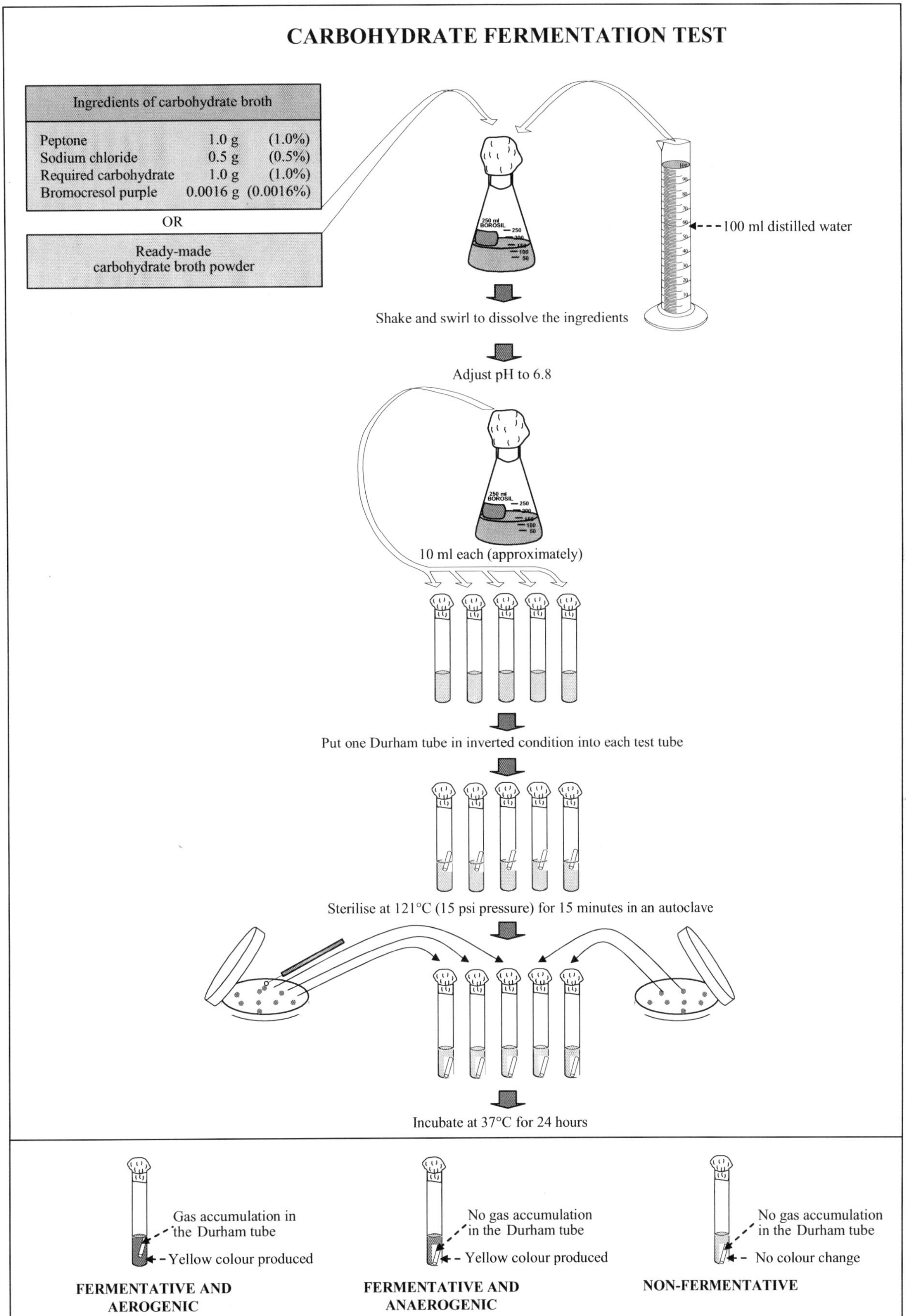

Figure 7.8: Carbohydrate fermentation test

Observations

1. *Colour of broth changes to yellow and gas accumulates in Durham tube*: Fermentative for the carbohydrate and aerogenic.
2. *Colour of broth changes to yellow, but no gas accumulates in Durham tube*: Fermentative for the carbohydrate and anaerogenic.
3. *Colour of broth does not change*: Non-fermentative for the carbohydrate.

Experiment 33

(7) Oxidation-Fermentation Test (O/F Test)

***Aim*: To perform oxidation-fermentation test (O/F test), to find out the ability of a bacteria to utilise glucose aerobically (oxidatively) or anaerobically (fermentatively).**

Principle

Some bacteria have the ability to utilise glucose. Some of them utilise it only in presence of oxygen (oxidatively or aerobically), while the others, besides utilising aerobically, can also utilise it in absence of oxygen (fermentatively or anaerobically). Thus, a bacteria, able to ferment glucose must be able to oxidise it, but a bacteria able to oxidise glucose may not ferment it. If glucose is utilised in either way, acid is produced, which reduces the pH changing the colour of bromocresol purple from purple to yellow.

In the oxidation-fermentation test (O/F Test), the test bacteria is grown aerobically and anaerobically separately, in semisolid agar tubes containing glucose and bromocresol purple. If the bacteria has the ability to utilise glucose, the colour of the medium changes from purple to yellow. If it utilises glucose aerobically, it is oxidative and if it utilises glucose anaerobically, it is fermentative.

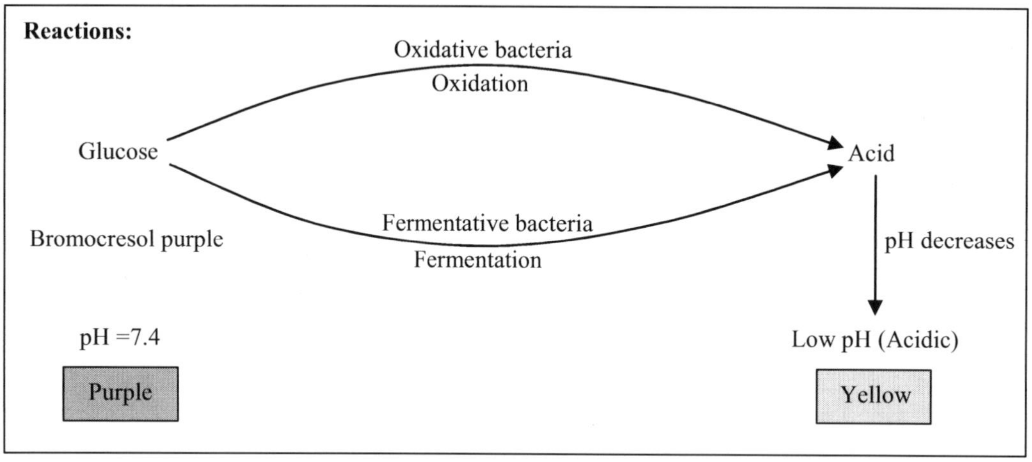

Materials Required

Test tubes, conical flask, cotton plugs, inoculating loop, autoclave, bunsen burner, laminar flow chamber, dispose jar, incubator, Hugh-Leifson glucose broth (*See* Appendix I at page 247), liquid paraffin, isolated colonies or pure cultures of bacteria.

Procedure

1. The ingredients of Hugh-Leifson glucose broth medium (HLGB) (*See* Appendix I at page 247) (containing glucose and bromocresol purple as the main components) or its ready-made powder required for 100 ml of the broth is weighed and dissolved in 100 ml of distilled water in a 250 ml conical flask by shaking and swirling (Figure 7.9).

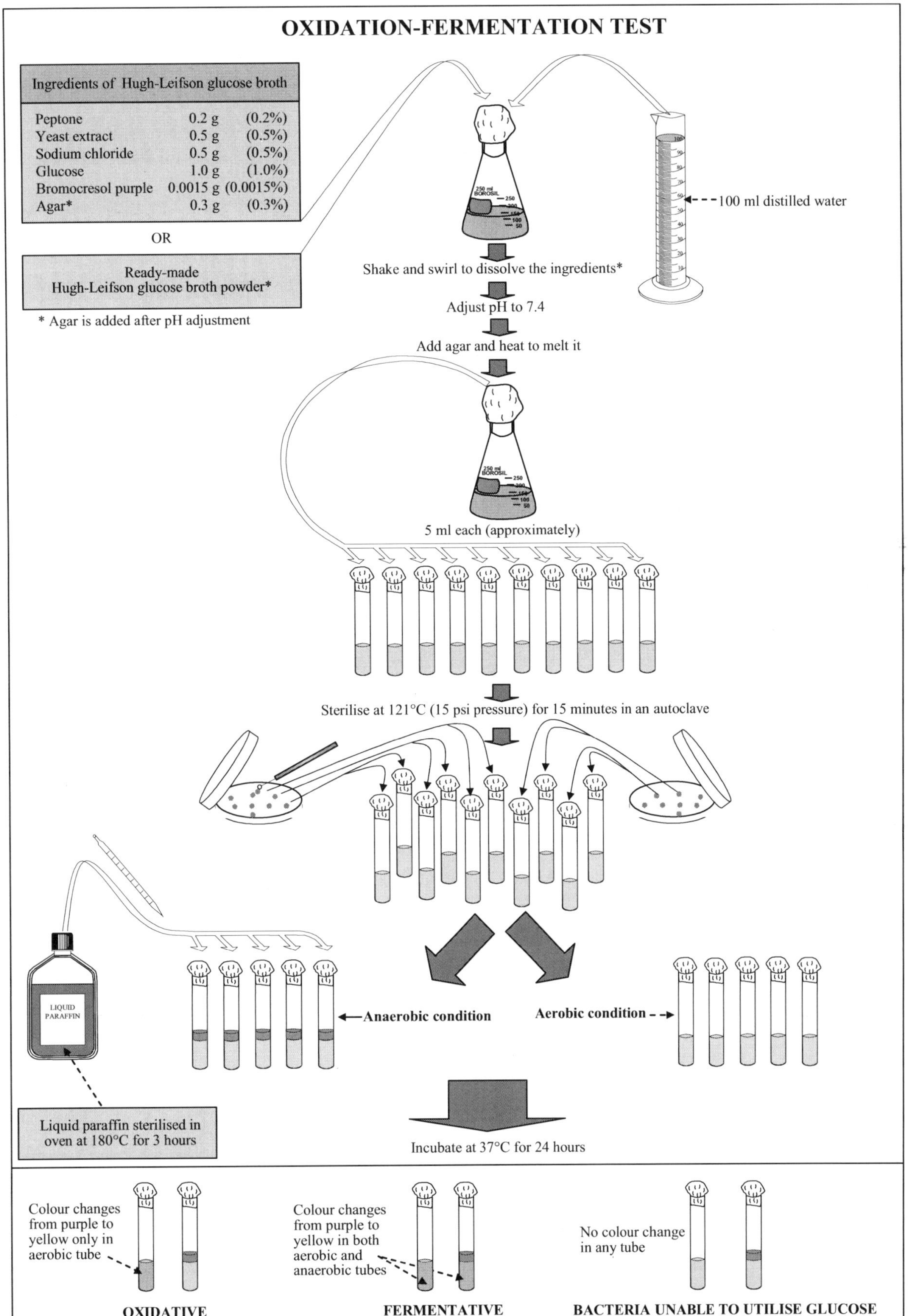

Figure 7.9: Oxidation-fermentation test (O/F test)

2. Its pH is determined using a pH paper or pH meter and adjusted to 7.4 using 0.1N HCl if it is more or using 0.1N NaOH if it is less.
3. After adjusting pH, agar is added. Less agar is used here to get a semisolid medium, so as to facilitate stab.
4. The flask is heated to dissolve the agar in the medium completely.
5. Before it solidifies, the medium in warm molten condition, is distributed into two sets of test tubes (approximately 5 ml each); each set having five test tubes.
6. The test tubes are cotton-plugged, covered with craft paper and tied with thread or rubber band.
7. The broth tubes are sterilised at 121°C (15 psi pressure) for 15 minutes in an autoclave.
8. The broth tubes are allowed to cool to room temperature.
9. Liquid paraffin is sterilised by heating at 180°C for 3 hours in a hot air oven.
10. The test bacteria is inoculated aseptically, preferably in a laminar flow chamber, into all the sterilised semisolid broth tubes by stabbing with the help of a flame-sterilised inoculating loop. The loop is sterilised after each inoculation.
11. The sterilised liquid paraffin is gently poured aseptically into one set of inoculated tubes, (about 1 cm high on the medium) to provide anaerobic condition.
12. All the inoculated broth tubes are incubated at 37°C for 24 hours in an incubator.

Observations

1. *Colour changes from purple to yellow in both tubes*: Fermentative.
2. *Colour changes only in tubes without paraffin*: Oxidative.
3. *No colour change in any tube*: Bacteria cannot utilise glucose.

Experiment 34

(8) Nitrate Reduction Test

***Aim* : To perform nitrate reduction test, to find out the ability of a bacteria to reduce nitrates.**

Principle

Some bacteria have the ability to reduce nitrates, as they can produce the enzyme 'nitrate reductase'. This enzyme, in presence of suitable electron donor, reduces nitrates (NO_3^-) to nitrites (NO_2^-). The presence of NO_2^- is indicated by sulphanilic acid and α-naphthylamine, which change the colour to red.

In the nitrate reduction test, the test bacteria is grown in a broth medium containing nitrate (NO_3^-). If the bacteria has the ability to reduce nitrates, the broth acquires a red colour upon addition of sulphanilic acid and α-naphthylamine. If red colour is not produced, it indicates that either NO_3^- is not reduced by the bacteria at all or the bacteria produces highly potent nitrate reductase enzyme, which rapidly reduces NO_3^- beyond NO_2^- to NH_3 and N_2. To confirm this, a small amount of zinc dust is added, which reduces NO_3^-, if available in the medium, to NO_2^-, thereby producing red colour. Thus, if red colour is produced, it indicates that NO_3^- is present in the medium unchanged and the bacteria does not have the ability to reduce nitrates. If red colour is not produced, it indicates that, the NO_3^- has been reduced beyond NO_2^- to NH_3 and N_2 and the bacteria has the ability to reduce nitrates.

Reactions:

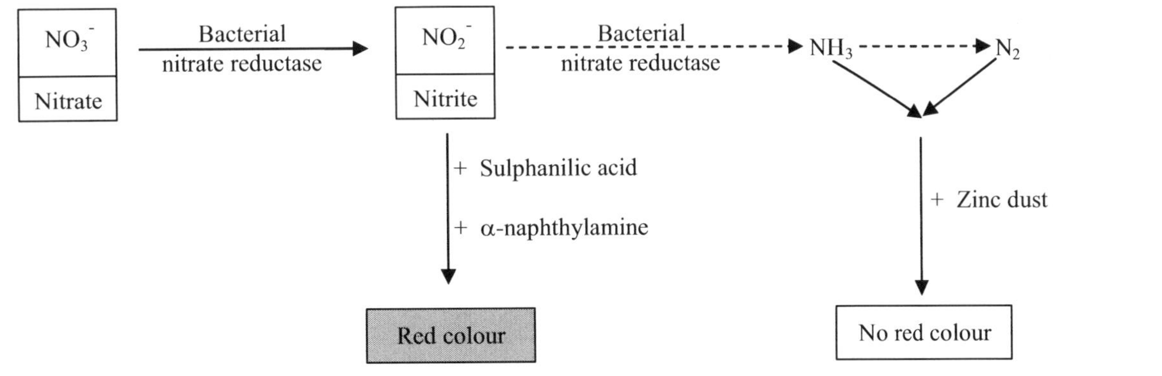

Materials Required

Test tubes, conical flask, cotton plugs, inoculating loop, autoclave, bunsen burner, laminar flow chamber, dispose jar, incubator, nitrate broth (*See* Appendix I at page 247), zinc dust, nitrate reagent Solution A, nitrate reagent Solution B (*See* Appendix II at page 251), isolated colonies or pure cultures of bacteria.

Procedure

1. The ingredients of nitrate broth medium (*See* Appendix I at page 247) (containing nitrate as the main component) or its ready-made powder required for 100 ml of the broth is weighed and dissolved in 100 ml of distilled water in a 250 ml conical flask by shaking and swirling (Figure 7.10).
2. Its pH is determined using a pH paper or pH meter and adjusted to 7.2 using 0.1N HCl if it is more or using 0.1N NaOH if it is less. The flask is heated, if required, to dissolve the ingredients completely.
3. The broth is distributed into five test tubes (approximately 10 ml each), cotton-plugged, covered with craft paper and tied with thread or rubber band.
4. The broth tubes are sterilised at 121°C (15 psi pressure) for 15 minutes in an autoclave.
5. The broth tubes are allowed to cool to room temperature.
6. The test bacteria is inoculated aseptically, preferably in a laminar flow chamber, into the broth with the help of an inoculating loop sterilised over bunsen flame. The loop is sterilised after each inoculation.
7. The inoculated broth tubes are incubated at 37°C for 48 hours in an incubator.
8. 0.5 ml each of the nitrate reagent Solution A (containing sulphanilic acid) and nitrate reagent Solution B (containing α-naphthylamine) (*See* Appendix II at page 251) are added into each test tube, shaken well and colour change is observed after 15 minutes.

Observations

1. *Red colour produced*: Nitrate reduction positive.
2. *Red colour not produced*: Zinc dust is added.
   (*a*) *Red colour produced*: Nitrate reduction negative.
   (*b*) *Red colour not produced*: Nitrate reduction positive.

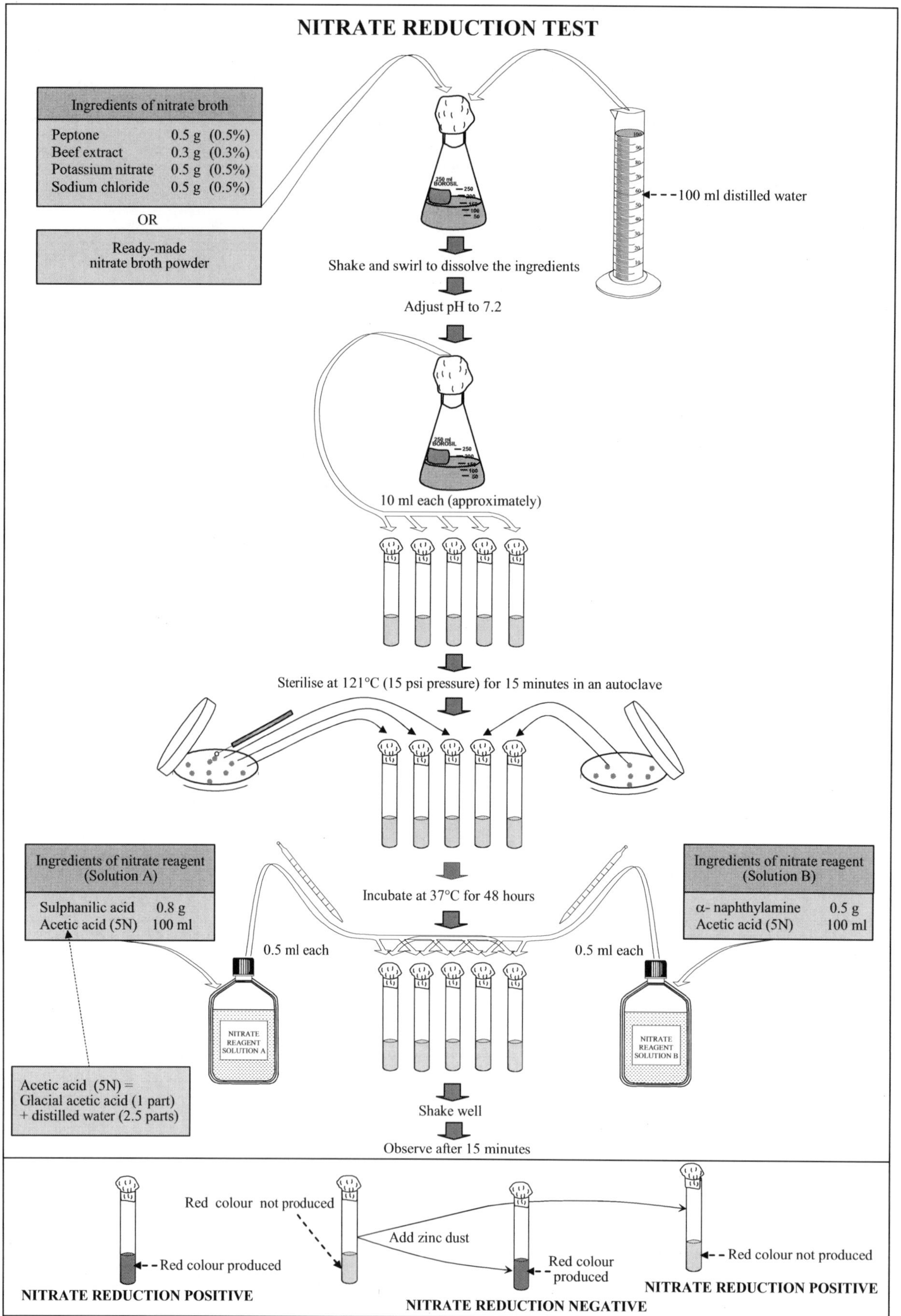

Figure 7.10: Nitrate reduction test

Experiment 35

(9) Amino Acid Decarboxylase Test

***Aim*: To perform amino acid decarboxylase test, to find out the ability of a bacteria to decarboxylate different amino acids by producing respective amino acid decarboxylase enzymes.**

Principle

Some bacteria have the ability to decarboxylate[7] different amino acids to corresponding amines and CO_2 as they can produce respective 'amino acid decarboxylase' enzymes. Among them, each bacteria can decarboxylate only some of the amino acids, while it cannot decarboxylate the others. Thus, the amino acids, which a bacteria can decarboxylate and the amino acids, which it cannot is the characteristic of the bacteria. The amino acid decarboxylase test is performed to test, separately, the ability of a bacteria to decarboxylate amino acids like lysine, ornithine and arginine with production of CO_2 and respective amines like cadaverine, putrescine and agmatine. If the bacteria can decarboxylate any one or more of the amino acids, respective amines are produced, which are alkaline (basic) and therefore, increase the pH changing the colour of bromocresol purple from yellow to purple.

In the amino acid decarboxylase test, the test bacteria is grown anaerobically in a broth medium containing glucose, bromocresol purple and one of the amino acids. The colour of the broth initially changes from purple to yellow due to the fall in pH resulting from the acids produced by fermentation of glucose. If the bacteria has the ability to decarboxylate the amino acid, the colour of the broth changes from yellow back to purple.

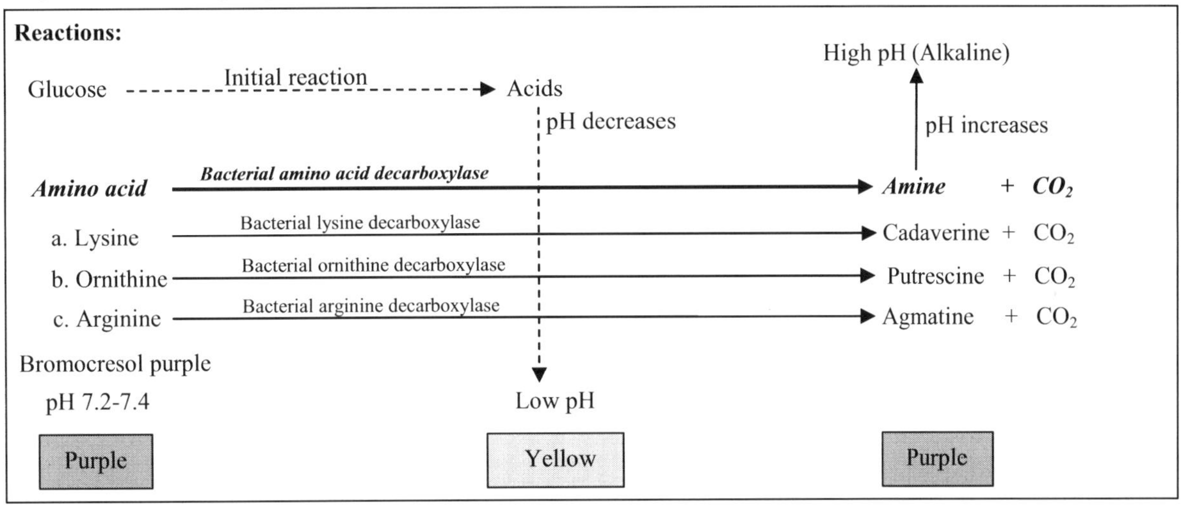

Materials Required

Test tubes, conical flask, cotton plugs, inoculating loop, autoclave, bunsen burner, laminar flow chamber, dispose jar, incubator, amino acid decarboxylase broth (*See* Appendix I at page 247), amino acids (lysine, ornithine, arginine), liquid paraffin, isolated colonies or pure cultures of bacteria.

Procedure

1. The ingredients of amino acid decarboxylase broth medium (*See* Appendix I at page 247) (containing glucose and bromocresol purple as the main components) or its ready-made powder required for 400 ml of the broth is weighed and dissolved in 400 ml of distilled water in a 500 ml conical flask by shaking and swirling (Figure 7.11).

---

7 Each amino acid has two essential components such as (1) A carboxylic group (-COOH) and (2) An amino group ($-NH_2$). The removal of these essential groups is of two types as follows.

(1) Decarboxylation: Removal of the carboxylic group (-COOH) with production of CO_2.

(2) Deamination: Removal of the amino group ($-NH_2$) with production of NH_3.

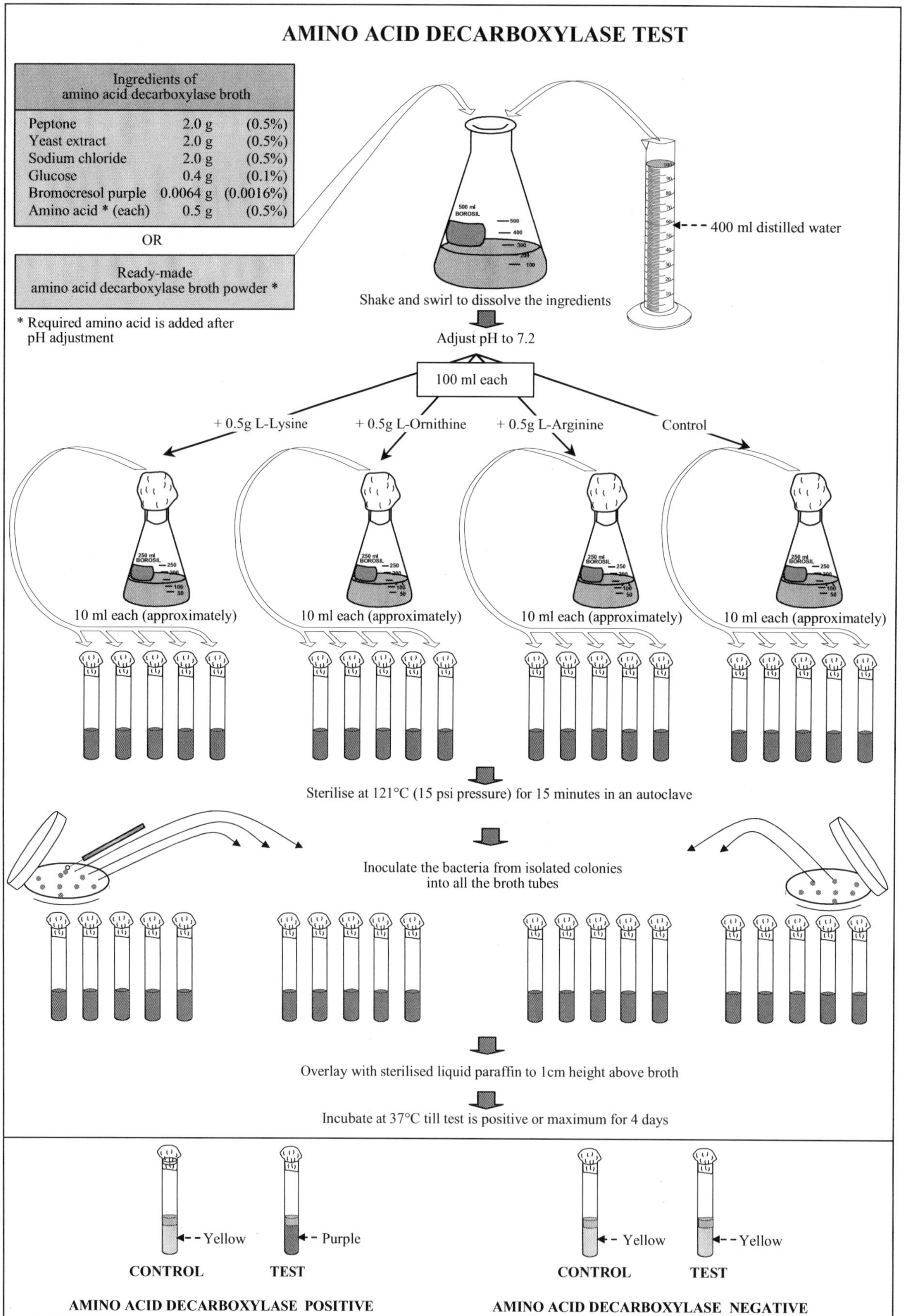

Figure 7.11: Amino acid decarboxylase test

2. Its pH is determined using a pH paper or pH meter and adjusted to 7.2 using 0.1N HCl if it is more or using 0.1N NaOH if it is less. The flask is heated, if required, to dissolve the ingredients completely.
3. The 400 ml broth is distributed into four 250 ml conical flasks, so that each flask contains 100 ml of the broth.
4. To three of these flasks, three amino acids, such as, lysine, ornithine and arginine are added separately (0.5 gram each) and one is kept without any amino acid to serve as control. The control is used for distinguishing between the two-step colour changes in the test medium (*i.e.* from purple to yellow and from yellow back to purple).
5. The broths in the four conical flasks are distributed into four separate sets of test tubes (approximately 10 ml each), cotton-plugged, covered with craft paper and tied with thread or rubber band.
6. The broth tubes are sterilised at 121°C (15 psi pressure) for 15 minutes in an autoclave.
7. The broth tubes are allowed to cool to room temperature.
8. Liquid paraffin is sterilised by heating at 180°C for 3 hours in a hot air oven.
9. The test bacteria is inoculated aseptically, preferably in a laminar flow chamber, into the broth with the help of an inoculating loop sterilised over bunsen flame. The loop is sterilised after each inoculation.
10. The sterilised liquid paraffin is gently poured aseptically into the inoculated tubes, (about 1 cm high on the medium) to provide anaerobic condition.
11. The inoculated broth tubes are incubated at 37°C in an incubator and observed daily till the test is positive or for a maximum period of 4 days.

Observations

Amino Acids	Observation		Result
	Test	*Control*	
Lysine	Purple → Yellow → Purple Purple → Yellow	Purple → Yellow Purple → Yellow	Lysine positive Lysine negative
Ornithine	Purple → Yellow → Purple Purple → Yellow	Purple → Yellow Purple → Yellow	Ornithine positive Ornithine negative
Arginine	Purple → Yellow → Purple Purple → Yellow	Purple → Yellow Purple → Yellow	Arginine positive Arginine negative
Control	Purple → Yellow Purple		Experiment is correct Experiment is wrong

Experiment 36

(10) Litmus Milk Test

***Aim*: To perform litmus milk test, to find out the ability of a bacteria to transform different milk components into varied end products.**

Principle

Some bacteria have the ability to grow in milk and transform different milk components into varied end products. Milk is a complex mixture of several components. The major components capable of transformation by bacteria are the milk sugar lactose and the milk proteins casein, lactoalbumin and lactoglobulin. Different bacteria have different enzyme systems, due to which they act on different components and transform them into varied metabolic end products, which are characteristics of the bacteria. The litmus milk test is performed to find out the ability of a bacteria to transform different milk components, which is manifested as change in colour of litmus, production of gas, curd formation etc. Litmus is a pH indicator and oxidation-reduction indicator, which changes colour depending on the condition of the broth.

In the litmus milk test, the test bacteria is grown in a broth medium containing milk and litmus. If the bacteria has the ability to transform different milk components into varied end products, it grows in the broth and transforms the components in different ways depending on its enzyme systems. The six most important transformations, which can be observed in the litmus milk as a result of bacterial activities, are as follows.

(*i*) Lactose fermentation
(*ii*) Gas formation
(*iii*) Litmus reduction
(*iv*) Curd formation
(*v*) Proteolysis (Peptonisation)
(*vi*) Alkaline reaction

(i) Lactose Fermentation

Bacteria capable of using lactose as a carbon source for energy production utilise the inducible enzyme β-galactosidase and degrade lactose to glucose and galactose. Glucose is further degraded through the Embden-Meyerhof pathway to pyruvic acid, which in turn is converted to lactic acid. Accumulation of lactic acid reduces the pH of the medium to about 4.0, due to which the colour of litmus changes from purple at a neutral pH to pink at the acidic pH.

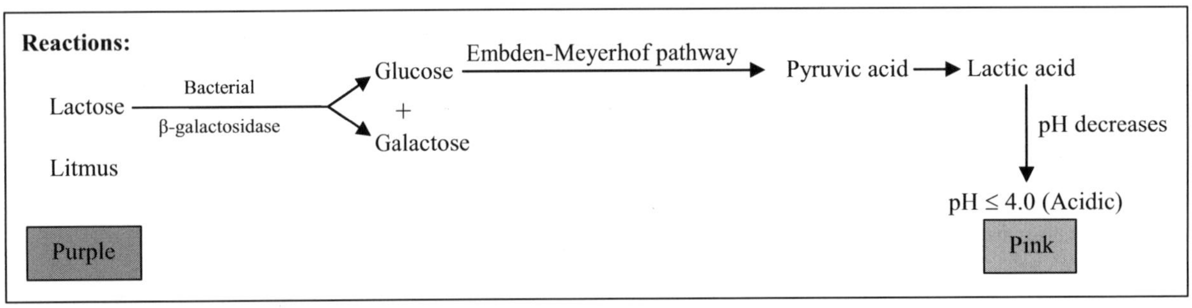

(ii) Gas Formation

The end products of the bacterial fermentation of lactose may include gases like carbon dioxide and hydrogen. The presence of these gases may be seen as separations of the curd or by the development of tracks or fissures within the curd, as the gases rise to the surface.

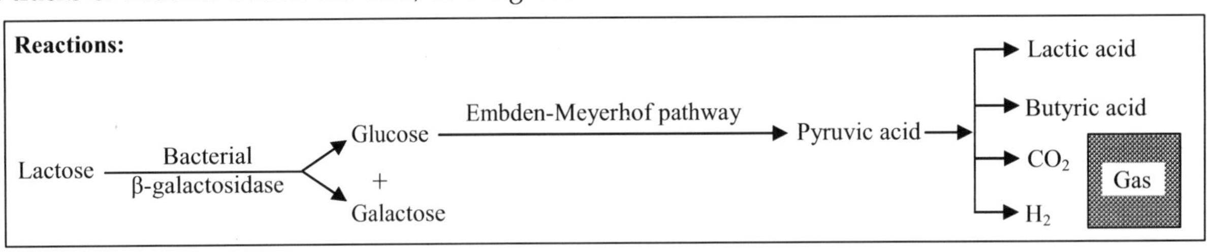

(iii) Litmus Reduction

Fermentation is an anaerobic process involving oxidation that occurs in the absence of molecular oxygen. Oxidation can occur either by addition of oxygen or removal of hydrogen ion. Lactose fermentation, being an anaerobic process, involves the removal of hydrogen ion from it. Since hydrogen ion cannot exist in the free state, there must be an acceptor of hydrogen ion. In the litmus milk test, litmus acts as the acceptor of the hydrogen ion. Litmus is purple in the oxidised state, but when it accepts hydrogen, it becomes reduced and turns white or milk-coloured.

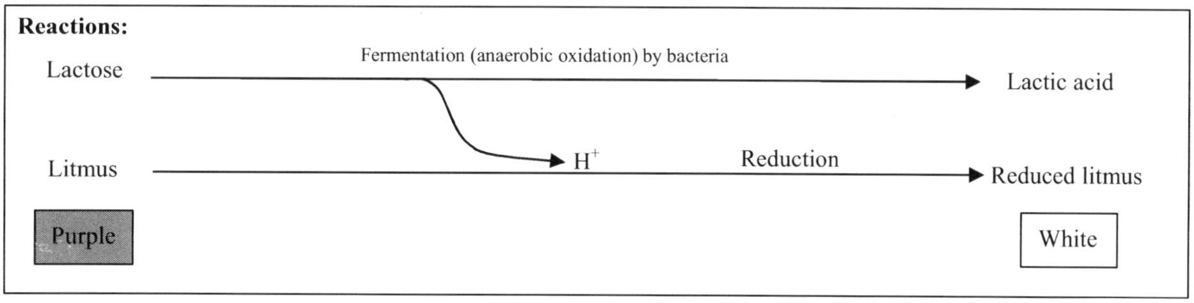

(iv) Curd Formation

The biochemical activities of different bacteria grown in litmus milk may result in the production of two distinct types of curds (clots). Curd is designated either as 'acid curd' or as 'rennet curd' depending on the biochemical mechanism responsible for its formation. In case of acid curd, lactic acid or other organic acids, in presence of calcium ions, cause precipitation of the milk protein, casein as calcium caseinate to form an insoluble clot. The clot is hard and does not retract from the wall of the test tube. An acid curd is easily identified if the test tube is inverted and the clot remains immobile. In case of rennet curd, some bacteria produce rennin, an enzyme that acts on casein to form paracasein, which, in presence of calcium ions, is precipitated as calcium paracaseinate and forms an insoluble clot. Unlike the acid curd, this is a soft semisolid clot that flows slowly, when the test tube is tilted.

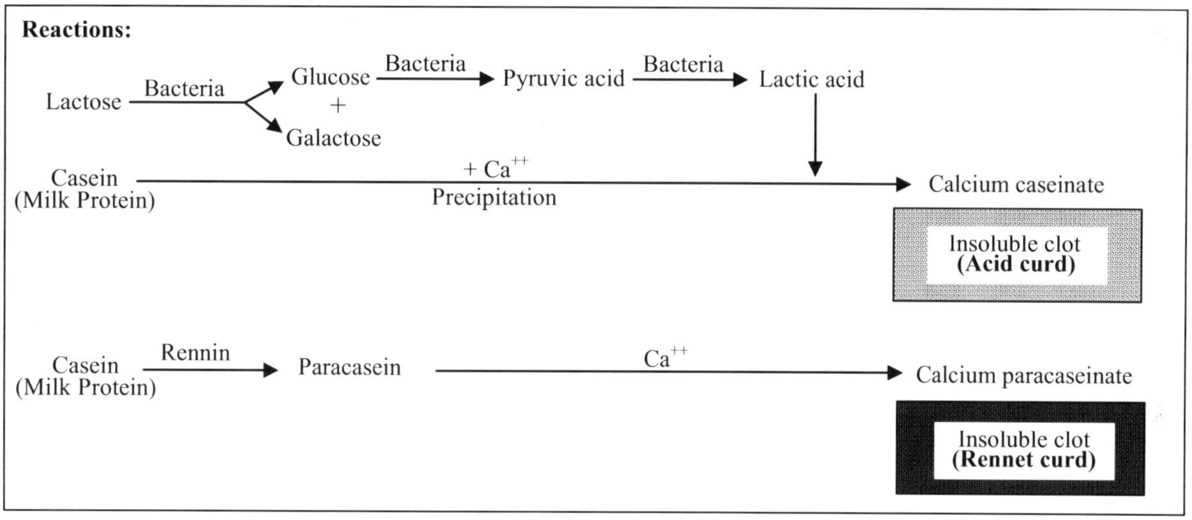

(v) Proteolysis (Peptonisation)

Some bacteria, which do not have the ability to obtain energy by lactose fermentation, use other nutritional sources such as proteins for this purpose. By means of proteolytic enzymes, these bacteria hydrolyse the milk proteins, primarily casein, to their basic building blocks, namely amino acids. The litmus turns deep purple in the upper portion of the tube, while the medium begins to lose body and produces translucent, brown, whey-like appearance, as the proteins are hydrolysed to amino acids.

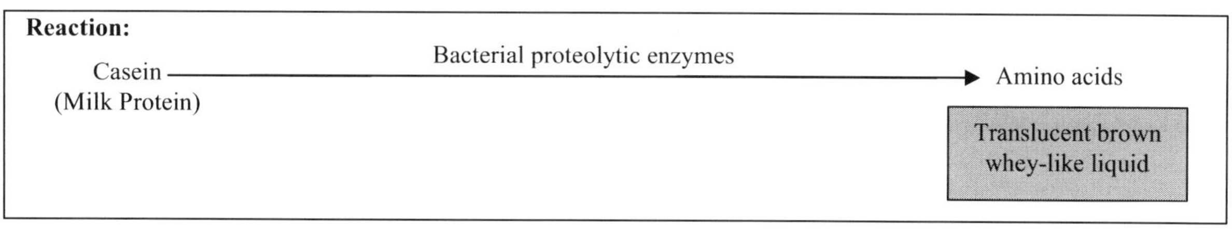

(vi) Alkaline Reaction

An alkaline reaction is evident, when the colour of the medium remains unchanged or changes to deep blue. This reaction is indicative of the partial degradation of casein by bacteria into shorter polypeptide chains, with the simultaneous release of alkaline end products that are responsible for the observable colour change.

Reaction:

Casein (Milk Protein) —Bacteria→ Shorter polypeptides + Alkaline end products

Deep blue (or remains unchanged)

Materials Required

Test tubes, conical flask, cotton plugs, inoculating loop, autoclave, bunsen burner, laminar flow chamber, dispose jar, incubator, litmus milk broth (*See* Appendix I at page 247), isolated colonies or pure cultures of bacteria.

Procedure

1. The ingredients of litmus milk broth medium (*See* Appendix I at page 247) or its ready-made powder required for 100 ml of the broth is weighed and dissolved in 100 ml of distilled water in a 250 ml conical flask by shaking and swirling (Figure 7.12).
2. Its pH is determined using a pH paper or pH meter and adjusted to 6.8 using 0.1N HCl if it is more or using 0.1N NaOH if it is less. The flask is heated, if required, to dissolve the ingredients completely.
3. The broth is distributed into five test tubes (approximately 10 ml each), cotton-plugged, covered with craft paper and tied with thread or rubber band.
4. The broth tubes are sterilised at 121°C for 15 minutes in an autoclave.
5. The broth tubes are allowed to cool to room temperature.
6. The test bacteria is inoculated aseptically, preferably in a laminar flow chamber, into the broth with the help of an inoculating loop sterilised over bunsen flame. The loop is sterilised after each inoculation.
7. The inoculated broth tubes are incubated at 37°C for 24 to 48 hours in an incubator.

Observations

1. *Colour of the broth changes to pink*: Lactose fermentation.
2. *Broth becomes solid curd with fissures in it*: Gas formation.
3. *Colour of the broth changes to white with purple ring at top*: Litmus reduction.
4. *Broth becomes white solid curd with purple ring at top*: Curd formation.
5. *Broth becomes whey-like brownish translucent with deep purple ring at top*: Proteolysis.
6. *Broth colour remains unchanged or changes to deep blue*: Alkaline reaction.

Experiment 37

(11) Hydrogen Sulphide Test (H_2S Test)

***Aim*: To perform hydrogen sulphide test (H_2S test), to find out the ability of a bacteria to produce hydrogen sulphide by reduction of sulphur compounds.**

Principle

Some bacteria have the ability to reduce sulphur to hydrogen sulphide. It is a colourless gas, which reacts with iron (ferrous salts) to produce black precipitates of ferrous sulphide. It also reacts with lead acetate to produce black precipitates of lead sulphide. Hydrogen sulphide test (H_2S test) can be done in two ways, based on the source of sulphur. They are as follows.

(*i*) H_2S test using inorganic source of sulphur

(*ii*) H_2S test using organic source of sulphur

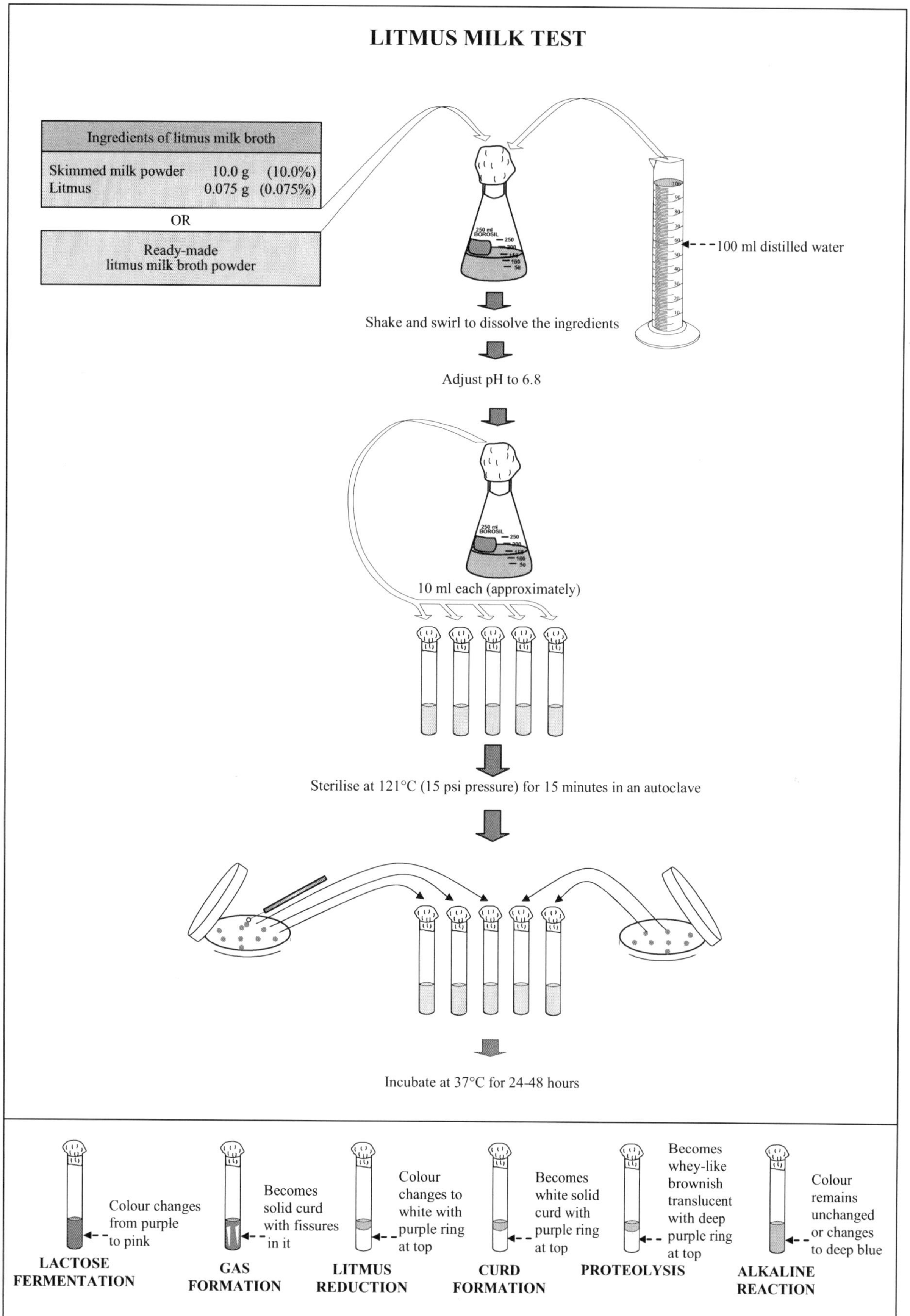

Figure 7.12: Litmus milk test

(i) H_2S Test Using Inorganic Source of Sulphur

In this test, the test bacteria is grown on triple sugar iron agar slants (TSI agar slants), which contain glucose, sucrose, lactose, phenol red, sodium thiosulphate and ferrous sulphate. If the bacteria utilises the inorganic sulphur (sodium thiosulphate) used in the medium, H_2S is produced, which combines with the ferrous sulphate in the medium to form black precipitates of ferrous sulphide resulting in a change in the colour of the butt to black. Besides utilising inorganic sulphur, if the bacteria can utilise any of the three sugars (glucose, sucrose or lactose), acid is produced, which reduces the pH of the medium. As a result, the colour of the slant changes from red to yellow.

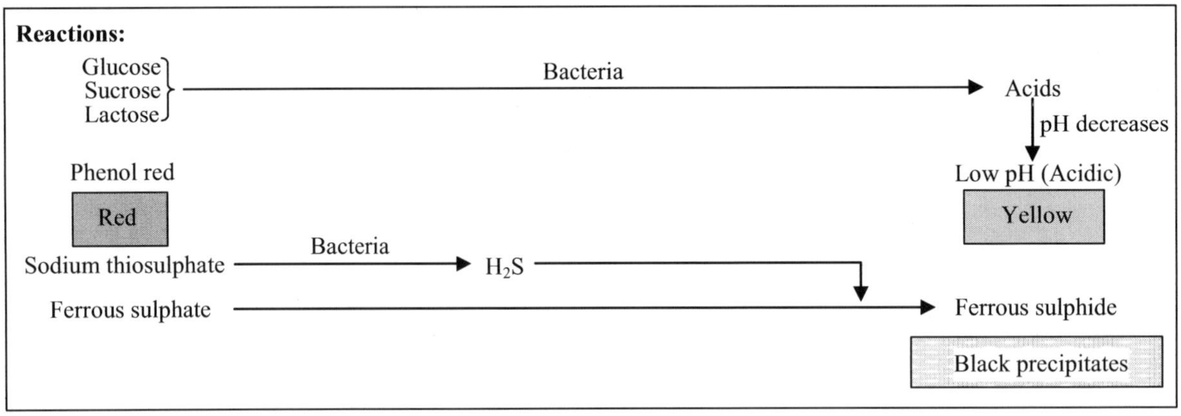

Materials Required

Test tubes, conical flask, cotton plugs, inoculating needle, autoclave, bunsen burner, laminar flow chamber, dispose jar, incubator, triple sugar iron agar (TSI agar) (*See* Appendix I at page 247), isolated colonies or pure cultures of bacteria.

Procedure

1. The ingredients of TSI agar medium (*See* Appendix I at page 247) (containing the 3 sugars and iron as the main components) or its ready-made powder required for 100 ml of the medium is weighed and dissolved in 100 ml of distilled water in a 250 ml conical flask by shaking and swirling (Figure 7.13).
2. Its pH is determined using a pH paper or pH meter and adjusted to 7.4 using 0.1N HCl if it is more or using 0.1N NaOH if it is less.
3. The flask is heated to dissolve the agar in the medium completely.
4. Before it solidifies, the medium in warm molten condition, is distributed into 5 test tubes (approximately 20 ml each).
5. The test tubes are cotton-plugged, covered with craft paper and tied with thread or rubber band.
6. They are sterilised at 121°C (15 psi pressure) for 15 minutes in an autoclave.
7. After sterilisation, they are removed from the autoclave and kept in a slanting position to cool and solidify the medium, so as to get TSI agar slants.
8. The test bacteria is inoculated aseptically, preferably in a laminar flow chamber, into the slants by stabbing into the butt and streaking on the surface of the slants with the help of a flame-sterilised needle. The needle is sterilised after each inoculation.
9. The inoculated slants are incubated at 37°C for 24 hours in an incubator.

Observations

1. *Colour of butt changes to black*: H_2S positive.
2. *Colour of butt does not change to black*: H_2S negative.

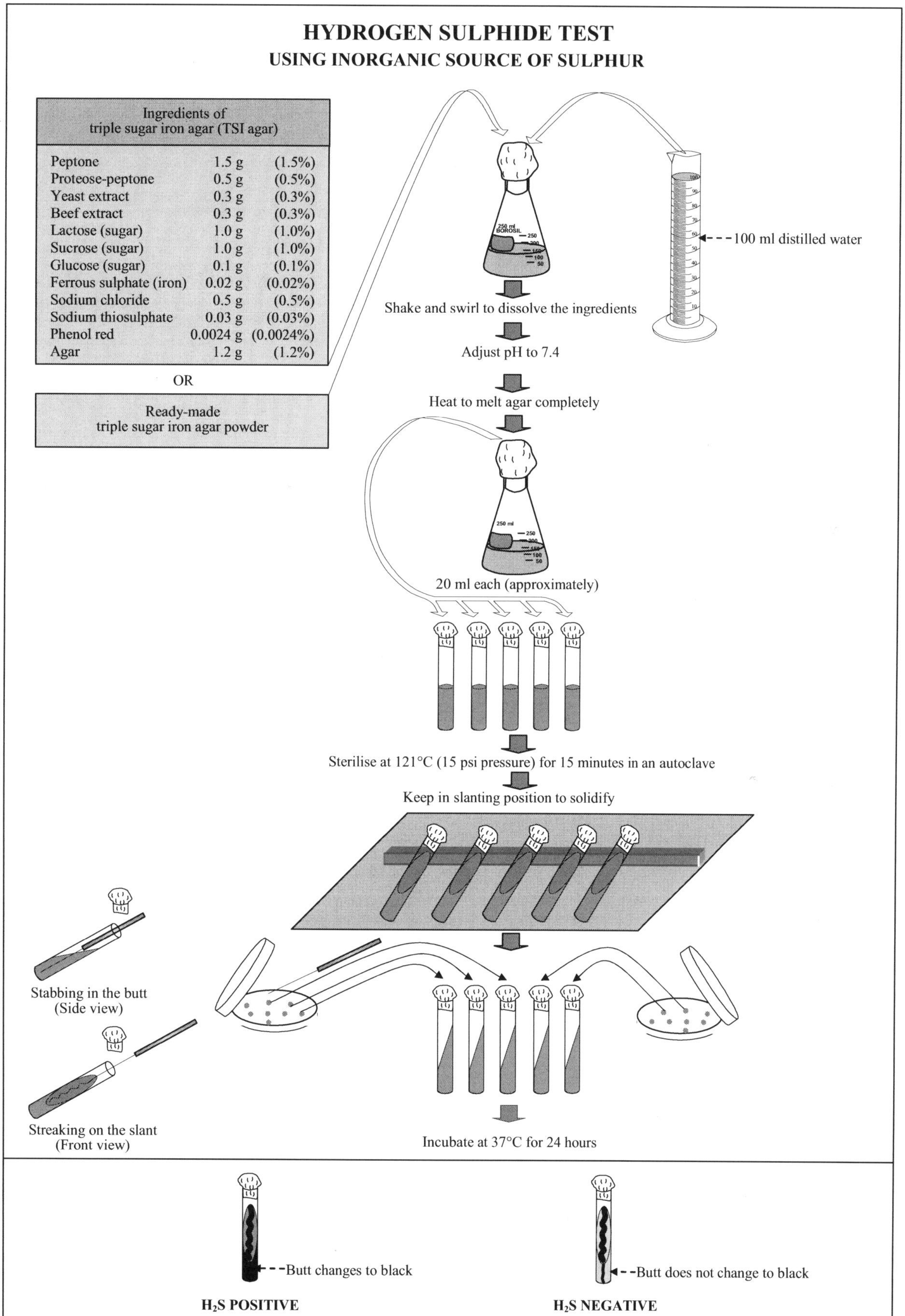

Figure 7.13: Hydrogen sulphide test (H_2S test) using inorganic source of sulphur

(ii) H_2S Test Using Organic Source of Sulphur

In this test, the test bacteria is grown in cysteine broth, which contains cysteine as the organic source of sulphur. If the bacteria utilises the organic sulphur (cysteine) used in the medium with the help of its enzyme 'cysteine desulphurase', H_2S is produced. This H_2S combines with the lead acetate soaked in a paper to form black precipitates of lead sulphide resulting in a change in the colour of the paper strip to black.

Reactions:

$$\text{Cysteine} \xrightarrow{\text{Bacterial cysteine desulphurase}} H_2S + NH_3 + \text{Pyruvic acid}$$

$$H_2S + \text{Lead acetate} \longrightarrow \text{Lead sulphide} + \text{Acetic acid}$$

Black precipitates

Materials Required

Test tubes, conical flask, cotton plugs, inoculating loop, autoclave, bunsen burner, laminar flow chamber, dispose jar, incubator, cysteine broth (*See* Appendix I at page 247), Whatman filter paper strips, lead acetate solution (saturated), isolated colonies or pure cultures of bacteria.

Procedure

1. The ingredients of cysteine broth medium (*See* Appendix I at page 247) (containing cysteine as the main component) or its ready-made powder required for 100 ml of the broth is weighed and dissolved in 100 ml of distilled water in a 250 ml conical flask by shaking and swirling (Figure 7.14).
2. Its pH is determined using a pH paper or pH meter and adjusted to 7.5 using 0.1N HCl if it is more or using 0.1N NaOH if it is less. The flask is heated, if required, to dissolve the ingredients completely.
3. The broth is distributed into five test tubes (approximately 10 ml each), cotton-plugged, covered with craft paper and tied with thread or rubber band.
4. The broth tubes are sterilised at 121°C (15 psi pressure) for 15 minutes in an autoclave.
5. The broth tubes are allowed to cool to room temperature.
6. The test bacteria is inoculated aseptically, preferably in a laminar flow chamber, into the broth with the help of an inoculating loop sterilised over bunsen flame. The loop is sterilised after each inoculation.
7. A small strip of paper soaked in lead acetate solution (saturated) is fixed at the mouth of each test tube in such a way that a long portion of it remains inside the test tube and a small portion remains outside.
8. The inoculated broth tubes are incubated at 37°C for 48 hours in an incubator.

Observations

1. *Colour of lead acetate strip changes to black*: H_2S positive.
2. *Colour of lead acetate strip does not change to black*: H_2S negative.

Experiment 38

(12) Urease Test

***Aim*: To perform urease test, to find out the ability of a bacteria to hydrolyse urea by producing the enzyme urease.**

Principle

Some bacteria have the ability to hydrolyse (breakdown in presence of water) urea to NH_3 and CO_2, as they can produce the enzyme 'urease'. NH_3 is alkaline (basic), due to which, it increases the pH changing the colour of phenol red from yellow to pink.

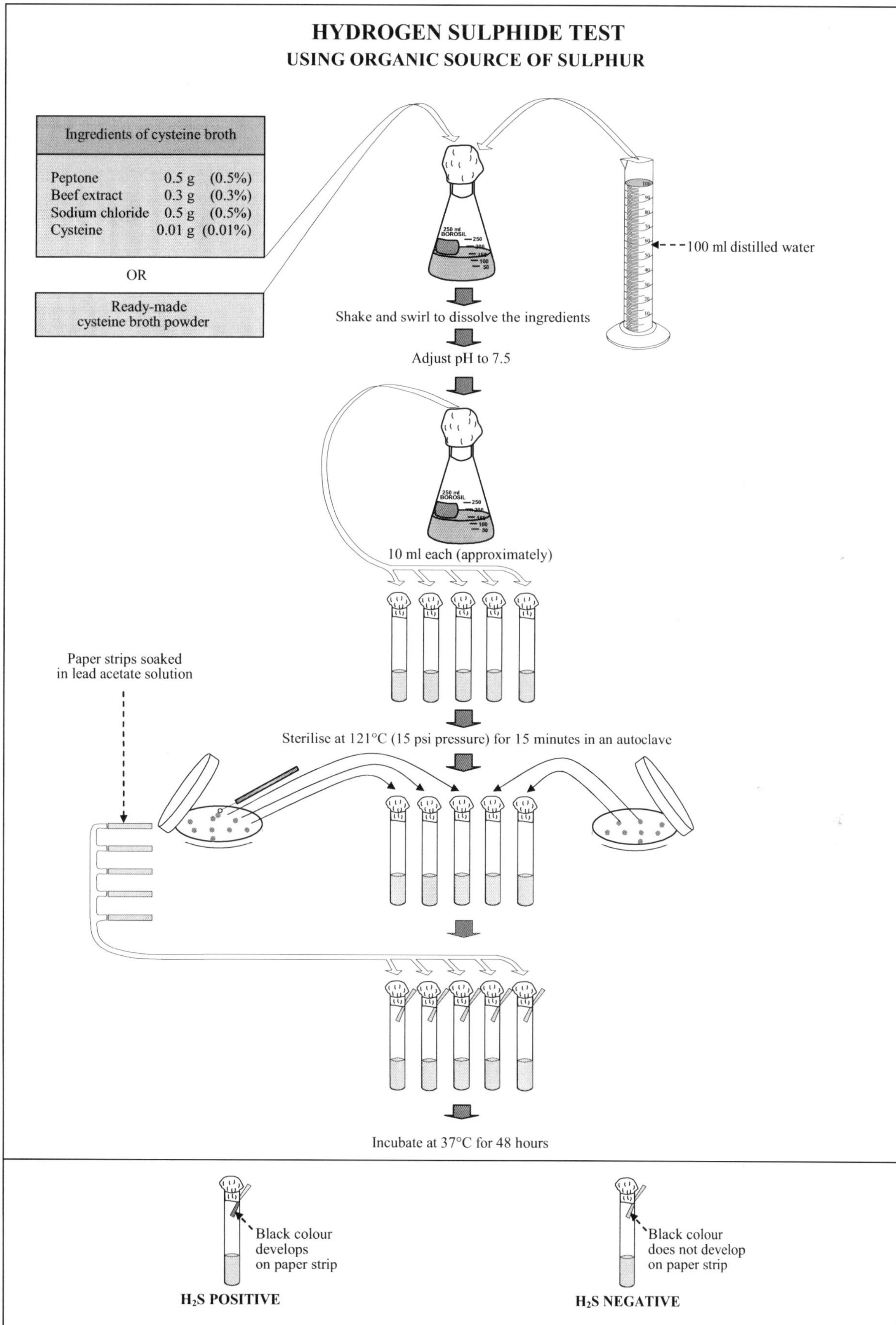

Figure 7.14: Hydrogen sulphide test (H_2S test) using organic source of sulphur

In the urease test, the test bacteria is grown on agar slants containing urea and phenol red. If the bacteria has the ability to hydrolyse urea, the colour of the medium changes from yellow to pink. Some bacteria may produce NH_3 by breaking down the peptones in the medium. In such cases false positive result is obtained.

Reactions:

$$\text{Urea} + 2H_2O \xrightarrow{\text{Bacterial urease}} 2\,NH_3 + CO_2 + H_2O$$

Urea: Phenol red, pH=6.9 — Yellow

NH_3: pH increases → pH ≥ 8.1 (Alkaline) — Pink

Materials Required

Test tubes, conical flask, cotton plugs, inoculating needle, autoclave, bunsen burner, laminar flow chamber, dispose jar, incubator, membrane filtration apparatus, urea agar (*See* Appendix I at page 247), isolated colonies or pure cultures of bacteria.

Procedure

1. Five test tubes are cotton-plugged, covered with craft paper and tied with thread or rubber band (Figure 7.15).
2. The ingredients of urea agar medium (*See* Appendix I at page 247) (containing urea as the main component) or its ready-made powder (except urea) required for 100 ml of the medium is weighed and dissolved in 90 ml of distilled water in a 250 ml conical flask by shaking and swirling.
3. Its pH is determined using a pH paper or pH meter and adjusted to 6.9 using 0.1N HCl if it is more or using 0.1N NaOH if it is less.
4. The flask is heated to dissolve the agar in the medium completely.
5. The flask is cotton-plugged, covered with craft paper and tied with thread or rubber band.
6. The five test tubes and the conical flask containing urea agar (except urea) are sterilised at 121°C (15 psi pressure) for 15 minutes in an autoclave.
7. After sterilisation, they are removed from the autoclave and allowed to cool for sometime without allowing the medium to solidify. Cooling of the medium prevents condensation and accumulation of water droplets on the slants. If the medium has already been prepared and solidified during storage, it has to be liquefied by heating carefully till it melts completely.
8. 20% urea solution is prepared by dissolving 20 grams of urea in 100 ml of distilled water and is sterilised by membrane filtration apparatus, because urea cannot be sterilised by heat, as it decomposes upon heating.
9. 10 ml of the sterilised urea solution is aseptically mixed thoroughly with 90 ml of the sterilised cooled liquefied medium (liquefied by heating).
10. Before it solidifies, the medium, in warm molten condition, is distributed aseptically into the 5 cotton-plugged sterilised test tubes (approximately 20 ml each).
11. The test tubes are kept in a slanting position to cool and solidify the medium, so as to get urea agar slants.

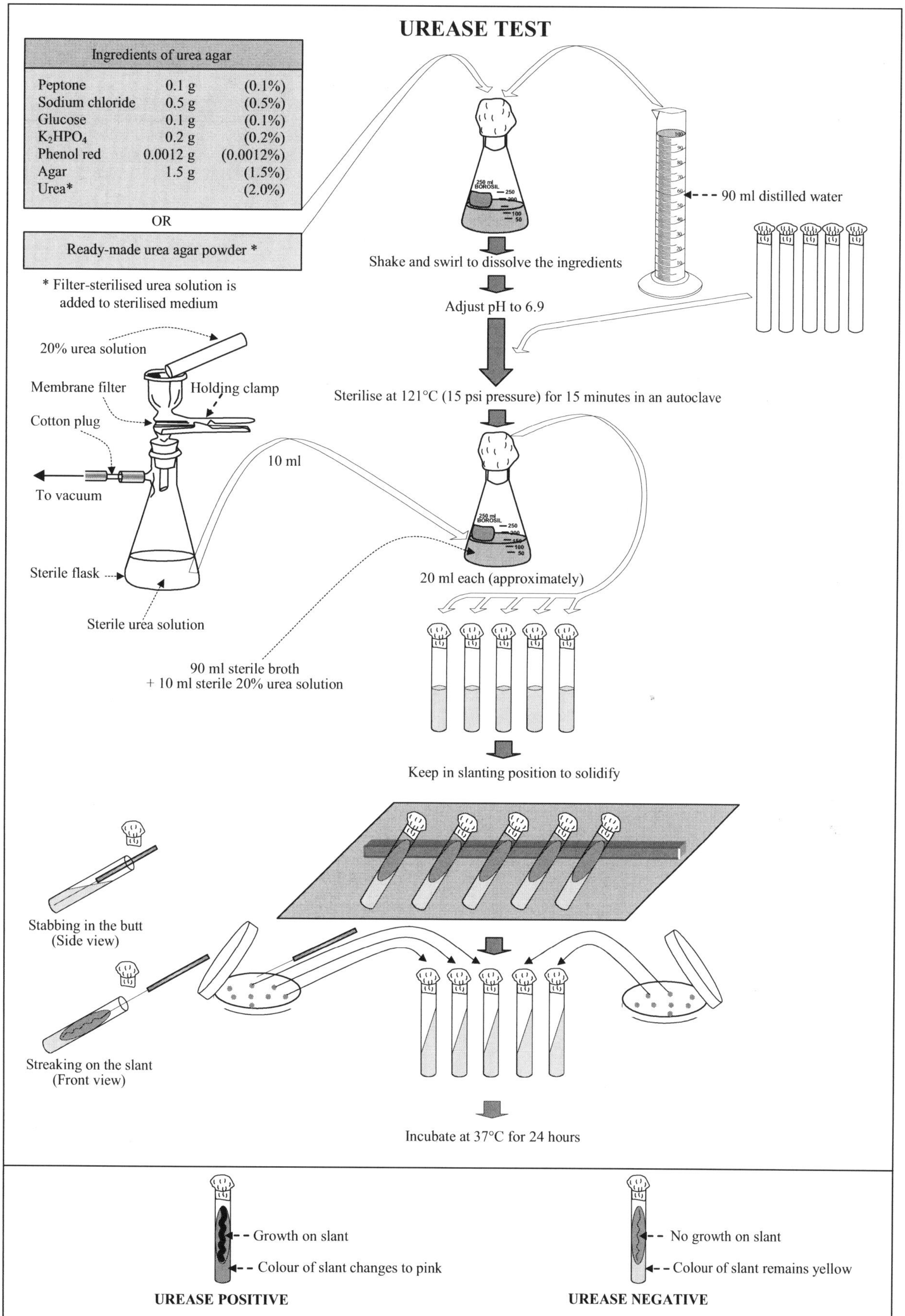

Figure 7.15: Urease test

12. The test bacteria is inoculated aseptically, preferably in a laminar flow chamber, into the slants by stabbing into the butt and streaking on the surface of the slants with the help of a flame-sterilised needle. The needle is sterilised after each inoculation.
13. The inoculated slants are incubated at 37°C for 24 hours in an incubator.

Observations

1. *Pink colour produced*: Urease positive.
2. *Pink colour not produced*: Urease negative.

Experiment 39

(13) Ortho-Nitrophenyl Galactoside Test (ONPG Test)

Aim: **To perform ortho-nitrophenyl galactoside test (ONPG test), to find out the ability of a lactose-non-fermenting bacteria to hydrolyse ortho-nitrophenyl-β-D-galactoside, by producing the enzyme β-galactosidase.**

Principle

Some bacteria have the ability to ferment lactose. They are called 'lactose-fermenting bacteria' or 'lactose-fermenters'. The others, which cannot ferment lactose are called 'lactose-non-fermenting bacteria' or 'lactose-non-fermenters'. The lactose-fermenting bacteria can produce two enzymes, namely 'permease' and 'β-galactosidase', which are involved in the fermentation of lactose. Permease helps in the entry of lactose into the bacteria cells, while β-galactosidase hydrolyses lactose to glucose and galactose. β-galactosidase is an intracellular inducible enzyme, whose production is induced by the presence of lactose in the environment of the bacteria cells. While lactose-fermenting bacteria can produce both permease as well as β-galactosidase, lactose-non-fermenting bacteria cannot produce permease, but may or may not produce β-galactosidase. The ONPG test is performed to find out the ability of a lactose-non-fermenting bacteria to produce β-galactosidase. For this, the cell membrane of the lactose-non-fermenting bacteria cells is dissolved by adding toluene, so as to release all the intracellular enzymes including β-galactosidase, if present. The enzyme, β-galactosidase, hydrolyses the substrate ortho-nitrophenyl-β-D-galctoside[8] (ONPG) to ortho-nitrophenol, which is yellow in colour.

In the ortho-nitrophenyl galactoside test (ONPG test), the test bacteria is grown on triple sugar iron agar (TSI agar) slants, which contain lactose. If the bacteria is a lactose-non-fermenter, as indicated by red butt and red slant, a thick suspension of the bacteria is made in saline, to which is added toluene followed by ONPG solution. If the bacteria has the ability to produce the enzyme β-galactosidase, the colour of the bacteria suspension changes to yellow.

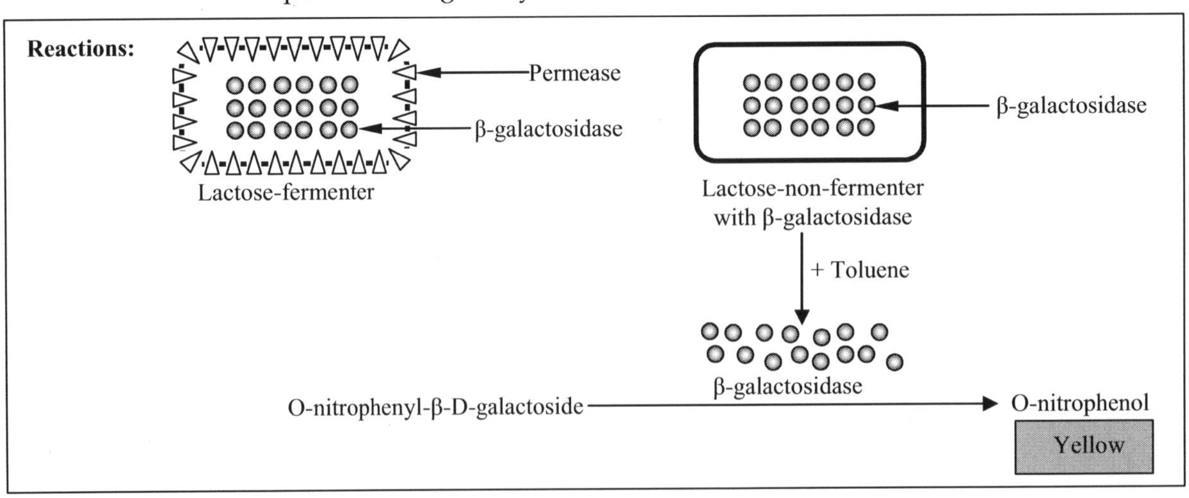

8 Ortho-nitrophenyl-β-D-galactoside = o-nitrophenyl-β-D-galactoside = o-nitrophenol-β-D-galactoside = o-nitrophenyl-β-D-galactopyranoside

Materials Required

Test tubes, conical flask, cotton plugs, inoculating loop, inoculating needle, autoclave, bunsen burner, laminar flow chamber, dispose jar, incubator, TSI agar (*See* Appendix I at page 247), toluene, o-nitrophenyl-β-D-galactoside (ONPG) solution, isolated colonies or pure cultures of bacteria.

Procedure

1. The ingredients of TSI agar medium (*See* Appendix I at page 247) (containing the 3 sugars and iron as the main components) or its ready-made powder required for 100 ml of the medium is weighed and dissolved in 100 ml of distilled water in a 250 ml conical flask by shaking and swirling (Figure 7.16).
2. Its pH is determined using a pH paper or pH meter and adjusted to 7.4 using 0.1N HCl if it is more or using 0.1N NaOH if it is less.
3. The flask is heated to dissolve the agar in the medium completely.
4. Before it solidifies, the medium in warm molten condition, is distributed into 5 test tubes (approximately 20 ml each).
5. The test tubes are cotton-plugged, covered with craft paper and tied with thread or rubber band.
6. They are sterilised at 121°C (15 psi pressure) for 15 minutes in an autoclave.
7. After sterilisation, they are removed from the autoclave and kept in a slanting position to cool and solidify the medium, so as to get TSI agar slants.
8. The test bacteria is inoculated aseptically, preferably in a laminar flow chamber, into the slants by stabbing into the butt and streaking on the surface of the slants with the help of a flame-sterilised needle. The needle is sterilised after each inoculation.
9. The inoculated slants are incubated at 37°C for 24 hours in an incubator.
10. If the bacteria is a lactose-fermenter, it is not selected for ONPG test. If the bacteria is lactose-non-fermenter, as indicated by red butt and red slant, it is selected for ONPG test.
11. To a test tube containing 0.25 ml of saline, a thick culture of the bacteria is put by means of a flame-sterilised loop, so as to make a thick suspension of the bacteria.
12. One drop of toluene is added, mixed and incubated for 5 minutes at 37°C.
13. O-nitrophenyl galactoside solution (ONPG solution) is added and incubated at 37°C for 30 minutes. Then the colour change is observed. Again colour change is observed after 24 hours.

Observations

1. *Yellow colour produced*: ONPG positive.
2. *Remains colourless*: ONPG negative.

Experiment 40

(14) Phenylalanine Deaminase Test

Aim: **To perform phenylalanine deaminase test, to find out the ability of a bacteria to deaminate the amino acid phenylalanine by producing the enzyme phenylalanine deaminase.**

Principle

Some bacteria have the ability to deaminate[9] the amino acid phenylalanine, as they can produce the enzyme 'phenylalanine deaminase'. This enzyme deaminates phenylalanine by removing its amino group, thereby producing phenylpyruvic acid (a keto acid) and ammonia (NH_3). Phenylpyruvic acid forms green colour with ferric chloride solution.

---

9 Deaminate: To remove the amino group ($-NH_2$) of an amino acid with production of NH_3 (*See* footnote at page 153).

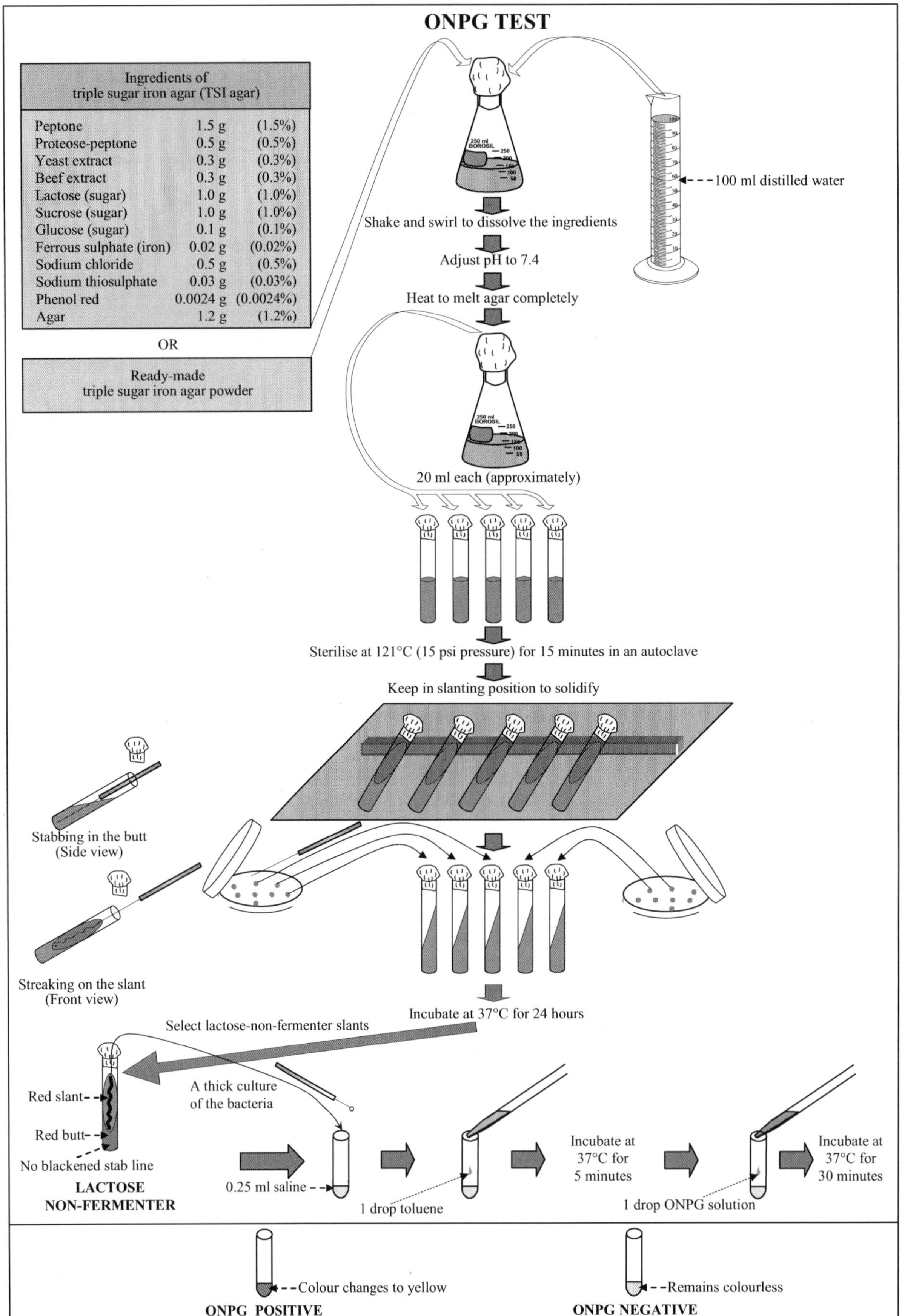

Figure 7.16: Ortho-nitrophenyl galactoside test (ONPG test)

In the phenylalanine deaminase test, the test bacteria is grown on agar slants containing phenylalanine. If the bacteria has the ability to deaminate phenylalanine, the colour of the slants changes from yellow to green, upon dropping of ferric chloride solution onto it.

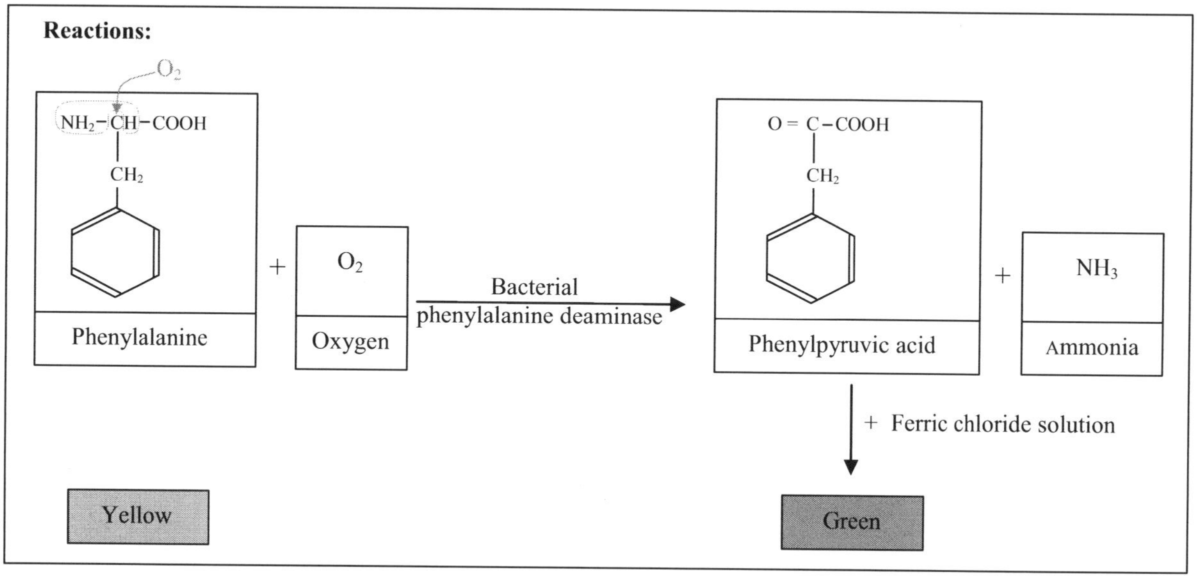

Materials Required

Test tubes, conical flask, cotton plugs, inoculating loop, autoclave, bunsen burner, laminar flow chamber, dispose jar, incubator, phenylalanine agar (*See* Appendix I at page 247), ferric chloride solution (10%) (*See* Appendix II at page 251), isolated colonies or pure cultures of bacteria.

Procedure

1. The ingredients of phenylalanine agar medium (*See* Appendix I at page 247) (containing phenylalanine as the main components) or its ready-made powder required for 100 ml of the medium is weighed and dissolved in 100 ml of distilled water in a 250 ml conical flask by shaking and swirling (Figure 7.17).
2. Its pH is determined using a pH paper or pH meter and adjusted to 7.2 using 0.1N HCl if it is more or using 0.1N NaOH if it is less.
3. The flask is heated to dissolve the agar in the medium completely.
4. Before it solidifies, the medium in warm molten condition, is distributed into 5 test tubes (approximately 20 ml each).
5. The test tubes are cotton-plugged, covered with craft paper and tied with thread or rubber band.
6. They are sterilised at 121°C (15 psi pressure) for 15 minutes in an autoclave.
7. After sterilisation, they are removed from the autoclave and kept in a slanting position to cool and solidify the medium, so as to get phenylalanine agar slants.
8. The test bacteria is inoculated aseptically, preferably in a laminar flow chamber, by streaking on surface of the slants with the help of a flame-sterilised loop. The loop is sterilised after each inoculation.
9. The inoculated slants are incubated at 37°C for 24 to 48 hours in an incubator.
10. 4–5 drops of ferric chloride solution (10%) (*See* Appendix II at page 251) is added to each slant.

Observations

1. *Colour of slant changes to green*: Phenylalanine deaminase positive.
2. *Colour of slant remains yellow*: Phenylalanine deaminase negative.

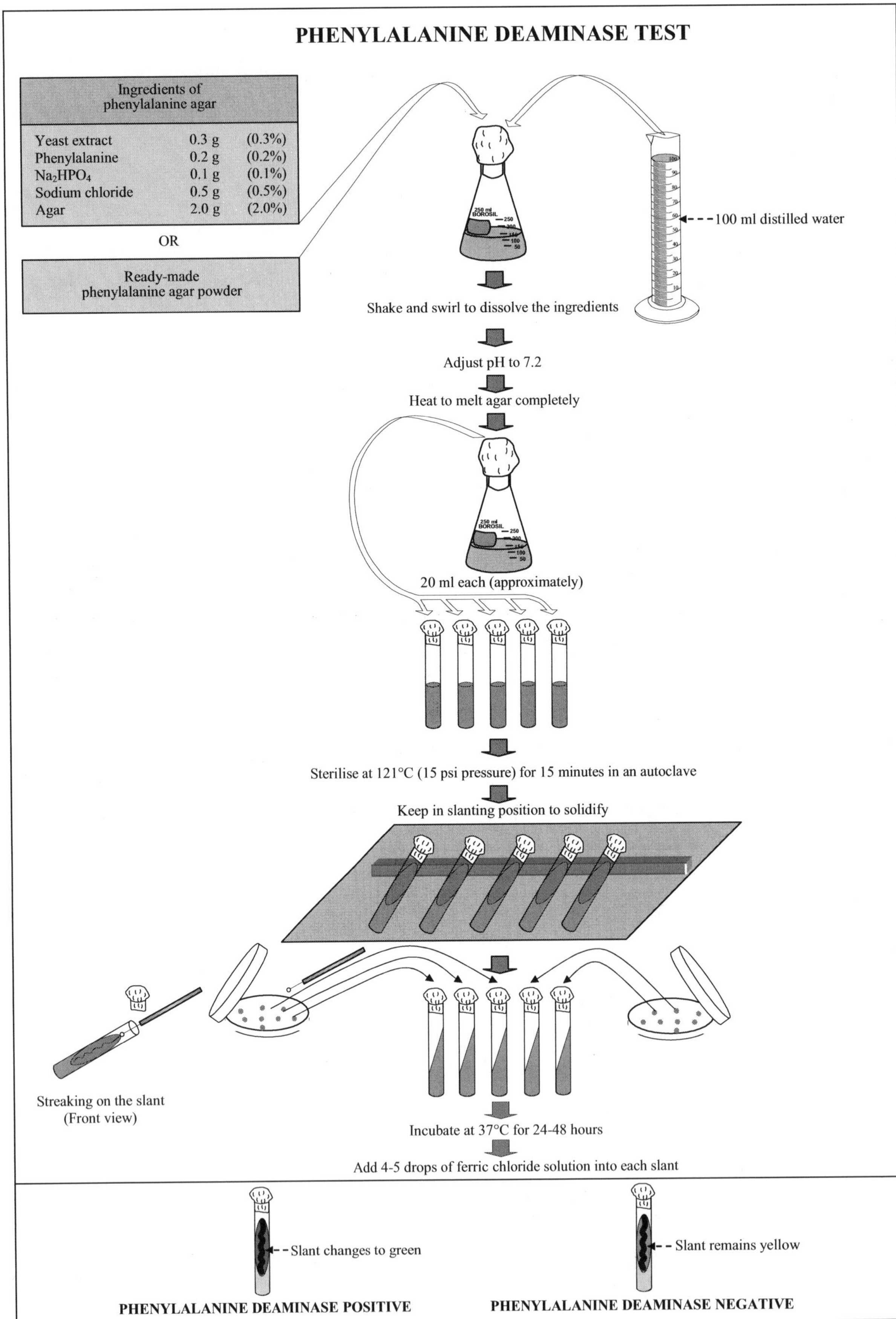

Figure 7.17: Phenylalanine deaminase test

Experiment 41

(15) Catalase Test

***Aim*: To perform catalase test, to find out the ability of a bacteria to degrade hydrogen peroxide (H_2O_2) by producing the enzyme catalase.**

Principle

Some bacteria have the ability to degrade hydrogen peroxide (H_2O_2) to water (H_2O) and oxygen ($O_2\uparrow$), as they can produce the enzyme 'catalase'. The breakdown of hydrogen peroxide by catalase is indicated by bubbles of free oxygen gas ($O_2\uparrow$).

In the catalase test, a loop of the test bacteria is put into a drop of hydrogen peroxide taken on a slide. If the bacteria has the ability to produce catalase, it breaks hydrogen peroxide (H_2O_2) to water and oxygen. Production of oxygen results in bubbling or foaming, which can be noticed in the drop.

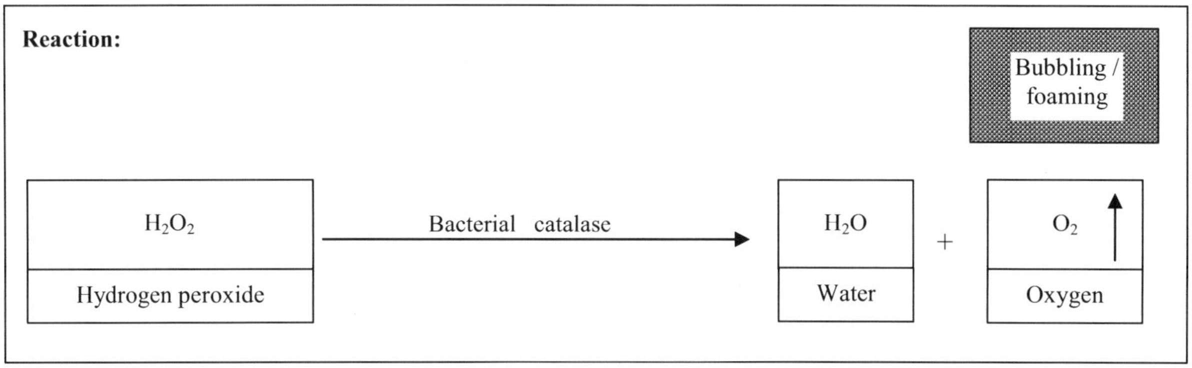

Materials Required

Slides, bibulous paper, inoculating loop, bunsen burner, laminar flow chamber, hydrogen peroxide (3%), isolated colonies or pure cultures of bacteria.

Procedure

1. A slide is cleaned under tap water (Figure 7.18).
2. The slide is wiped with bibulous paper and air-dried.
3. A drop of hydrogen peroxide (3%) is taken at the center of the slide.
4. A loop of the test bacteria is taken aseptically, preferably in a laminar flow chamber, with the help of a flame-sterilised loop and is put into the drop of hydrogen peroxide on the slide. The loop is sterilised after each inoculation.

Observations

1. *Bubbling or foaming occurs in the drop*: Catalase positive.
2. *Bubbling or foaming does not occur in the drop*: Catalase negative.

Precautions

A culture of bacteria from blood agar medium cannot be used for catalase test, as blood contains catalase and it always gives positive result. Catalase negative bacteria tend to die in sugar free media either because they produce H_2O_2 or because H_2O_2 accumulates in the media, when they are exposed to air and light. Therefore, stock cultures of such bacteria should be stored in the dark and where access to air is limited. Catalase is found in almost all bacteria that can grow aerobically. As the enzyme is produced only by viable bacteria, cultures over 24 hours old cannot be used for catalase test.

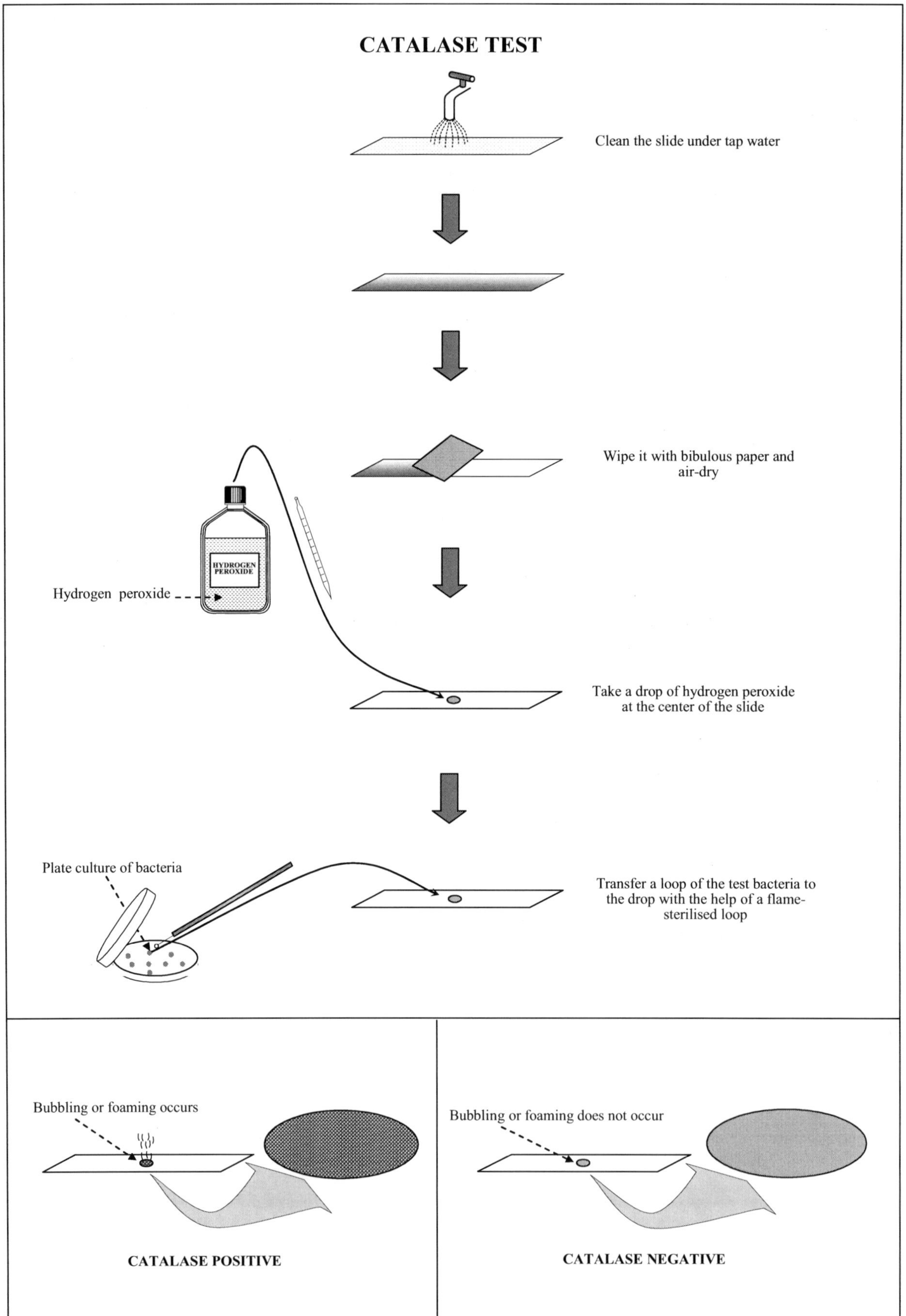

Figure 7.18: Catalase test

Experiment 42

(16) Oxidase Test

***Aim*: To perform oxidase test, to find out the ability of a bacteria to oxidise reduced cytochrome C by producing the enzyme cytochrome oxidase.**

Principle

Some bacteria have the ability to oxidase 'reduced cytochrome C′ present in their cells to 'oxidised cytochrome C′, as they can produce the enzyme 'cytochrome oxidase'. The oxidised cytochrome C produces purple colour (Wurster's purple) with the dye N-tetramethyl-para-phenylenediamine (*i.e.* oxidase reagent).

In the oxidase test, nutrient agar plates containing the colonies of the test bacteria are flooded with the solution of oxidase reagent. If the bacteria has the ability to produce the enzyme cytochrome oxidase, the colour of the colonies on the plates changes to purple. If the bacteria does not have the ability to produce cytochrome oxidase, the colonies retain the original pink colour of the oxidase reagent.

Reactions:

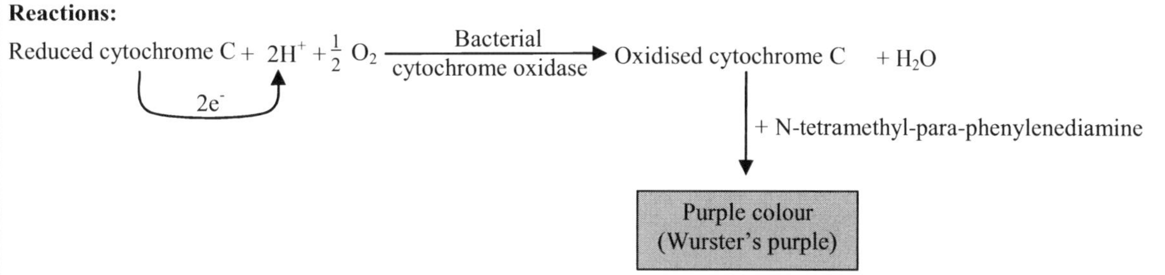

Materials Required

Petri dishes, conical flask, cotton plugs, platinum wire inoculating loop, autoclave, bunsen burner, laminar flow chamber, dispose jar, incubator, Whatman filter paper strip, oxidase reagent (N-tetramethyl-para-phenylenediamine) (*See* Appendix II at page 251), nutrient agar (*See* Appendix I at page 247), isolated colonies or pure cultures of bacteria.

Procedure

(a) Plate Method

1. Two petri dishes are cleaned, covered with craft paper and tied with thread or rubber band (Figure 7.19). This step as well as the sterilisation of the petri dishes at step 6 are omitted, if oven-sterilised petri dishes are used directly.
2. The ingredients of nutrient agar medium (*See* Appendix I at page 247) or its ready-made powder required for 100 ml of the medium is weighed and dissolved in 100 ml of distilled water in a 250 ml conical flask by shaking and swirling.
3. Its pH is determined using a pH paper or pH meter and adjusted to 7.0 using 0.1N HCl if it is more or using 0.1N NaOH if it is less.
4. The flask is heated to dissolve the agar in the medium completely.
5. The flask is cotton-plugged, covered with craft paper and tied with thread or rubber band.
6. The two petri dishes and the conical flask containing nutrient agar medium are sterilised at 121°C (15 psi pressure) for 15 minutes in an autoclave.
7. After sterilisation, they are removed from the autoclave and allowed to cool for sometime, without allowing the medium to solidify. Cooling of the medium prevents condensation and accumulation of water droplets inside the plates. If the medium has already been prepared and solidified during storage, it has to be liquefied by heating carefully till it melts completely.

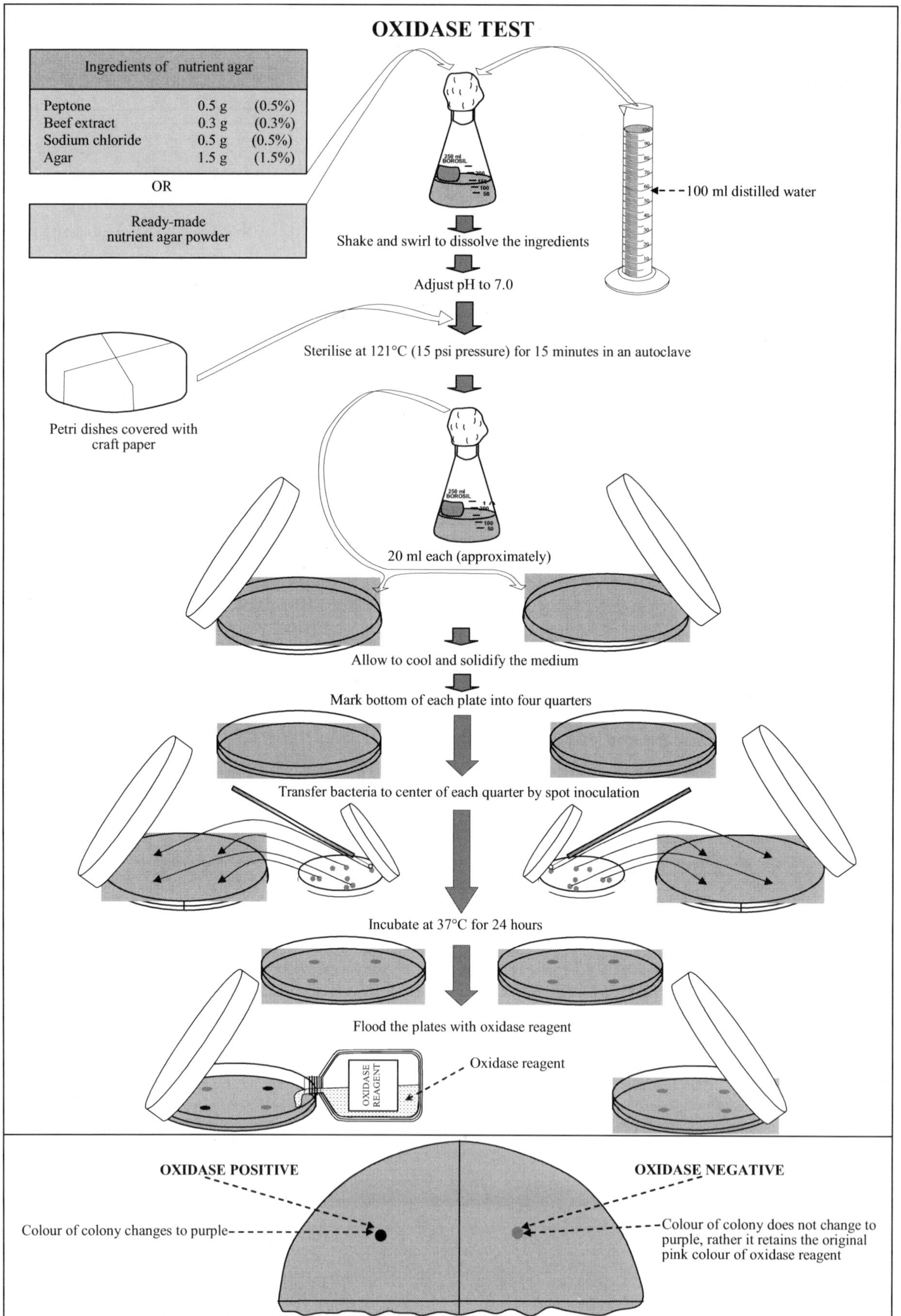

Figure 7.19: Oxidase test

8. To prepare nutrient agar plates, before the sterilised nutrient agar medium cools and solidifies, in warm molten condition, it is poured aseptically, preferably inside a laminar flow chamber, into the two sterilised petri dishes (approximately 20 ml each), so that the molten medium covers the bottom of the petri dishes completely. Then, the plates are covered with their lids and allowed to cool, so as to solidify the medium in them. Water vapour that may condense on the inner surface of the plates and lids is evaporated by keeping the plates and lids in inverted position in an incubator at 37°C for about 1 hour.
9. Each plate is marked on the bottom side into four quarters.
10. "Spot inoculation" of the test bacteria is done aseptically, preferably in a laminar flow chamber, on the center of each quarter by making a spot (or small smear) of the bacteria with the help of a flame-sterilised loop. The loop is sterilised after each inoculation.
11. The inoculated plates are incubated in inverted position, top down, at 37°C for 24 hours in an incubator till colonies of the bacteria are visible.
12. The plates are flooded with oxidase reagent (*See* Appendix II at page 251).

(b) Paper Method

1. A Whatman filter paper strip, dipped in 1% oxidase reagent (*See* Appendix II at page 251) is dried and kept in darkness.
2. Before use, it is moistened and a loop of the test bacteria is put on it as a spot with the help of a platinum wire loop. Nichrome loop can oxidise the reagent. Therefore, platinum loop has to be used.
3. The spot is observed after 10 seconds.

Observations

(a) Plate Method

1. *Purple colour develops on colonies of bacteria*: Oxidase positive.
2. *Purple colour does not develop on colonies*
   (Pink colour of the oxidase reagent is retained): Oxidase negative.

(b) Paper Method

1. *Purple colour develops on the spot*: Oxidase positive.
2. *Purple colour does not develop on the spot*: Oxidase negative.

Experiment 43

(17) Gelatinase Test

Aim: **To perform gelatinase test, to find out the ability of a bacteria to hydrolyse gelatin by producing the enzyme gelatinase.**

Principle

Some bacteria have the ability to hydrolyse gelatin[10], as they can produce the proteolytic enzyme 'gelatinase'. While the gelatin gets precipitated by mercuric chloride producing translucence, its hydrolysed end products do not gets precipitated by mercuric chloride, for which they do not produce such translucence, rather produce transparency.

In the gelatinase test, the test bacteria is grown on agar plates containing gelatin. After colonies of the bacteria are visible, the plates are flooded with a solution of mercuric chloride. If the bacteria has

10 Gelatin is a protein produced by the hydrolysis of collagen, a major component of connective tissues and tendons in human and other animals. Below 25°C, gelatin maintains its gel properties and exists as a solid, but above 25°C it is a liquid.

the ability to hydrolyse gelatin, its colonies hydrolyse the gelatin in the medium in the areas surrounding them, while the rest of the areas of the plates retain unhydrolysed gelatin. As a result, when flooded with a solution of mercuric chloride, transparent clear zones are formed around the colonies, as the hydrolysed products formed around them do not form precipitates with the mercuric chloride. On the other hand, the rest of the areas of the plates become translucent, as the unhydrolysed gelatin in these areas form precipitates with mercuric chloride.

Reactions:

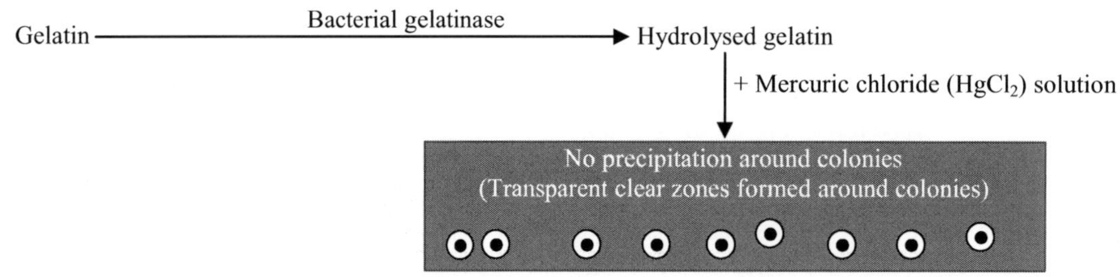

Materials Required

Petri dishes, conical flask, cotton plugs, inoculating loop, autoclave, bunsen burner, laminar flow chamber, dispose jar, incubator, Fraizer's gelatin agar (*See* Appendix I at page 247), mercuric chloride solution (*See* Appendix II at page 251), isolated colonies or pure cultures of bacteria.

Procedure

1. Two petri dishes are cleaned, covered with craft paper and tied with thread or rubber band (Figure 7.20). This step as well as the sterilisation of the petri dishes at step 6 are omitted, if oven-sterilised petri dishes are used directly
2. The ingredients of Fraizer's gelatin agar medium (*See* Appendix I at page 247) (containing gelatin as the main component) or its ready-made powder required for 100 ml of the medium is weighed and dissolved in 100 ml of distilled water in a 250 ml conical flask by shaking and swirling.
3. Its pH is determined using a pH paper or pH meter and adjusted to 7.2 using 0.1N HCl if it is more or using 0.1N NaOH if it is less.
4. The flask is heated to dissolve the agar in the medium completely.
5. The flask is cotton-plugged, covered with craft paper and tied with thread or rubber band.
6. The two petri dishes and the conical flask containing Fraizer's gelatin agar medium are sterilised at 121°C (15 psi pressure) for 15 minutes in an autoclave.
7. After sterilisation, they are removed from the autoclave and allowed to cool for sometime without allowing the medium to solidify. Cooling of the medium prevents condensation and accumulation of water droplets inside the plates. If the medium has already been prepared and solidified during storage, it has to be liquefied by heating carefully till it melts completely.
8. To prepare gelatin agar plates, before the sterilised Frazier's gelatin agar medium cools and solidifies, in warm molten condition, it is poured aseptically, preferably inside a laminar flow chamber, into the two sterilised petri dishes (approximately 20 ml each), so that the molten medium covers the bottom of the petri dishes completely. Then, the plates are covered with their lids and allowed to cool, so as to solidify the medium in them. Water vapour that may condense on the inner surface of the plates and lids is evaporated by keeping the plates and lids inverted position in an incubator at 37°C for about 1 hour.
9. Each plate is marked on the bottom side into four quarters.

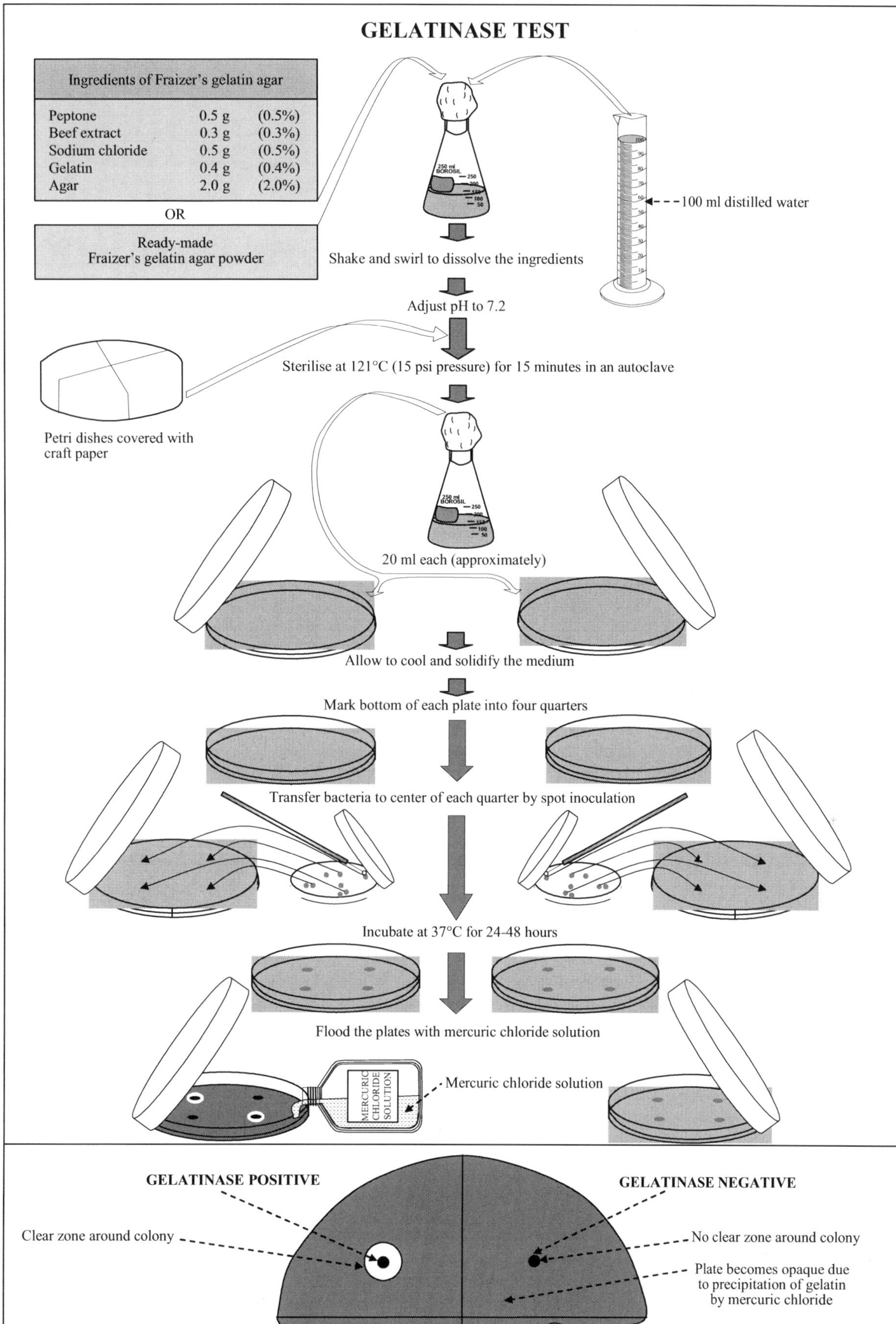

Figure 7.20: Gelatinase test

10. "Spot inoculation" of the test bacteria is done aseptically, preferably inside a laminar flow chamber, on the center of each quarter by making a spot (or small smear) of the bacteria with the help of a flame-sterilised loop. The loop is sterilised after each inoculation.
11. The inoculated plates are incubated in inverted position, top down, at 37°C for 24 to 48 hours in an incubator till colonies of the bacteria are visible.
12. The plates are flooded with solution of mercuric chloride ($HgCl_2$) (*See* Appendix II at page 251).

Observations

1. *Transparent clear zones formed around colonies of bacteria*: Gelatinase positive.
2. *Transparent clear zones not formed around colonies of bacteria*: Gelatinase negative.

Experiment 44

(18) Starch Hydrolysis Test

***Aim*: To perform starch hydrolysis test, to find out the ability of a bacteria to hydrolyse starch.**

Principle

Some bacteria have the ability to hydrolyse starch, as they can produce the saccharolytic enzyme, 'α-amylase'. While the starch forms dark blue colour with iodine, its hydrolysed end products do not acquire such dark blue colour with iodine.

In the starch hydrolysis test, the test bacteria is grown on agar plates containing starch. After colonies of the bacteria are visible, the plates are flooded with iodine solution. If the bacteria has the ability to hydrolyse starch, its colonies hydrolyse the starch in the medium in the areas surrounding them, while the rest of the areas of the plates contain unhydrolysed starch. As a result, when flooded with iodine solution, transparent clear zones are formed around the colonies, as the hydrolysed products formed around them do not form dark blue colour with iodine. On the other hand, the rest of the areas of the plates become dark blue, as iodine forms dark blue colour with the unhydrolysed starch in these areas.

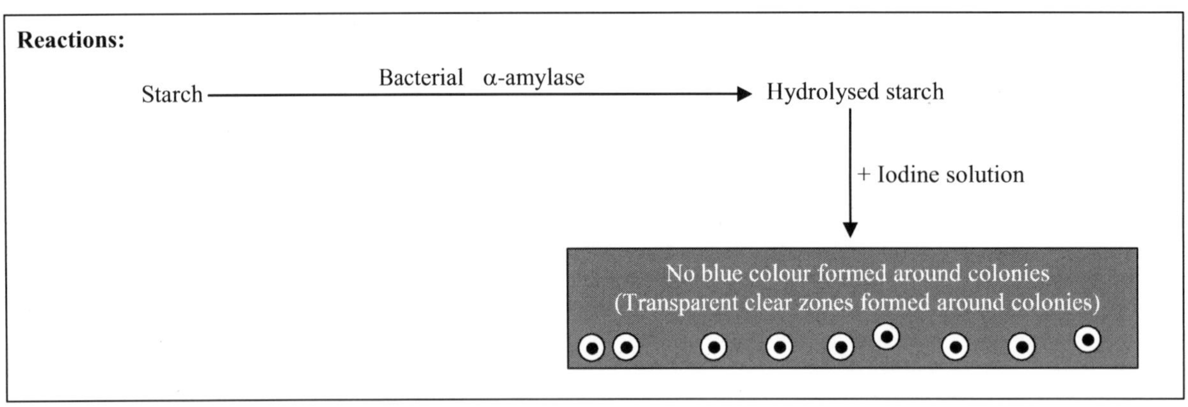

Materials Required

Petri dishes, conical flask, cotton plugs, inoculating loop, autoclave, bunsen burner, laminar flow chamber, dispose jar, incubator, starch agar (*See* Appendix I at page 247), Lugol's iodine solution (*See* Appendix II at page 251), isolated colonies or pure cultures of bacteria.

Procedure

1. Two petri dishes are cleaned, covered with craft paper and tied with thread or rubber band (Figure 7.21). This step as well as the sterilisation of the petri dishes at step 6 are omitted, if oven-sterilised petri dishes are used directly.

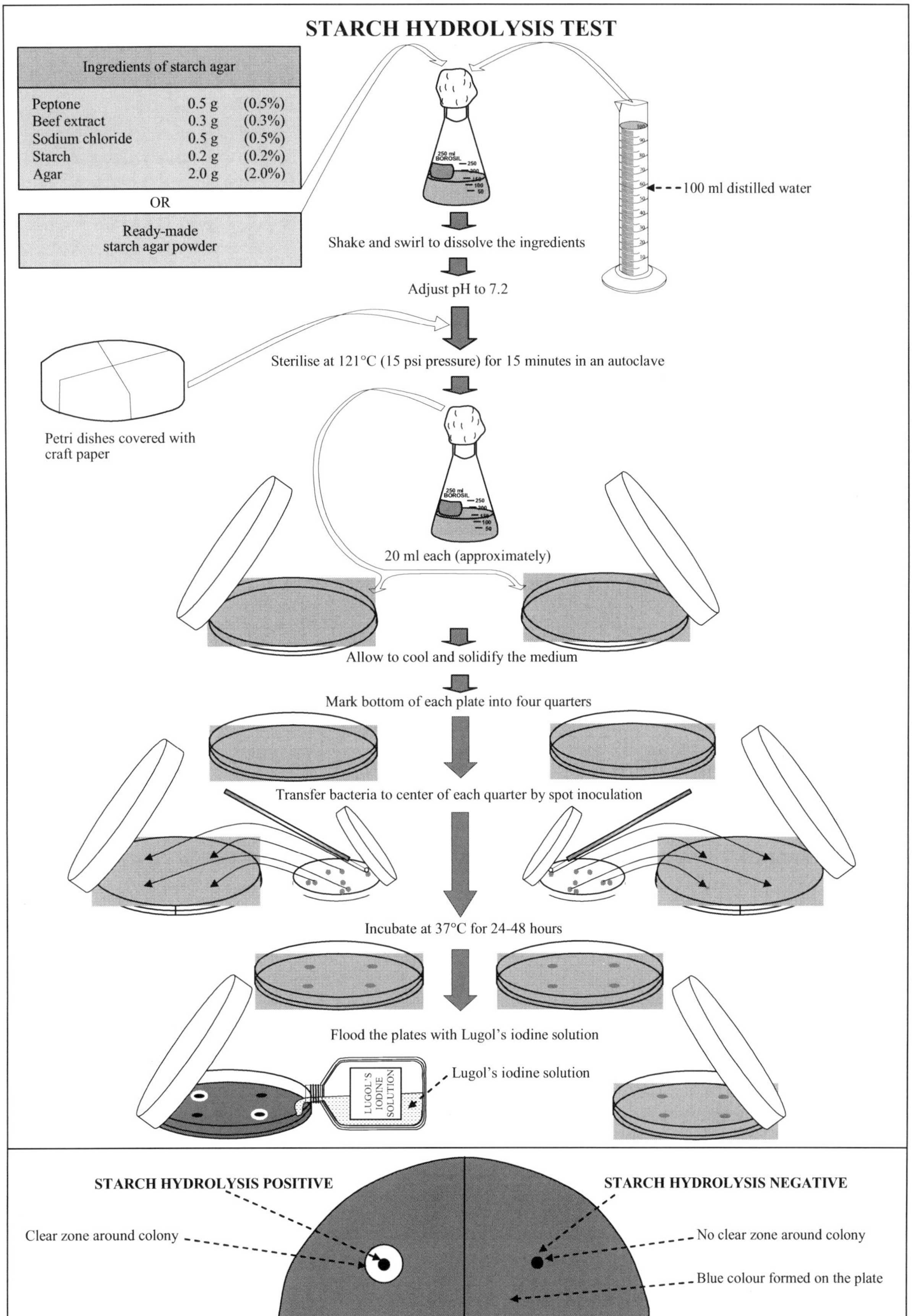

Figure 7.21: Starch hydrolysis test

2. The ingredients of starch agar medium (*See* Appendix I at page 247) (containing starch as the main component) or its ready-made powder required for 100 ml of the medium is weighed and dissolved in 100 ml of distilled water in a 250 ml conical flask by shaking and swirling.
3. Its pH is determined using a pH paper or pH meter and adjusted to 7.2 using 0.1N HCl if it is more or using 0.1N NaOH if it is less.
4. The flask is heated to dissolve the agar in the medium completely.
5. The flask is cotton-plugged, covered with craft paper and tied with thread or rubber band.
6. The two petri dishes and the conical flask containing starch agar medium are sterilised at 121°C (15 psi pressure) for 15 minutes in an autoclave.
7. After sterilisation, they are removed from the autoclave and allowed to cool for sometime, without allowing the medium to solidify. Cooling of the medium prevents condensation and accumulation of water droplets inside the plates. If the medium has already been prepared and solidified during storage, it has to be liquefied by heating carefully till it melts completely.
8. To prepare starch agar plates, before the sterilised starch agar medium cools and solidifies, in warm molten condition, it is poured aseptically, preferably inside a laminar flow chamber, into the two sterilised petri dishes (approximately 20 ml each), so that the molten medium covers the bottom of the petri dishes completely. Then, the plates are covered with by their lids and allowed to cool, so as to solidify the medium in them. Water vapour that may condense on the inner surface of the plates and lids is evaporated by keeping the plates and lids in an inverted position in an incubator at 37°C for about 1 hour.
9. Each plate is marked on the bottom side into four quarters.
10. "Spot inoculation" of the test bacteria is done aseptically, preferably inside a laminar flow chamber, on the center of each quarter by making a spot (or small smear) of the bacteria with the help of a flame-sterilised loop. The loop is sterilised after each inoculation.
11. The inoculated plates are incubated in inverted position, top down, at 37°C for 24 to 48 hours in an incubator till colonies of the bacteria are visible.
12. The plates are flooded with Lugol's iodine solution (*See* Appendix II at page 251).

Observations

1. *Transparent clear zones formed around colonies of bacteria*: Starch hydrolysis positive.
2. *Transparent clear zones not formed around colonies of bacteria*: Starch hydrolysis negative.

Experiment 45

(19) Lipid Hydrolysis Test

***Aim*: To perform lipid hydrolysis test, to find out the ability of a bacteria to hydrolyse lipids (fats).**

Principle

Some bacteria have the ability to hydrolyse lipids (fats) to glycerol and fatty acids, as they possess the lipolytic enzyme 'lipase'. These bacteria are called lipolytic bacteria. While the lipids form an emulsion, when dispensed in agar, producing opacity, their hydrolysed end products, glycerol and fatty acids, do not form such emulsion with agar, for which they do not produce such opacity; rather produce transparency.

In the lipid hydrolysis test, the test bacteria is grown on agar plates containing tributyrin as the lipid substrate. Tributyrin forms an emulsion, when dispensed in the agar, producing an opaque medium. If the bacteria has the ability to hydrolyse lipids, its colonies hydrolyse the tributyrin in the medium in the areas surrounding them to soluble glycerol and fatty acids (butyric acid), while the rest of the areas of the plates contain unhydrolysed tributyrin. As a result, transparent clear zones are formed around the colonies, as the hydrolysed products, glycerol and fatty acids, formed around them do not form emulsion with the agar. On the other hand, the rest of the areas of the plates remain opaque, as the unhydrolysed tributyrin in these areas forms an emulsion with the agar.

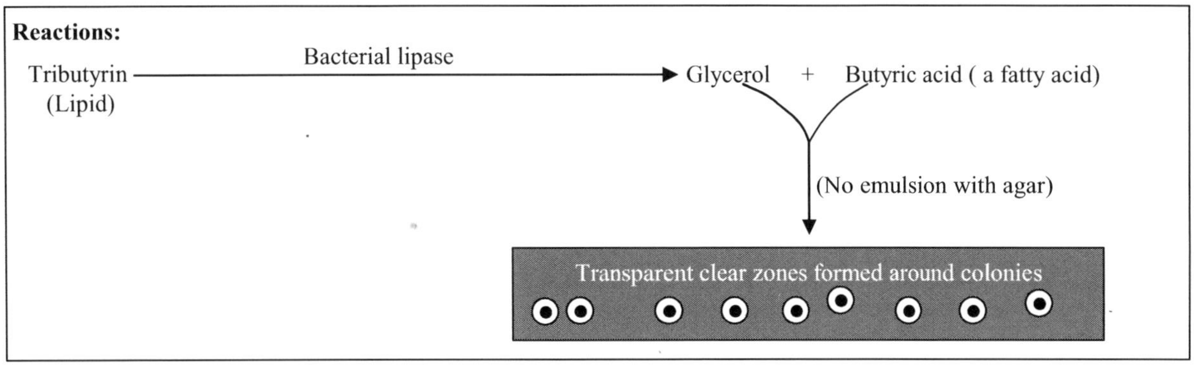

Materials Required

Petri dishes, conical flask, cotton plugs, inoculating loop, autoclave, bunsen burner, laminar flow chamber, dispose jar, incubator, tributyrin agar (*See* Appendix I at page 247), isolated colonies or pure cultures of bacteria.

Procedure

1. Two petri dishes are cleaned, covered with craft paper and tied with thread or rubber band (Figure 7.22). This step as well as the sterilisation of the petri dishes at step 6 are omitted, if oven-sterilised petri dishes are used directly.
2. The ingredients of tributyrin agar medium (*See* Appendix I at page 247) (excluding tributyrin, which is the lipid component) or its ready-made powder required for 100 ml of the medium is weighed and dissolved in 100 ml of distilled water in a 250 ml conical flask by shaking and swirling.
3. Its pH is determined using a pH paper or pH meter and adjusted to 7.2 using 0.1N HCl if it is more or using 0.1N NaOH if it is less.
4. The flask is heated to dissolve the agar in the medium completely.
5. After cooling to about 90°C, tributyrin is added and emulsified in a Waring blender.
6. The flask is cotton-plugged, covered with craft paper and tied with thread or rubber band.
7. The two petri dishes and the conical flask containing tributyrin agar medium are sterilised at 121°C (15 psi pressure) for 15 minutes in an autoclave.
8. After sterilisation, they are removed from the autoclave and allowed to cool for sometime, without allowing the medium to solidify. Cooling of the medium prevents condensation and accumulation of water droplets inside the plates. If the medium has already been prepared and solidified during storage, it has to be liquefied by heating carefully till it melts completely.
9. To prepare tributyrin agar plates, before the sterilised tributyrin agar medium cools and solidifies, in warm molten condition, it is poured aseptically, preferably inside a laminar flow chamber, into the two sterilised petri dishes (approximately 20 ml each), so that the molten medium covers the bottom of the petri dishes completely. Then, the plates are covered with their lids and allowed to cool, so as to solidify the medium in them. Tributyrin forms an emulsion, when dispensed in agar, producing an opaque medium. Water vapour that may condense on the inner surface of the plates and lids is evaporated by keeping the plates and lids in inverted position in an incubator at 37°C for about 1 hour.
10. Each plate is marked on the bottom side into four quarters.
11. "Spot inoculation" of the test bacteria is done aseptically, preferably inside a laminar flow chamber, on the center of each quarter by making a spot (or small smear) of the bacteria with the help of a flame-sterilised loop. The loop is sterilised after each inoculation.

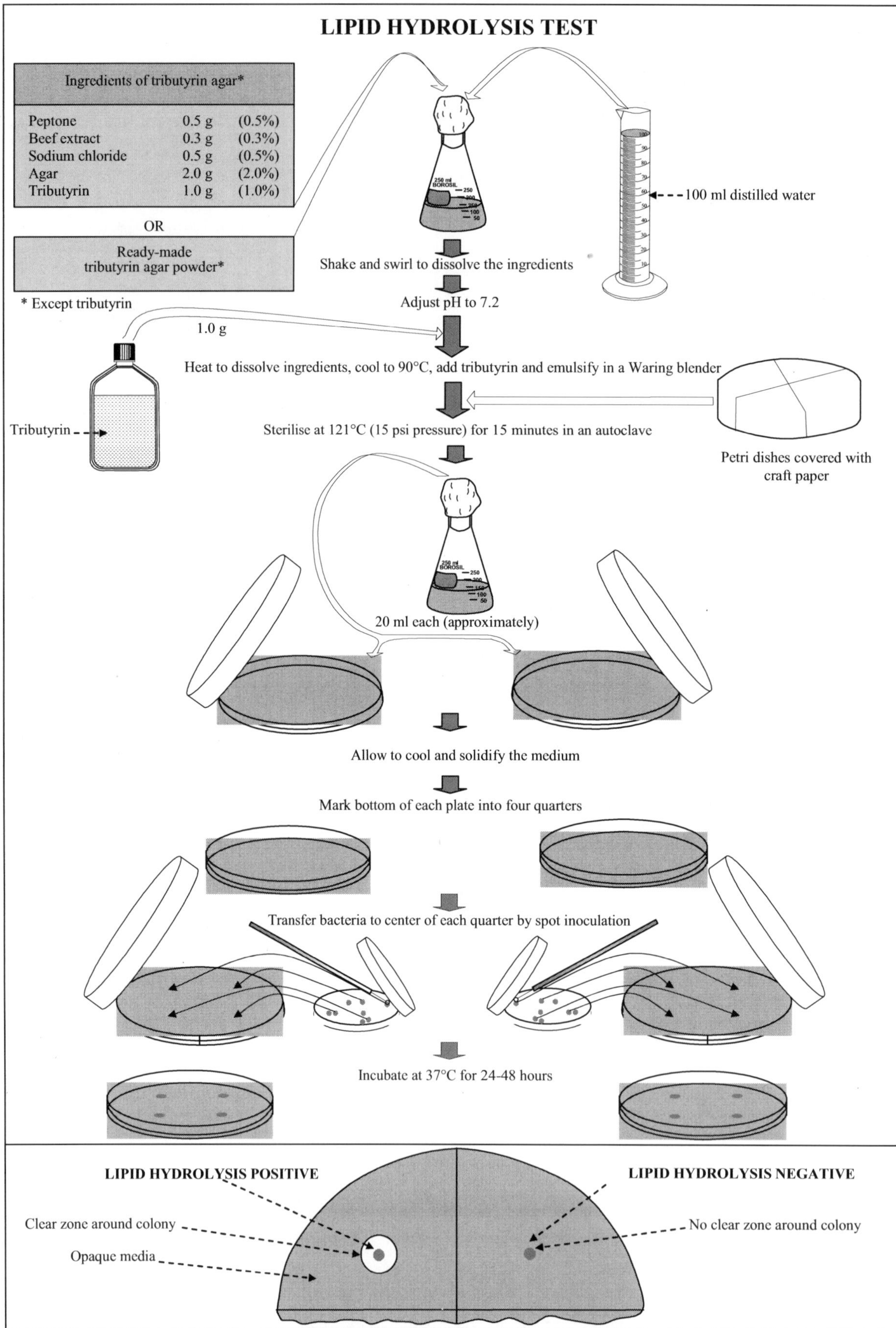

Figure 7.22: Lipid hydrolysis test

12. The inoculated plates are incubated in inverted position, top down, at 37°C for 24 to 48 hours in an incubator till colonies of the bacteria are visible.

Observations

1. *Transparent clear zones formed around colonies of bacteria*: Lipid hydrolysis positive.
2. *Transparent clear zones not formed around colonies of bacteria*: Lipid hydrolysis negative.

Experiment 46

(20) Deoxyribonuclease Test (DNase Test)

***Aim*: To perform deoxyribonuclease test (DNase test), to find out the ability of a bacteria to hydrolyse deoxyribonucleic acid (DNA) by producing the enzyme deoxyribonuclease (DNase).**

Principle

Some bacteria have the ability to hydrolyse deoxyribonucleic acid (DNA) to oligonucleotides, as they can produce the extracellular hydrolytic enzyme 'deoxyribonuclease' (DNase). While the DNA gets precipitated by hydrochloric acid producing opacity, its hydrolysed end products, oligonucleotides, do not get precipitated by hydrochloric acid, for which they do not produce such opacity; rather produce transparency.

In the DNase test, the test bacteria is grown on agar plates containing DNA. After colonies of the bacteria are visible, the plates are flooded with hydrochloric acid. If the bacteria has the ability to hydrolyse DNA, its colonies hydrolyse the DNA in the medium in the areas surrounding them, while the rest of the areas of the plates contain unhydrolysed DNA. As a result, when flooded with hydrochloric acid, transparent clear zones are formed around the colonies, as the hydrolysed products, oligonucleotides, formed around them do not form precipitates with the hydrochloric acid. On the other hand, the rest of the areas of the plates become opaque, as the unhydrolysed DNA in these areas form precipitates with the hydrochloric acid. If toluidine blue is used instead of hydrochloric acid, a rose pink halo is produced only around the colonies.

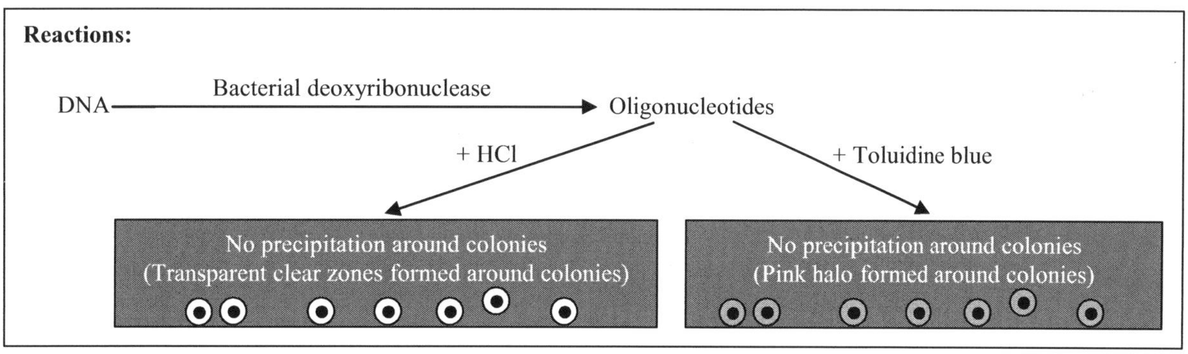

Materials Required

Petri dishes, conical flask, cotton plugs, inoculating loop, autoclave, bunsen burner, laminar flow chamber, dispose jar, incubator, DNase agar (*See* Appendix I at page 247), 1N hydrochloric acid (or 0.1% toluidine blue) (*See* Appendix II at page 251), isolated colonies or pure cultures of bacteria.

Procedure

1. Two petri dishes are cleaned, covered with craft paper and tied with thread or rubber band (Figure 7.23). This step as well as the sterilisation of the petri dishes at step 6 are omitted, if oven-sterilised petri dishes are used directly.
2. The ingredients of DNase agar medium (*See* Appendix I at page 247) (containing DNA as the main component) or its ready-made powder required for 100 ml of the medium is weighed and dissolved in 100 ml of distilled water in a 250 ml conical flask by shaking and swirling.

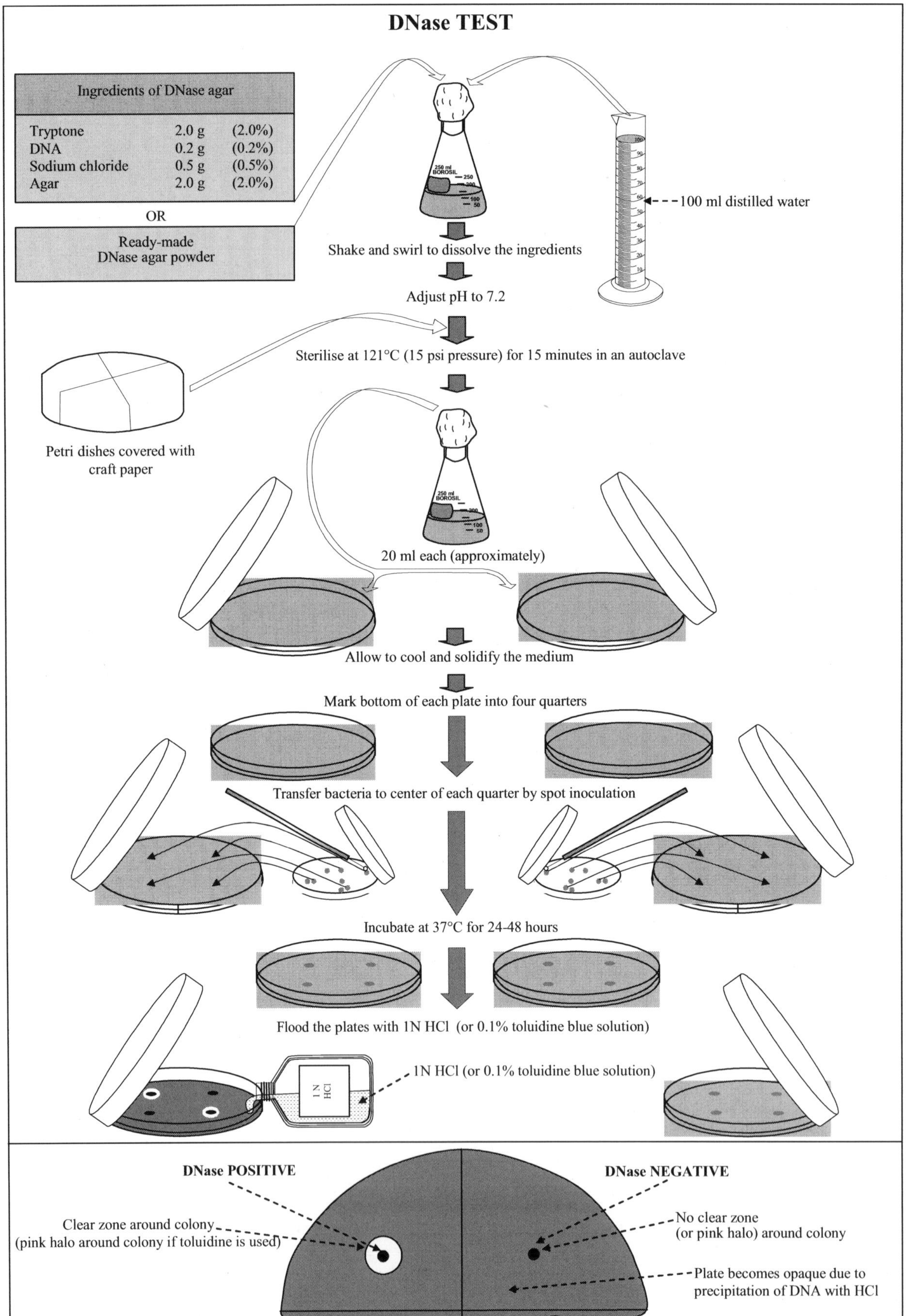

Figure 7.23: DNase test

3. Its pH is determined using a pH paper or pH meter and adjusted to 7.2 using 0.1N HCl if it is more or using 0.1N NaOH if it is less.
4. The flask is heated to dissolve the agar in the medium completely.
5. The flask is cotton-plugged, covered with craft paper and tied with thread or rubber band.
6. The two petri dishes and the conical flask containing DNase agar medium are sterilised at 121°C (15 psi pressure) for 15 minutes in an autoclave.
7. After sterilisation, they are removed from the autoclave and allowed to cool for sometime, without allowing the medium to solidify. Cooling of the medium prevents condensation and accumulation of water droplets inside the plates. If the medium has already been prepared and solidified during storage, it has to be liquefied by heating carefully till it melts completely.
8. To prepare DNase agar plates, before the sterilised DNase agar medium cools and solidifies, in warm molten condition, it is poured aseptically, preferably inside a laminar flow chamber, into the two sterilised petri dishes (approximately 20 ml each), so that the molten medium covers the bottom of the petri dishes completely. Then, the plates are covered with their lids and allowed to cool, so as to solidify the medium in them. Water vapour that may condense on the inner surface of the plates and lids is evaporated by keeping the plates and lids in inverted position in an incubator at 37°C for about 1 hour.
9. Each plate is marked on the bottom side into four quarters.
10. "Spot inoculation" of the test bacteria is done aseptically, preferably inside a laminar flow chamber, on the center of each quarter by making a spot (or small smear) of the bacteria with the help of a flame-sterilised loop. The loop is sterilised after each inoculation.
11. The inoculated plates are incubated in inverted position, top down, at 37°C for 24 to 48 hours in an incubator till colonies of the bacteria are visible.
12. The plates are flooded with solution of 1 N hydrochloric acid (or 0.1% toluidine blue) (*See* Appendix II at page 251).

Observations

1. *Transparent clear zones (or pink halo) formed around colonies*: DNase positive.
2. *Transparent clear zones (or pink halo) not formed around colonies*: DNase negative.

Experiment 47

(21) Coagulase Test

***Aim*: To perform coagulase test, to find out the ability of a bacteria to coagulate blood by producing the enzyme coagulase.**

Principle

The pathogenic strains of the bacteria *Staphylococcus* contain the enzyme coagulase, which acts within host tissues to convert fibrinogen to fibrin. The fibrin meshwork that is formed surrounds the bacteria cells or the infected tissues, protecting the bacteria from non-specific host resistance mechanisms, such as phagocytosis and the anti-staphylococcal activity of normal serum. This enzyme also helps in the coagulation of blood in the host by being a precursor of the thrombin-like substance, which coagulates or clots blood. The coagulase test is performed to distinguish between coagulase positive (pathogenic or virulent)) and coagulase negative (non-pathogenic or avirulent) *Staphylococcus*.

In the coagulase test, a suspension of the test species of *Staphylococcus* is mixed with blood plasma and the inoculated plasma is then periodically examined for fibrin formation or coagulation. Clot formation within four hours is interpreted as a positive result and indicative of a virulent (pathogenic) *Staphylococcus* strain. The absence of coagulation after 24 hours of incubation is a negative result, indicative of an avirulent (non-pathogenic) strain.

Reactions:

Blood - Blood cells (RBC, WBC etc) = Plasma

↓ + Coagulase from pathogenic *Staphylococcus* strain

Coagulation of plasma into clumps

Materials Required

Laboratory animal (rabbit or guinea pig), syringe, anticoagulant (sodium citrate or heparin), blood collection tubes, centrifuge, test tubes, slide, inoculating loop, bunsen burner, laminar flow chamber, dispose jar, isolated colonies or pure cultures of bacteria of the genus *Staphylococcus*.

Procedure

1. The syringe and the blood collection tubes are washed with solution of sodium citrate or heparin, so as to prevent clotting of blood immediately after collection (Figure 7.24).
2. With the help of the syringe, blood is collected from laboratory animals like rabbit or guinea pig and put into the collection tubes.
3. The blood is centrifuged at 3000 rpm for 15 minutes in a centrifuge.
4. The supernatant (plasma) is collected into another citrated test tube and the residue (blood cells) discarded.

(a) Slide Method

1. Two drops of a suspension of the test bacteria belonging to the genus *Staphylococcus,* is put on two equally divided halves of a slide with the help of an inoculating loop. One drop is used as 'control' to see if the bacteria itself is in clumps and the other drop is used as 'test'.
2. To the 'test drop', a drop of collected plasma is added, mixed and incubated at room temperature.
3. The drops are observed at hourly intervals upto 4 hours.

(b) Tube Method

1. Two small test tubes are taken. One test tube is marked 'test' and the other 'control'. In each test tube, 0.5 ml of the bacterial suspension is taken.
2. To the 'test' tube, 1 ml of plasma is added, mixed and incubated
3. The tubes are observed at hourly intervals upto 4 hours.

Observations

1. *Clumps are formed*: Coagulase positive *Staphylococcus.*
2. *Clumps are not formed*: Coagulase negative *Staphylococcus.*

Experiment 48

D. Identification of Unknown Bacteria

***Aim*: To identify an unknown bacteria.**

Principle

Identification of unknown bacteria is one of the major responsibilities of the microbiologists. Samples of blood, tissue, food, water and cosmetics are examined daily in laboratories throughout the world for the presence of contaminating microorganisms. In addition, industrial organisations are constantly screening materials to isolate new antibiotic-producing microbes or microbes that will increase the

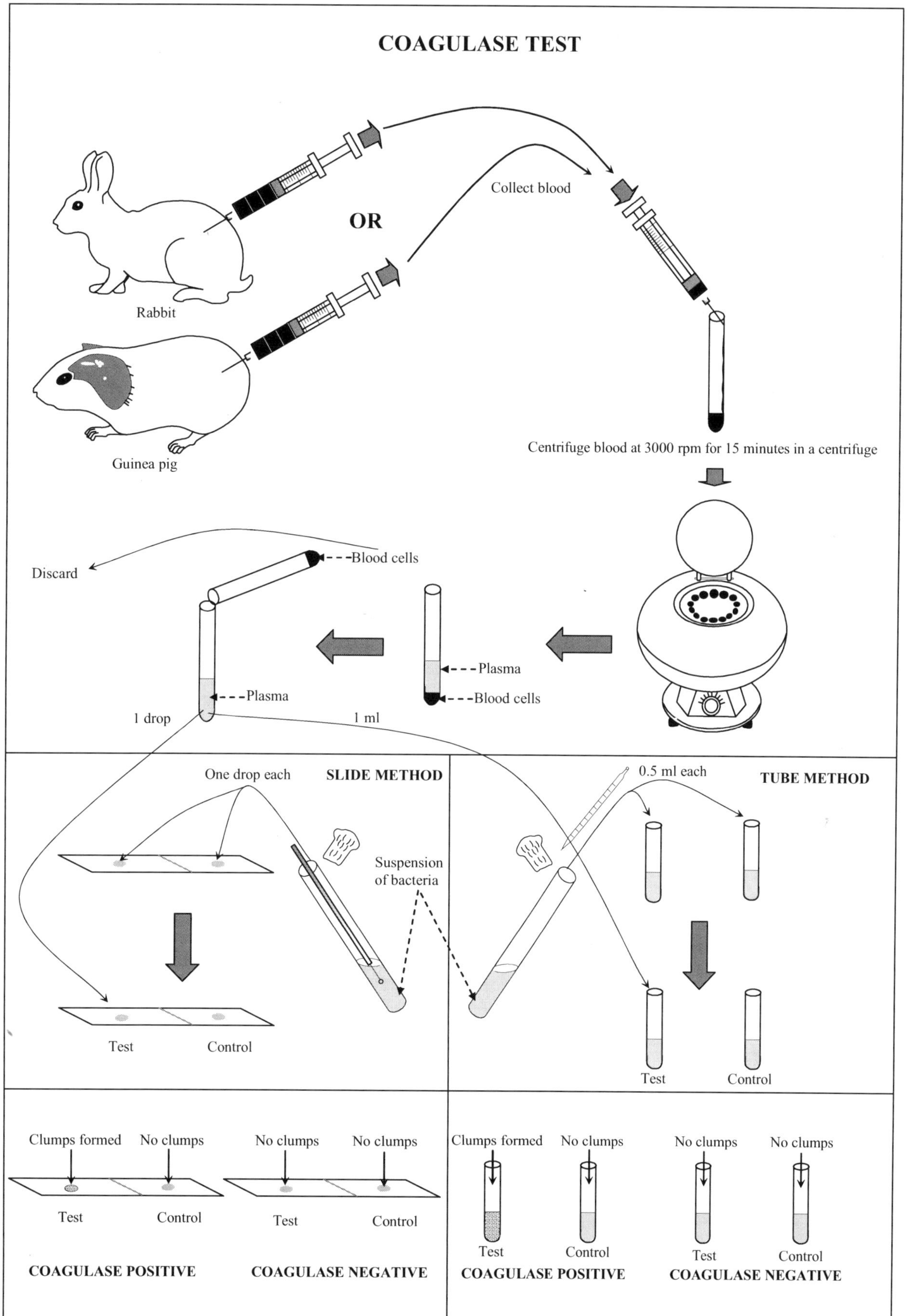

Figure 7.24: Coagulase test

yield of marketable products, such as vitamins, solvents and enzymes. Once isolated, these unknown microbes must be identified and classified. The science of classification is called taxonomy and deals with the separation of living organisms into interrelated groups. *Bergey's Manual of Determinative Bacteriology,* 8th edition, is the official taxonomic key containing the orders, families, genera and species of all known classified bacteria (Appendix III). With the fundamental knowledge in staining methods, isolation techniques, bacterial nutrition, biochemical activities and growth characteristics of bacteria, it becomes easier for identification of any unknown bacteria. Characteristics of few bacteria have been given in Table 7.2. Other bacteria can be identified in a similar way based on the observations and results obtained following the experimental procedures.

Materials Required

Slides, cavity slides, petri dishes, conical flasks, cotton plugs, inoculating loop, autoclave, bunsen burner, laminar flow chamber, dispose jar, incubator, nutrient broth, nutrient agar, gram staining reagents, media and reagents for biochemical tests, compound microscope, isolated colonies or pure cultures of bacteria.

Procedure

1. Gram staining of the unknown bacteria is performed. Besides gram staining, its morphology and arrangement is also recorded. Motility test of the bacteria is determined by hanging drop preparation (Figure 7.25).
2. Using sterile inoculating technique, the bacteria is inoculated into two nutrient agar slants, a nutrient broth tube and to a nutrient agar plate by means of streak inoculation. Following incubation, one slant culture is used to determine the cultural characteristics of the unknown bacteria. The second is used as a stock sub-culture, should it be necessary to repeat any of the tests. Growth characteristics are also observed in the broth tube and colony characteristics on the plate.
3. Exercising care in sterile technique, so as not to contaminate cultures and thereby obtain spurious results, the bacteria is inoculated into respective media to carry out the different biochemical tests.
4. The inoculated media are incubated at the required temperatures for the required lengths of time.

Observations

1. In gram staining, besides gram reaction, the morphology and arrangement of the bacteria are also recorded.
2. The cultural characteristics of the bacteria in nutrient broth, on agar slant and on nutrient agar plate are noted.
3. Results of the biochemical reactions are recorded.

Interpretation of Results

1. Using the above recorded data (For example, *see* Table 7.1) and with the help of the *Bergey's Manual of Determinative Bacteriology,* the bacteria is identified as to its genus and species. It should be kept in mind that, results might vary depending on the strains of each species used and the length of time the bacteria has been maintained in stock culture. The observed results may not be completely identical to the expected results. Therefore, the bacteria that best fits the results is chosen. The identifying characteristics of few bacteria have given in Table 7.2.
2. Alternatively, using the above-recorded data, code numbers are given for the recorded results (*See* Table 7.3) and the bacteria identified easily with the help of computer program available for Apple II, IBM PC or TRS-80. The program is designed to identify the unknown bacteria on

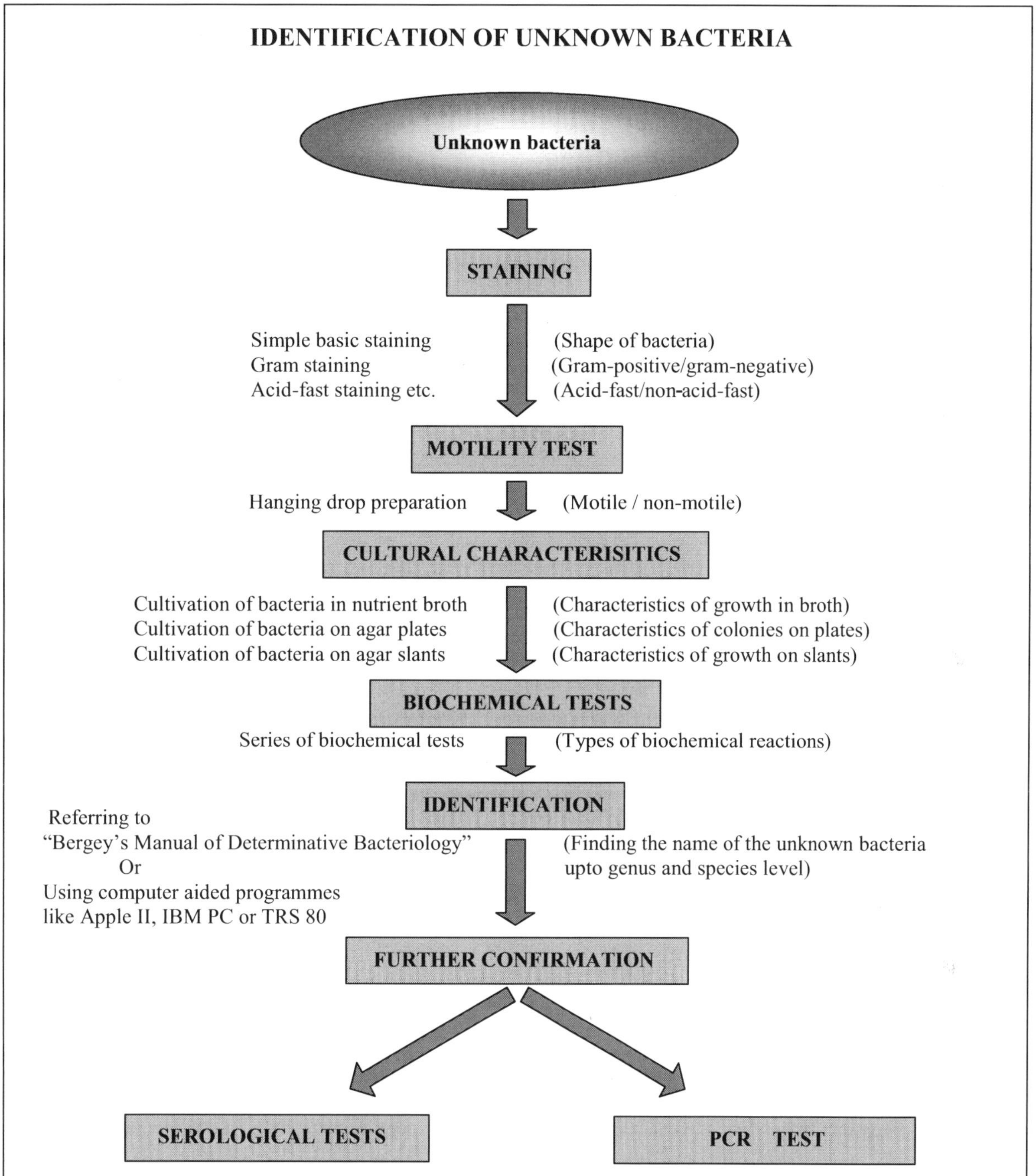

Figure 7.25: Identification of unknown bacteria

the basis of percentage of similarity between the unknown bacteria and the known bacteria with respect to the above observations.

To initiate the program for the *Apple II* or *IBM-PC*:

(*a*) The disc is inserted in the left drive.

(*b*) The computer is turned on.

(*c*) The program instructions are followed by typing the responses, unknown bacteria number and code numbers as the questions appear on the screen.

To initiate the program for the *TRS-80*:

(*a*) The computer is turned on.

(*b*) The disc is inserted in the bottom drive.

Table 7.1: Recording of data of unknown bacteria

DESCRIPTION OF UNKNOWN'S CHARACTERISTICS	*Student* ______ *Culture no.* ______ *Organism* ______		
Experimental Procedure	*Observations*	*Results*	*Computer Code No.*
Gram staining			
Acid-fast staining			
Shape (morphology)			
Cultural characteristics			
Litmus milk reactions			
Carbohydrate fermentation *Lactose* *Dextrose* *Sucrose* *Mannitol*			
H_2S production			
Nitrate reduction			
Indole production			
Methyl red test			
Voges-Proskauer test			
Citrate utilisation			
Urease activity			
Catalase activity			
Starch hydrolysis			
Lipid hydrolysis			

(*c*) The orange button is pressed.

(*d*) When asked, "date (MM/DD/YY)" is entered.

(*e*) Orange button is pressed again.

(*f*) Program instructions are followed by typing in the responses, unknown bacteria number and code numbers as the questions appear on the screen.

E. Automated Methods of Identification of Unknown Bacteria

Identification of unknown bacteria by the manual method using staining reactions, motility test, cultural characteristics and biochemical tests is a cumbersome, lengthy and time-consuming process. To make the process easy and short, automatic methods have been developed. These methods basically use the same biochemical tests as used in the manual methods, but here it is performed in an automatic manner and the interpretation is done with a computer-aided programme. Two such systems used at present for the automatic identification of bacteria are given as follows.

1. MINI API System (*See* page 56)
2. VITEK 2 System (*See* page 58)

F. Further Confirmation

(1) *Serological Tests*

Serological tests may be performed for further confirmation of the identified bacteria. To a suspension of the identified bacteria (*say* X), a drop of the antiserum (anti-X) against that bacteria is mixed. If it

Table 7.2: The identifying characteristics of few bacteria

Organism	Gram Stain	Agar slant cultural characteristics	Litmus milk reaction	Carbohydrate fermentation			H_2S production	Nitrate reduction	Indole production	MR reaction	VP reaction	Citrate utilisation	Urease activity	Catalase activity	Oxidase activity	Gelatin liquefaction	Starch hydrolysis	Lipid hydrolysis
				Lactose	Dextrose	Sucrose												
Escherichia coli	Rod −	White, moist, glistening growth	Acid, curd ±, gas ±, reduction ±	AG	AG	A ±	−	+	+	+	−	−	−	+	−	−	−	−
Enterobacter aerogenes	Rod −	Abundant, thick, white, glistening growth	Acid	AG	AG	AG ±	−	+	−	−	+	+	−	+	−	−	−	−
Klebsiella pneumoniae	Rod −	Slimy, white, somewhat–translucent, raised growth	Acid, gas, curd ±.	AG	AG	AG	−	+	−	−	±	+	+	+	−	−	−	−
Shigella dysenteriae	Rod −	Thin, even, grayish growth	Alkaline	−	A	A ±	−	+	+	+	−	−	−	+	−	−	−	−
Salmonella typhimurium	Rod −	Thin, even, grayish growth	Alkaline	−	AG ±	A ±	+	+	−	+	−	+	−	+	−	−	−	−
Proteus vulgaris	Rod −	Thin, blue–gray, spreading growth	Alkaline	−	AG	AG ±	+	+	+	+	−	−	+	+	−	+	−	−
Pseudomonas aeruginosa	Rod −	Abundant, thin, white growth, with medium turning green	Rapid peptoni-sation	−	−	−	−	+	−	−	−	+	−	+	+	+ Rapid	−	+
Alcaligens faecalis	Rod* −	Thin, white, spreading, viscous growth	Alkaline	−	−	−	−	−	−	−	−	−	−	+	+	−	−	−
Staphylococcus aureus	Coccus +	Abundant, opaque, golden growth	Acid, reduction, ±	A	A	A	−	+	−	+	±	−	−	+	−	+	−	+
Streptococcus lactis	Coccus +	Thin, even, growth	Acid, rapid reduction with curd	A	A	A	−	−	−	+	−	−	−	−	−	−	−	−
Micrococcus luteus	Coccus +	Soft, smooth, yellow growth	Alkaline	−	−	−	−	±	−	−	−	−	+	+	−	+ Slow	−	−
Corynebacterium xerosis	Rod +	Grayish, granular, limited growth	Alkaline	−	A ±	A ±	−	−	−	−	−	−	−	+	−	−	−	−
Bacillus cereus	Rod +	Abundant, opaque, white waxy growth	Peptoni-sation	−	A	A	−	+	−	−	±.	−	−	+	−	+ Rapid	+	+

Notes: AG: Acid and gas; ±: Variable reaction; Rod*: Coccobacillus.

results in the formation of clumps or precipitates (X-anti-X complex), then the identification is confirmed. The antisera for different bacteria are commercially available. They are produced commercially in different laboratories. The antiserum of a particular bacteria is produced by injecting killed or attenuated

Table 7.3: Code numbers for computer assisted identification of unknown bacteria

Test	Codes
Gram stain	0-not done 1-blue (Gram +) 2-red (Gram -)
Acid-fast stain	0-not done 1-red (acid-fast) 2-blue (non-acid fast)
Shape (morphology)	0-not done 1-straight rod 2-curved rod 3-spiral 4-spirochete 5-coccus 6-pleomorphic rod 7-coccobacillus
Cultural characteristics	0-not done 1-white, moist, glistening growth 2-abundant, white, thick, glistening growth 3-slimy, translucent, raised growth 4-thin, even, grayish growth 5-thin, bluish-gray, spreading growth 6-thin, transparent growth with medium turning green 7-thin, white, spreading, viscous growth 8-abundant, opaque, golden growth 9-thin, even, transparent growth 10-soft, smooth, yellow-pigmented growth 11-grayish, granular, united growth
Litmus milk reactions	0-not done 1-acid 2-acid, reduction 3-acid, reduction, curd 4-acid, reduction, curd, gas 5-peptonisation (proteolysis) 6-alkaline
Lactose fermentation **Dextrose fermentation** **Sucrose fermentation** **Mannitol fermentation**	0-not done 1-yellow medium (acid) 2-yellow medium + air bubble (acid + gas) 3-red medium (negative)
Hydrogen sulphide	0-not done 1-medium black (positive) 2-medium clear (negative)
Nitrate reduction	0-not done 1-red colour with solutions A + B (positive) 2-no colour change with solutions A + B + Zn (positive) 3-red colour with solutions A + B + Zn (negative)
Indole production	0-not done 1-red reagent layer (positive) 2-yellow reagent layer (negative)
Methyl red test	0-not done 1-red colouration of medium (positive) 2-yellow-orange colouration of medium (negative)
Voges-Proskauer test	0-not done 1-pink colouration of medium (positive) 2-no colour change in medium (negative)
Citrate utilization test	0-not done 1-growth, medium blue (positive) 2-no growth, medium green (negative)
Urease activity	0-not done 1-medium deep pink (positive) 2-no colour change in medium (negative)
Catalase activity	0--not done 1-evolution of oxygen bubbles (positive) 2-no evolution of oxygen bubbles (negative)
Starch hydrolysis	0-not done 1-clear zone with iodine (positive) 2-no clear zone with iodine (negative)
Lipid hydrolysis	0-not done 1-zone of lipolysis (positive) 2-no zone of lipolysis (negative)

cells of that bacteria (say X) into a laboratory animal. As a defense mechanism, the host animal produces antibodies (anti-X) against that bacteria, which remains in the blood. The blood is collected from this animal and its serum isolated by special techniques. This serum, containing antibody against that bacteria is called the antiserum of that bacteria.

(2) *PCR Test*

The Polymerase Chain Reaction (PCR) test is a rapid molecular method for confirmation of the identified bacteria. This technique is very often used for the detection of various bacteria and viruses quickly and precisely.

8

Cultivation of Viruses

A. Definition

Viruses are ultra-microscopic, non-cellular living particles, composed solely of a nucleic acid (DNA or RNA) core, surrounded by a protein envelope called capsid.

B. Characteristics of Viruses

The major distinguishing characteristics of viruses are given below.

1. They are non-cellular and very simple in structure, consisting mainly of a nucleic acid surrounded by a protein envelope called capsid. Therefore, a unit of virus is referred to as 'a virus particle' rather than 'a virus cell'.
2. They are devoid of the sophisticated enzymatic and biosynthetic machinery essential for independent activities of cellular life. Therefore, they can grow only inside suitable living cells. That is why, they are cultivated in the laboratory only inside living cells, unlike bacteria and fungi, which can be cultivated in the laboratory on non-living matter like nutrient agar.
3. They are ultra-microscopic and can only be visualised under electron microscope.
4. They do not increase in size.
5. They can pass through filters, through which bacteria cannot pass.
6. A virus is called either 'DNA virus' or 'RNA virus' depending on whether it contains the nucleic acid DNA or RNA. A virus cannot have both DNA and RNA

C. Structure of Viruses

Much of our knowledge about viruses has been gathered from the study of few viruses, which infect bacteria. These viruses, which infect bacteria, are called 'bacteriophages' or 'phages'. The bacteriophages were first described in 1915 almost simultaneously by Twort and d'Herelle. The name bacteriophage, which in Greek means *to eat bacteria,* was coined by d'Herelle because of the ability of these viruses to destroy the infected bacteria cells through lysis. Bacteriophages exhibit notable variability in their size, shape and complexity of structure. The T-even (T_2, T_4 and T_6) phages demonstrate the greatest morphological complexity (Figure 8.1). The functions of its structural components are as follows.

1. *Capsid (Protein Coat)*: Protection of nucleic acid from destruction by DNase.
2. *Nucleic Acid Core*: Phage genome carrying genetic information necessary for replication of new phage.

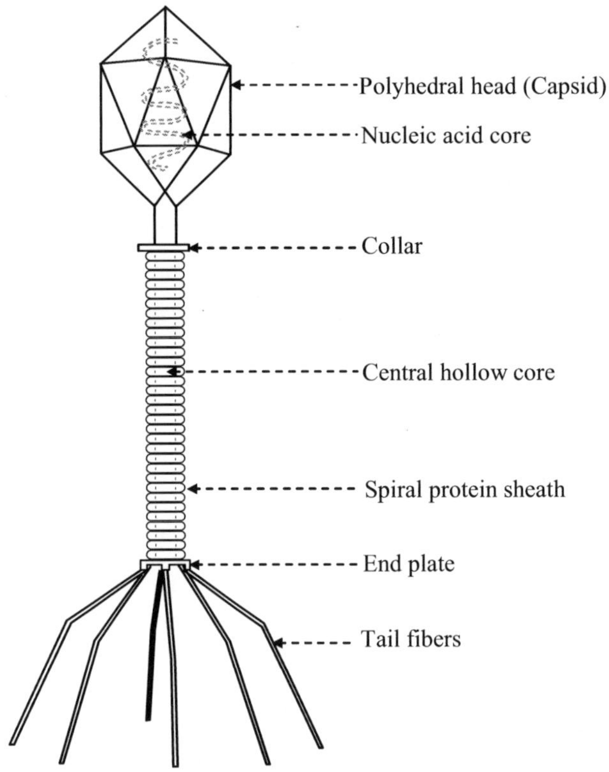

Figure 8.1: Structure of T-even bacteriophage

3. *Spiral Protein Sheath*: Retracts, so that nucleic acid can pass from capsid into host cell's cytoplasm.
4. *End Plate and Tail Fibers*: Attachment of phage to specific receptor sites on a susceptible host's cell wall.

D. Viral Infection

Phage replication depends on the ability of the phage particle to infect a suitable bacterial host cell. Infection consists of the following sequential events.

1. *Adsorption*: Tail portion of the phage particle binds to receptor sites on host's cell wall.
2. *Penetration (Infection)*: Spiral protein sheath retracts and an enzyme, early muramidase, perforates the bacterial cell wall enabling the phage nucleic acid to pass through the hollow core into the host cell's cytoplasm. The empty protein shell remains attached to the cell wall and is called the protein ghost.
3. *Replication*: The phage genome subverts the synthetic machinery, which is then used for the production of new phage components.
4. *Maturation*: The new phage components are assembled and form complete, mature virulent phage particles.
5. *Release*: Late muramidase lyses the cell wall, liberating infectious phage particles that are now capable of infecting new susceptible host cells, thereby starting the cycle over again.

E. Shape of Viruses

The shape of some of the important viruses has been revealed by electron microscope (Figure 8.2). All of them cause different diseases in plants and animals. The bacteriophages infect bacteria cells.

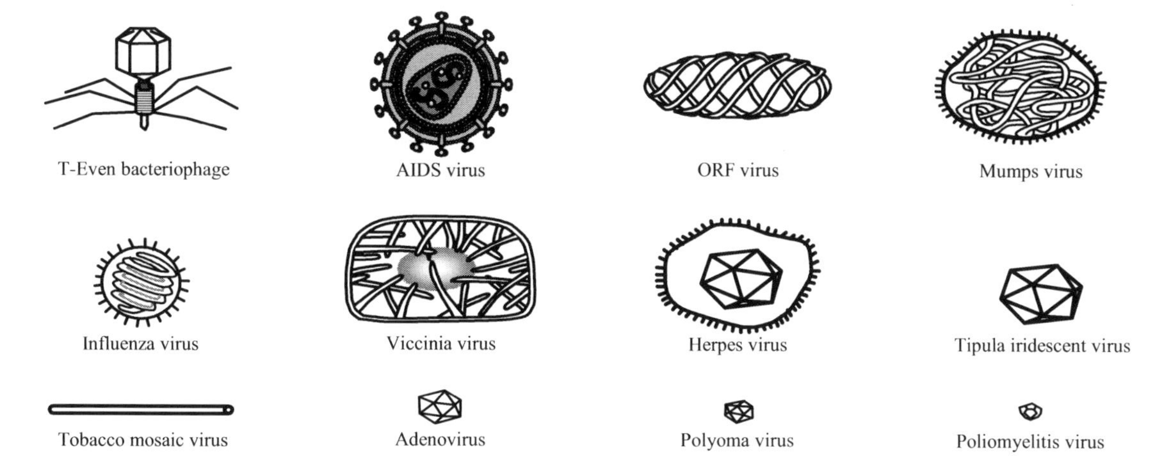

Figure 8.2: Shape of some common viruses

Experiment 49

F. Cultivation and Enumeration of Bacteriophages

***Aim*: To cultivate and enumerate a bacteriophage.**

Principle

A suspension of bacteria, susceptible to a bacteriophage (virus that infects bacteria) is seeded with that bacteriophage and allowed to grow as a confluent lawn on an agar plate. The bacteriophage particles grow within the bacteria cells and lyse them. Lysis of the bacteria cells results in the formation of clear zones in the confluent lawn of bacteria. These clear zones are called 'plaques'. Each clear zone is assumed to be formed by a single bacteriophage particle. Thus, the number of plaque forming units (PFUs) represents the number of the bacteriophage. Serial dilution technique is used in the enumeration of bacteriophages similar to that used in the enumeration of bacteria. The number of phage particles contained in a sample is determined by counting the number of plaques formed on the seeded agar plate and multiplying this by the dilution factor. To determine a valid phage count, the number of plaques per plate should not exceed 300 nor be less than 30. Plates showing greater than 300 PFUs are termed 'too numerous to count' (TNTC), while plates showing fewer than 30 PFUs are termed 'too few to count' (TFTC).

Materials Required

Tryptone broth, tryptone soft agar, tryptone hard agar (*See* Appendix I at page 247), conical flask, test tubes, sterilised petri dishes, cotton plugs, stock culture of bacteriophage (Ex: T_2coliphage), nutrient broth culture of the bacteria (Ex: *Escherichia coli B*), sterilised pipettes, autoclave, hot water bath, bunsen burner, laminar flow chamber, dispose jar, incubator.

Procedure

1. Fifteen pipettes (in a stainless steel pipette case) and five petri dishes are sterilised in a hot air oven at 180° C for 3 hours. Alternatively, they can be covered with craft paper, tied with thread or rubber band and sterilised in an autoclave along with the media (Figure 8.3).
2. The ingredients of tryptone broth medium (*See* Appendix I at page 247) or its ready-made powder, required for 100 ml of the broth is weighed and dissolved in 100 ml of distilled water in a 250 ml conical flask by shaking and swirling. Its pH is adjusted to 7.5 using 0.1N HCl or 0.1N NaOH as required. The flask is heated, if required, to dissolve the ingredients completely.
3. The broth is distributed into 10 test tubes (9 ml each), cotton-plugged, covered with craft paper and tied with thread or rubber band.

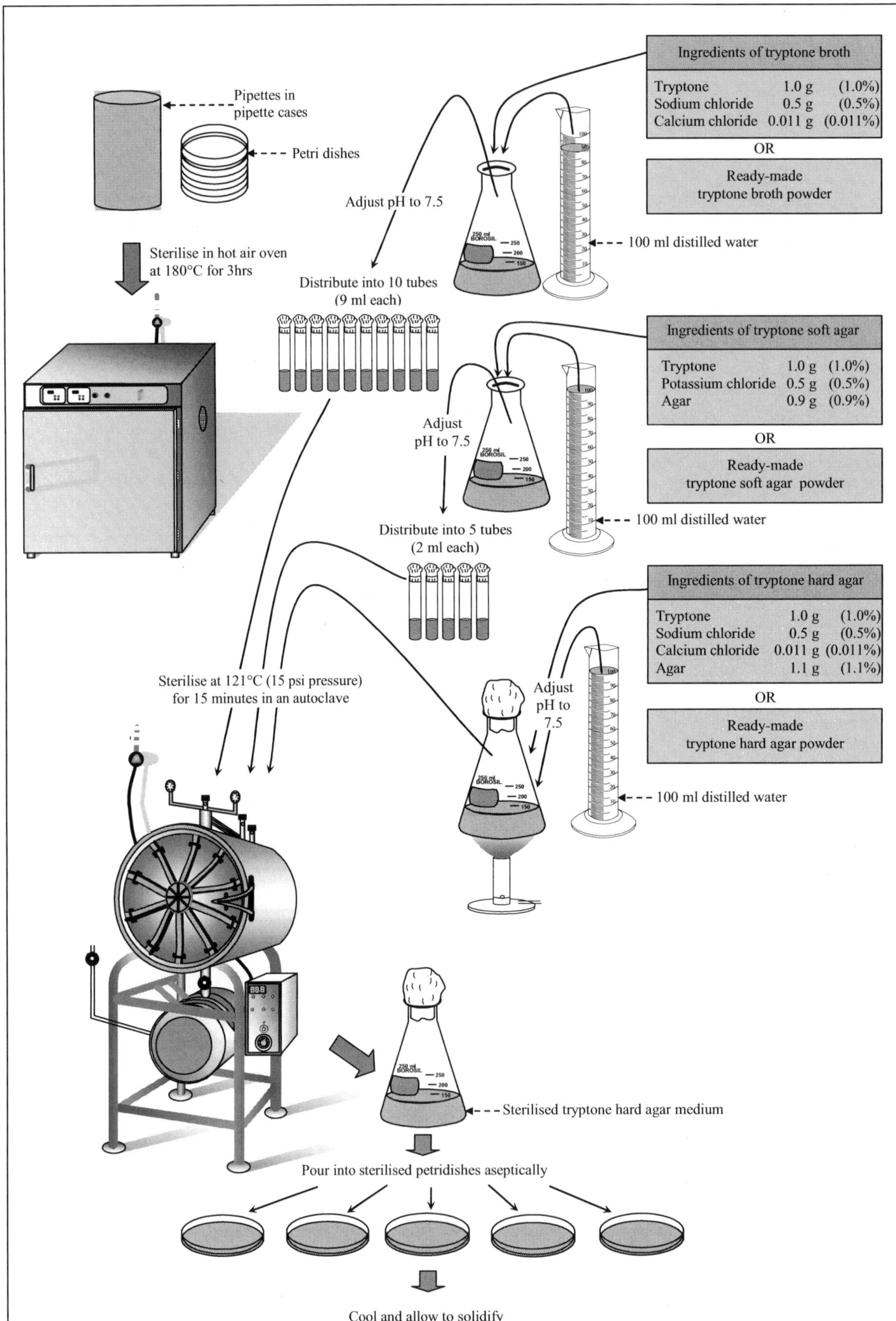

Figure 8.3: Cultivation and enumeration of bacteriophage: Preparation and sterilisation of media

4. The ingredients of tryptone soft agar medium (*See* Appendix I at page 247) or its ready-made powder, required for 100 ml of the medium is weighed and dissolved in 100 ml of distilled water in a 250 ml conical flask by shaking and swirling. Its pH is adjusted to 7.5 using 0.1N HCl or 0.1N NaOH as required. The flask is heated to dissolve the agar in the medium completely.
5. This liquid medium is distributed into 5 test tubes (2 ml each), cotton-plugged, covered with craft paper and tied with thread or rubber band.
6. The ingredients of tryptone hard agar medium (*See* Appendix I at page 247) or its ready-made powder required for 100 ml of the medium is weighed and dissolved in 100 ml of distilled water in a 250 ml conical flask by heating after pH adjustment to 7.5. The flask is cotton-plugged, covered with craft paper and tied with thread or rubber band.
7. The 10 tryptone broth tubes, the 5 tryptone soft agar tubes and the flask containing tryptone hard agar medium are sterilised at 121°C (15 psi pressure) for 15 minutes in an autoclave.
8. The sterilised tryptone hard agar medium in the conical flask is poured into 5 sterilised petri dishes aseptically to get 5 tryptone hard agar plates.
9. One ml of the stock culture of the bacteriophage (Ex: T_2 coliphage) is aseptically transferred, preferably in a laminar flow chamber, to a tryptone broth tube (9 ml) using a sterilised pipette. This becomes the 10 times dilution (*i.e.* 10^{-1}). This is aseptically diluted serially into the other nine broth tubes, so as to get a final dilution of 10^{-10} (Figure 8.4).
10. The 5 sterilised tryptone soft agar tubes are taken and heated on a water bath to 100°C, so as to melt the agar. The tubes are cooled and the molten soft soft tubes are maintained at 45°C.
11. From among the above 10 tubes containing phages at different concentrations, five tubes (*i.e.* 10^{-5}, 10^{-6}, 10^{-7}, 10^{-8} and 10^{-9}) are selected. From these tubes, aseptically 1 ml each is transferred to the five tryptone soft agar tubes using separate sterilised pipettes.
12. Two drops of nutrient broth culture of the bacteria (Ex: *Escherichia coli B*) is aseptically transferred, preferably in a laminar flow chamber, to each tryptone soft agar tube containing the bacteriophage at five different concentrations (10^{-5} to 10^{-9}).
13. The contents of the five tryptone soft agar tubes containing the bacteriophage and the bacteria are rapidly mixed by rotating between the palms of hands.
14. The contents are aseptically poured over the five tryptone hard agar plates labeled 10^{-5} to 10^{-9}, thereby forming a double layer plate culture preparation. The plates are swirled gently and allowed to harden.
15. The plates are incubated in inverted position at 37°C in an incubator.

Observations

1. All the plates are observed for plaque forming units (PFUs) that develop as clear zones on the lawn of bacteria.
2. Only those plates having PFUs between 30 and 300 are considered for enumeration of phage. The number of PFUs on each plate is counted. Plates showing greater than 300 PFUs are designated 'too numerous to count' (TNTC), while plates showing fewer than 30 PFUs are designated 'too few to count' (TFTC). Such plates are not considered.
3. Based on the observations, the number of bacteriophages per ml of the stock phage culture is calculated using following formula.

No. of phages/ml = No. of PFUs X dilution factor

For example, if the number of PFUs is 280 in a dilution of 10^{-7}, then the number of phage in the stock culture of phage is 280 X 10^7 phage/ml (= 2.80 X 10^9 phage/ml).

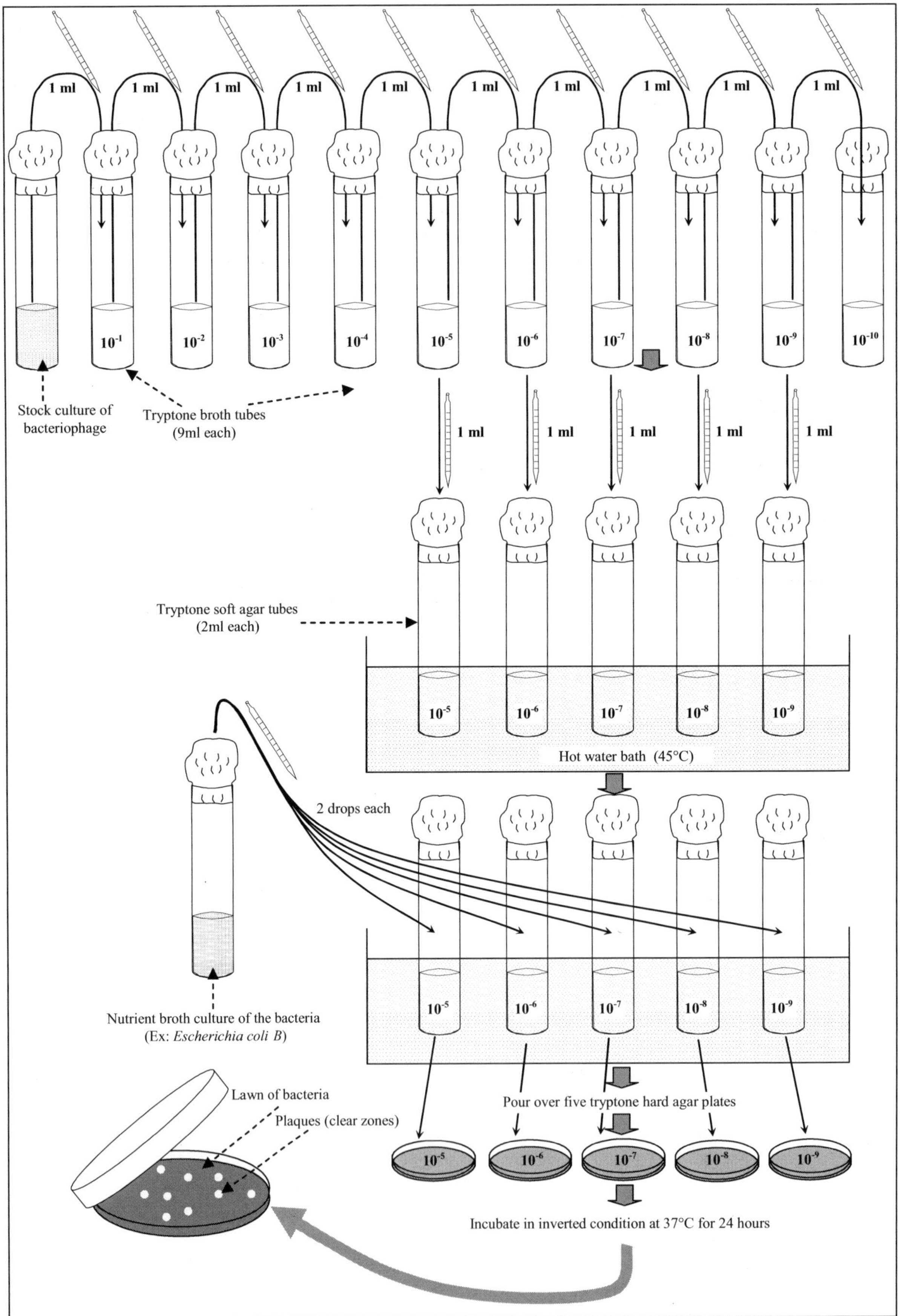

Figure 8.4: Cultivation and enumeration of bacteriophage: Inoculation and incubation

Experiment 50

G. Isolation of Coliphage

***Aim*: To isolate coliphage from a given sample.**

Principle

The bacteriophage or phage (virus) that infects the bacteria, *Escherichia coli* is called coliphage (*coli*: *E. coli*; *phage*: bacteriophage). It can be obtained from a variety of natural sources, such as soil, fecal matter and raw sewage. Its isolation from these sources is not very easy, as it is present in low concentration. Therefore, first its number is increased by an enrichment step, in which a rich culture of the host bacteria (*i.e. E. coli*) is added to the coliphage-containing sample and incubated. The coliphage infects *E. coli* and increases in number profusely. This coliphage-rich culture is centrifuged to settle down the particulate matter. The sediment is discarded and the supernatant is filtered through microbial filter to retain bacteria and other particles, while allowing the coliphage to pass through. The filtrate, rich in coliphage, is used to seed a suspension of *E. coli*, which is then allowed to grow as a confluent lawn on an agar plate. The coliphage grows within the *E. coli* cells and lyse them. Lysis of the bacteria cells results in the formation of clear zones on the confluent lawn of bacteria. These clear zones are called plaques. Each clear zone is assumed to be formed by a single coliphage.

Materials Required

Pipettes, conical flasks, petri dishes, test tubes, cotton plugs, bunsen burner, dispose jar, centrifuge, membrane filtration apparatus, laminar flow chamber, autoclave, incubator, bacteriophage broth, tryptone soft agar, tryptone hard agar (*See* Appendix I at page 247), nutrient broth culture of the bacteria *Escherichia coli* (*e.g., E. coli B*), sample (*e.g.,* raw sewage).

Procedure

1. Five pipettes (in a stainless steel pipette case) and five petri dishes are sterilised in a hot air oven at 180° C for 3 hours. Alternatively, they can be covered with craft paper, tied with thread or rubber band and sterilised in an autoclave along with the media (Figure 8.5).
2. The ingredients of bacteriophage broth medium (*See* Appendix I at page 247) or its ready-made powder, required for 100 ml of the medium is weighed, dissolved in 100 ml of distilled water in a 250 ml conical flask and pH adjusted to 7.6. The flask is cotton-plugged, covered with craft paper and tied with thread or rubber band.
3. The ingredients of tryptone soft agar medium or its ready-made powder, required for 100 ml of the medium is weighed, dissolved in 100 ml of distilled water in a 250 ml conical flask and pH adjusted to 7.5.
4. This liquid medium is distributed into 5 test tubes (2 ml each), cotton-plugged, covered with craft paper and tied with thread or rubber band.
5. The ingredients of tryptone hard agar medium or its ready-made powder required for 100 ml of the medium is weighed and dissolved in 100 ml of distilled water in a 250 ml conical flask by heating after pH adjustment to 7.5. The flask is cotton-plugged, covered with craft paper and tied with thread or rubber band.
6. The flask containing bacteriophage broth, the 5 tryptone soft agar tubes, the flask containing tryptone hard agar medium and an empty cotton-plugged 250 ml conical flask are sterilised at 121°C (15 psi pressure) for 15 minutes in an autoclave.
7. The sterilised tryptone hard agar medium in the conical flask is poured into the 5 sterilised petri dishes aseptically and allowed to cool, so as to get 5 tryptone hard agar plates.
8. Into the cotton-plugged sterilised empty 250 ml conical flask, 5 ml of sterilised bacteriophage broth, 5 ml of *E. coli B* broth culture and 45 ml of raw sewage are transferred aseptically, preferably in a laminar flow chamber (Figure 8.6).

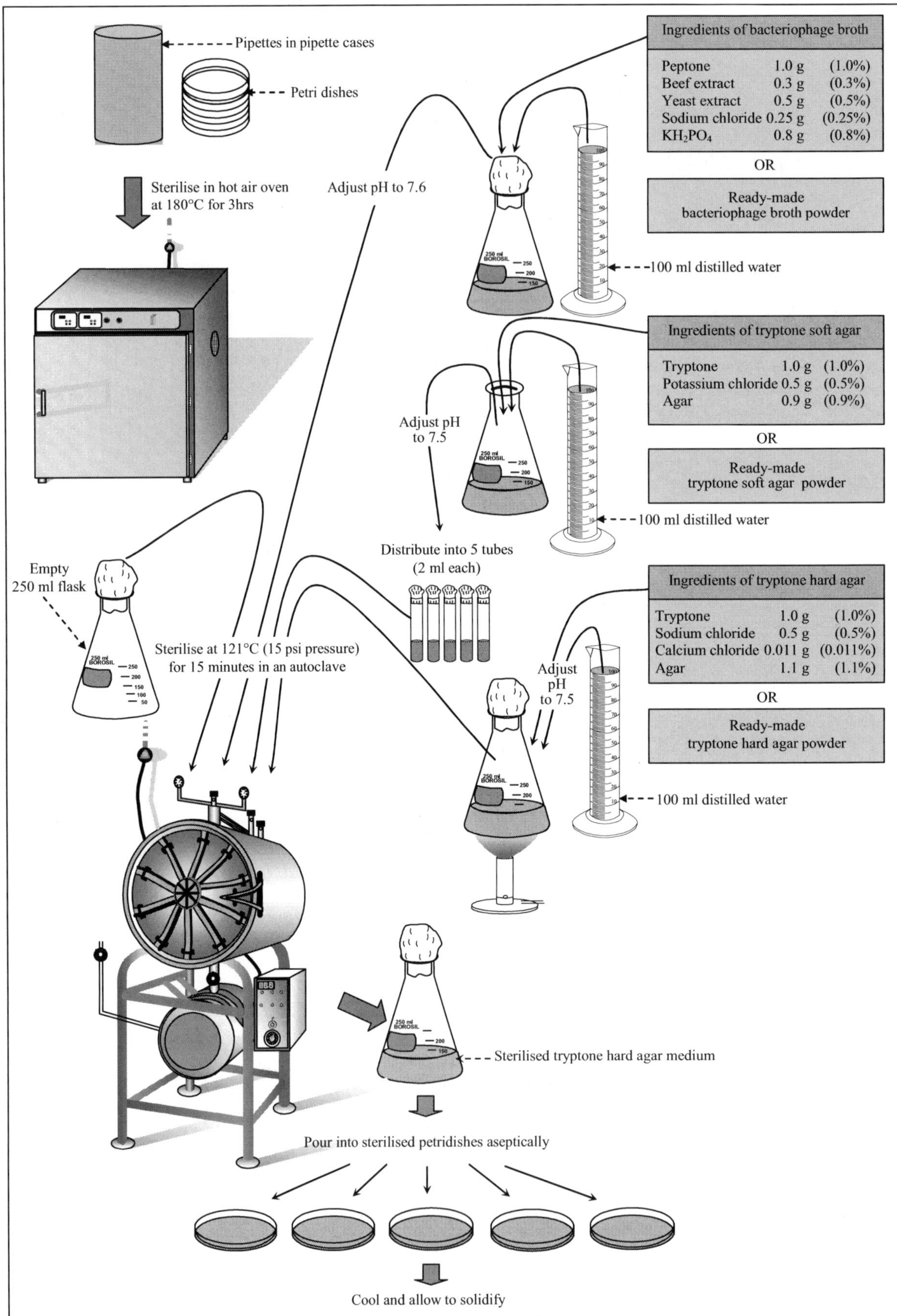

Figure 8.5: Isolation of coliphage: Preparation and sterilisation of media

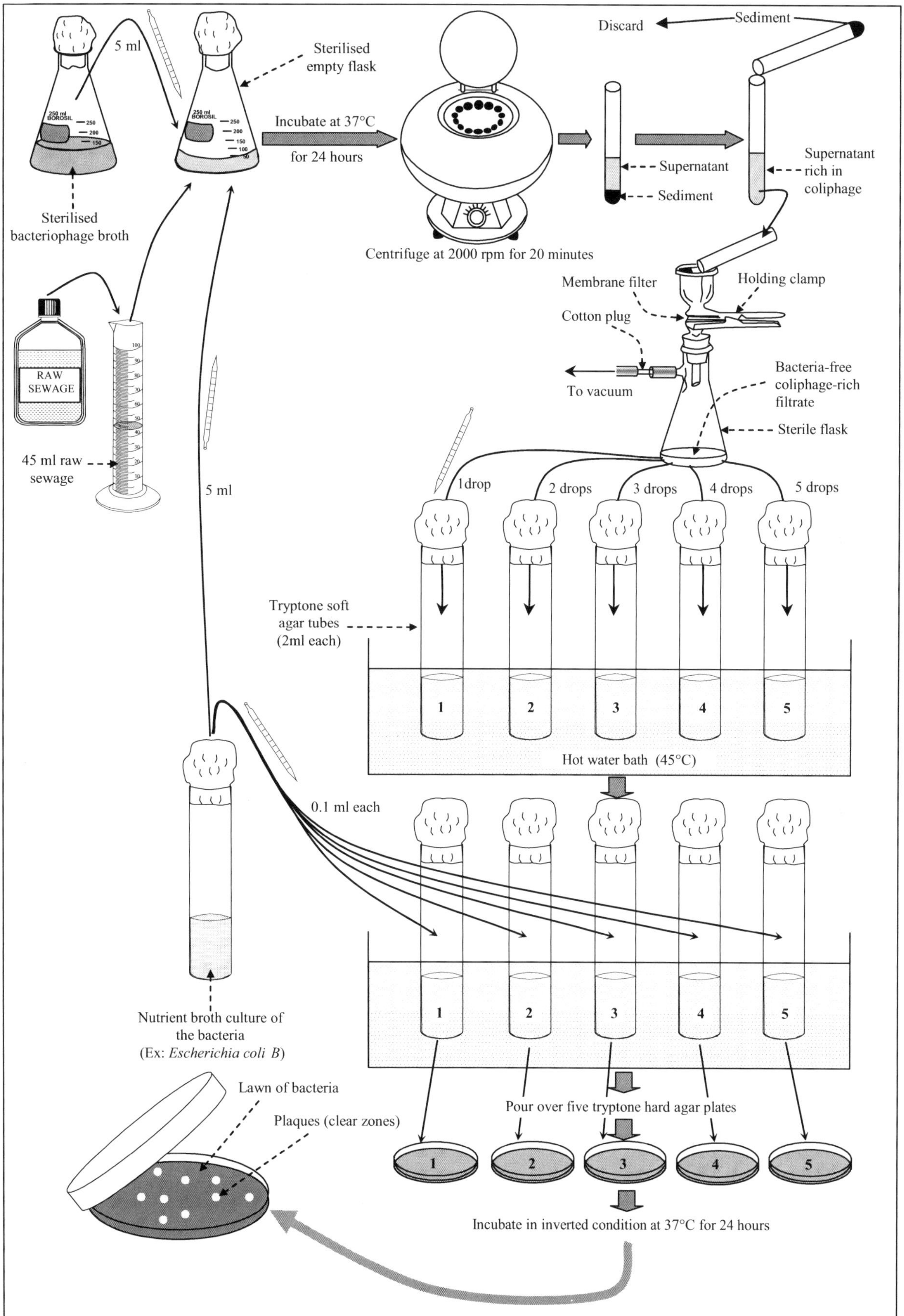

Figure 8.6: Isolation of coliphage: Inoculation, incubation and enumeration

9. The flask is incubated at 37°C for 24 hours, so as to allow the coliphage in the sewage to proliferate within the host bacteria cells (cells of *E. coli B*).
10. The contents of the flask is poured into 100 ml centrifuge tubes and centrifuged at 2500 rpm for 20 minutes in a centrifuge to settle down the particles. The sediment is discarded.
11. The supernatant, rich in coliphage, is filtered through a membrane filtration apparatus. The residue is discarded.
12. The five sterilised tryptone soft agar tubes are taken and heated on a water bath to 100°C, so as to melt the agar. The tubes are cooled and maintained at 45°C on a water bath.
13. Using a sterile pipette, 1, 2, 3, 4 and 5 drops of the bacteria-free filtrate, rich in coliphage is transferred aseptically to the five tryptone soft agar tubes.
14. To each tryptone soft agar tube, 0.1 ml of a nutrient broth culture of *Escherichia coli B* is transferred aseptically.
15. The contents of the five tryptone soft agar tubes having the virus, coliphage and the bacteria, *E. coli B* are rapidly mixed by rotating the tubes between the palms of hands.
16. The contents are poured over the five tryptone hard agar plates (labeled 1 to 5 drops), thereby forming a double layer plate culture preparation. The plates are swirled gently and allowed to harden.
17. The inoculated plates are incubated in an inverted position at 37°C for 24 hours in an incubator.

Observations

1. All the plates are observed for plaque forming units (PFUs) that develop as clear zones on the lawn of bacteria. Plaque formation is indicative of presence of coliphage in the culture.
2. Each plaque represents a rich growth of isolated coliphage.
3. The number of plaques is counted in all the plates and tabulated as follows (Table 8.1).

Table 8.1: Observations of the number of coliphage

Number of Drops	*Number of Plaques*
1 drop	
2 drops	
3 drops	
4 drops	
5 drops	

Experiment 51

H. Cultivation of Animal Virus in Embryonated Chick Egg

***Aim*: To cultivate animal virus in embryonated chick egg.**

Principle

Viruses can grow only in living systems. They cannot grow in non-living media like nutrient agar or nutrient broth. Therefore, their cultivation needs host cells susceptible to the specific virus. The virus such as bacteriophage, which infects and grows in bacteria cells are cultivated using cultures of bacteria cells as the living system. For example, the virus coliphage (a bacteriophage) is cultivated using the culture of the bacteria *E. coli*. In contrast, animal viruses, which infect and grow in the body of animals, require susceptible living animal systems. The three living animal systems used for cultivation of animal viruses in the laboratories are as follows.

1. *Susceptible Animals*

In this technique, the virus to be cultivated is allowed to grow in the body of a living animal such as mouse or guinea pig, which is susceptible to that virus. This technique is no longer used having been replaced by the following more recent, efficient and economic techniques.

2. *Tissue Culture*

It is a highly sophisticated technique. Here animal cells known to be susceptible to the virus to be cultivated and also known to multiply rapidly are first isolated from suitable living tissue of an animal. These cells are placed in a glass or plastic vessel containing an extremely rich nutritional medium. The cells attach to the surface of the vessel and continue dividing until the entire surface is covered with a confluent monolayer of cells. This is called tissue culture. Then, the virus to be cultivated is inoculated into the susceptible tissue culture. The virus infects the living cells of the tissue culture, subvert their metabolic machinery and replicate rapidly, thereby growing profusely in the cells.

3. *Embryonated Chick Eggs*

In this simple and economic technique, the virus to be cultivated is injected into an embryonated chick egg[1]. The virus grows within the living chick egg and causes disease in the embryo, manifested by several disease symptoms (cytopathogenic effects) specific to that virus. Presence of these symptoms indicates the growth of that virus within the egg.

Materials Required

Two embryonated chick eggs, candling device, tincture iodine, absorbent cotton, 70% alcohol, a small drill, 1:2 dilution of Newcastle virus, syringe, sterile vasper, sterile saline, petri dishes, bunsen burner, laminar flow chamber, dispose jar, incubator.

Procedure

1. Two embryonated chick eggs are candled using a candling device to demonstrate the viability of the embryo. The embryo is viable, if it shows movement in response to heat from light. Also the positions of the air sac and large blood vessels are determined and marked on the egg shell during candling (Figure 8.7).
2. The shell is disinfected over the air sac with tincture iodine and then allowed to dry. The same place is swabbed with absorbent cotton soaked with 70% alcohol.
3. The tip of a small drill is sterilised by dipping in 70% alcohol and then flaming it.
4. Using this drill, a small hole is made aseptically on the shell over the air sac in a region away from the blood vessels.
5. 0.2 ml of the 1:2 dilution of Newcastle virus is aseptically injected into the allantoic cavity of one of the two eggs using a sterilised syringe. This is done by holding the egg in a vertical position, inserting the needle of the syringe through the hole on the shell to its hilt at a 45° angle, piercing the air sac membrane and penetrating into the allantoic cavity. This virus-inoculated egg serves as the 'test egg'.
6. After inoculation, the needle is withdrawn and the hole on the shell is sealed with sterile hot vasper.
7. Using the same technique, 0.2 ml of sterile saline is inoculated into the other embryonated chick egg, which serves as the 'control egg'.
8. Both the eggs are incubated at 37°C for 3 to 4 days in an incubator with proper humidity.
9. The observations are noted everyday.

---

1 Chick eggs are of two types as follows.

(*i*) *Fertilized chick egg (embryonated chick eggs)*: These are produced after the fertilization of the egg present in the hen by the sperm from the cock, so that the egg contains an embryo. These eggs can hatch to chicks after proper incubation.

(*ii*) *Unfertilised eggs*: These are the eggs produced within the hens and released to outside without fertilization. These eggs cannot hatch to chicks. These are the eggs commercially available in the market and used as food.

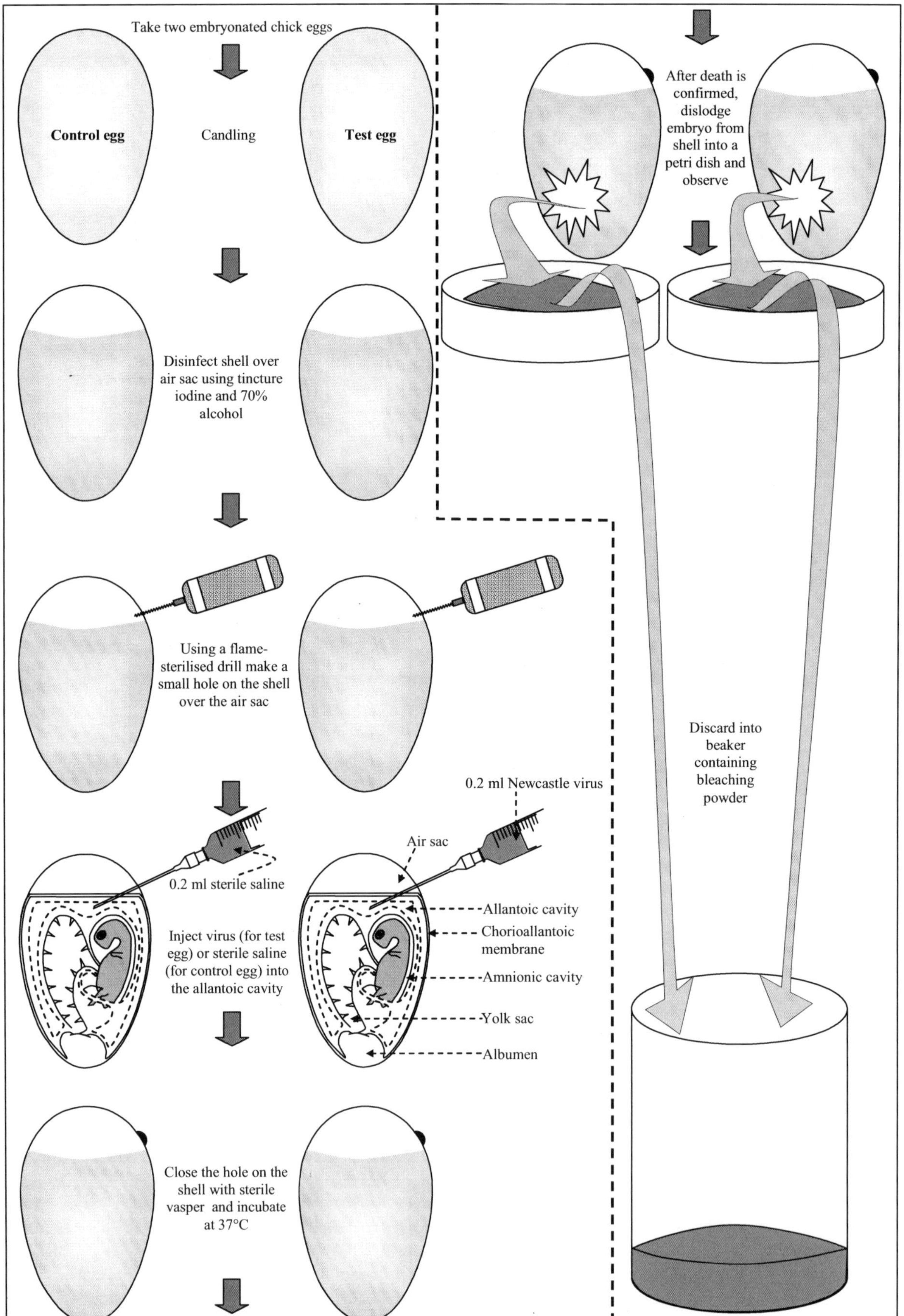

Figure 8.7: Cultivation of animal virus in embryonated chick egg

10. Once death has been determined, the embryo is dislodged from its shell and the contents poured into a petri dish and again observed.
11. All contaminated materials are discarded into a beaker containing bleaching powder.

Observations

1. The eggs are candled everyday during incubation and observed for embryonic death as evidenced by cessation of movement, which usually occurs 3 to 4 days following inoculation of the virus.
2. Once death has been determined, the embryo is dislodged from its shell and the contents poured into a petri dish. It is observed for necrotic lesions and evidence of hemorrhage.
3. The control egg is examined for evidence of cytopathogenic effects.
4. The observations are recorded in Table 8.2.

Table 8.2: Observations of the embryonated chick eggs (control and virus infected)

Symptoms	*Sample*	*Days of Incubation*			
		1st day	*2nd day*	*3rd day*	*4th day*
Movement (+ or –)	Virus infected				
	Control				
Viability (+ or –)	Virus infected				
	Control				
Presence of necrotic lesions (+ or –)	Virus infected				
	Control				
Hemorrhage (+ or –)	Virus infected				
	Control				

9

Identification of Protozoa

A. Definition

Protozoa are eukaryotic, unicellular microorganisms, which lack cell wall.

B. Characteristics of Protozoa

The major distinguishing characteristics of protozoa are given below.

1. They do not have cell wall; some however, possess a flexible layer, a pellicle, or a rigid shell of inorganic materials outside the cell membrane.
2. They have the ability during their entire life cycle or part of it to move by locomotor organelles or by a gliding mechanism.
3. They have heterotrophic mode of nutrition, whereby the free-living forms ingest particulates, such as bacteria, yeast and algae, while the parasitic forms derive nutrients from the body fluids of their hosts.
4. They reproduce primarily by asexual means, although in some groups sexual modes also occur.

C. Classification of Protozoa

The classification of protozoa is mainly based on their means of locomotion. They are subdivided into the following four classes (or subphyla by some taxonomists). Species marked with asterisks(*) have been described in details with illustrations.

1. Sarcodina

Motility is due to the streaming of ectoplasm, producing protoplasmic projections called pseudopodia (false feet). Examples: Free-living form like *Amoeba proteus** and parasitic form like *Entamoeba histolytica**.

2. Mastigophora

Locomotion is effected by one or more whip-like, thin structures called flagella. Examples: Free-living forms like *Euglena viridis**, *Cercomonas longicauda**, *Heteronema acus** and parasitic forms like *Trichomonas vaginalis*, *Trypanosoma gambiense**, *Giardia lamblia**.

3. Ciliophora

Locomotion is carried out by means of short hair-like projections called cilia, whose synchronous beating propels the organisms. Examples: Free-living forms like *Paramecium caudatum**, *Stentor polymorpha**, *Vorticella campanula** and parasitic form like *Balantidium coli**.

4. Sporozoa

Unlike the above three classess of protozoa, members of the class sporozoa do not have locomotor organelles in their mature stage; however, immature forms exhibit some type of movement. All the members of this group are parasites. Examples: *Plasmodium*, the malarial parasites of animals and human beings.

D. Types of Protozoa

Based on the mode of nutrition, protozoa are of the following two types.

1. Free-living protozoa: They ingest particulates, such as bacteria, yeast and algae.
2. Parasitic protozoa: They derive nutrients from the body fluids of their hosts.

Experiment 52

E. Identification of Free-living Protozoa

***Aim*: To identify an unknown free-living protozoa.**

Principle

There are more than 20,000 known species of free-living protozoa. They are identified with the help of their structural characteristics observed under microscope. The structural characteristics of few of the free-living protozoa and meaning of these structures have been given in Figure 9.1.

Materials Required

Pond water, sampling bottle, dropper, glass slide, methylcellulose, cover slip, compound microscope

Procedure

1. Pond water is collected in a bottle from the bottom layer of the pond.
2. A drop of the pond water is placed at the center of a clean slide.
3. A drop of methylcellulose is added to the water on the slide to slow down the movement of the protozoa.
4. One edge of a cover slip is placed against the outer edge of the drop of water.
5. After the drop of water spreads along the inner edge of the cover slip, the cover slip is gently lowered onto the slide.
6. The slide preparation is observed under low power and high power objectives of a compound microscope with diminished light.

Observations

Protozoa can be seen in the drop of water. Sketches of the protozoa are drawn as observed under the microscope. They are identified by comparing their structures with those of different protozoa available in the literature (Figure 9.1).

Experiment 53

F. Identification of Parasitic Protozoa

***Aim*: To identify an unknown parasitic protozoa.**

Principle

Unlike the free-living protozoa, the life cycle of parasitic protozoa vary greatly in complexity. Knowledge of the various developmental stages in their life cycles is essential in the diagnosis, clinical management and chemotherapy of parasitic infection. As they are parasitic, they are found only in the diseased individuals and therefore, cannot be demonstrated directly. Therefore, prepared slides are used to acquaint the students with these parasites. Any parasitic protozoa is identified based on its

<table>
<tr>
<td>

Class Sarcodina

AMOEBA

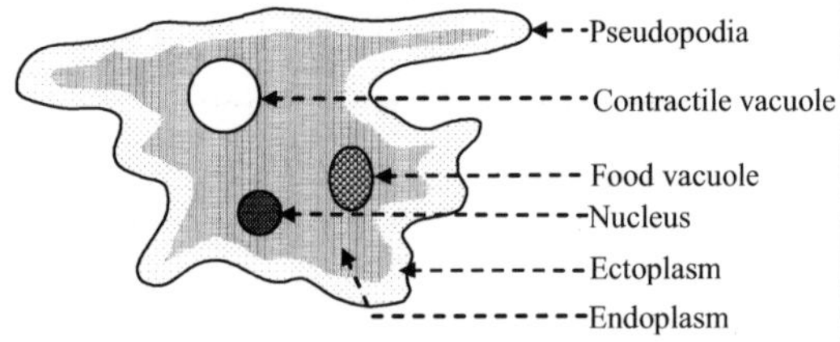

Amoeba proteus

</td>
<td>

1. **Pseudopodia:** These are protoplasmic projections that function for the locomotion of *Amoeba*.
2. **Ectoplasm:** It is the outer layer of cytoplasm clear in appearance.
3. **Endoplasm:** It is the inner cytoplasmic region with granular appearance.
4. **Nucleus:** The cell has one nucleus.
5. **Food vacuoles:** These are membrane-bound organelles, which contain engulfed food undergoing digestion.
6. **Contractile vacuoles:** These are large, clear circular membrane-bound organelles that regulate internal water pressure.

</td>
</tr>
<tr>
<td>

Class Mastigophora

EUGLENA
CERCOMONAS
HETERON

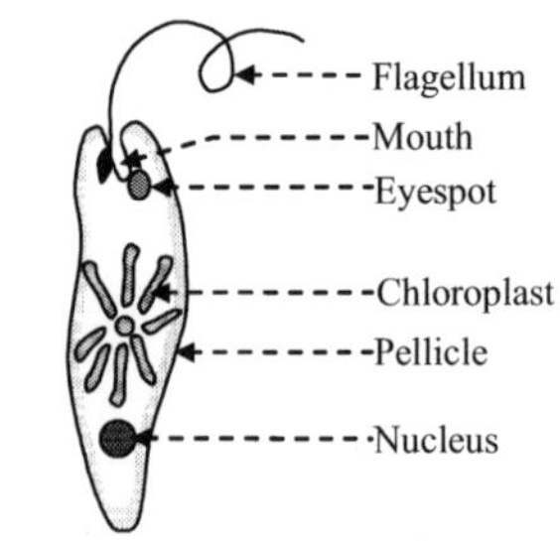

Euglena viridis

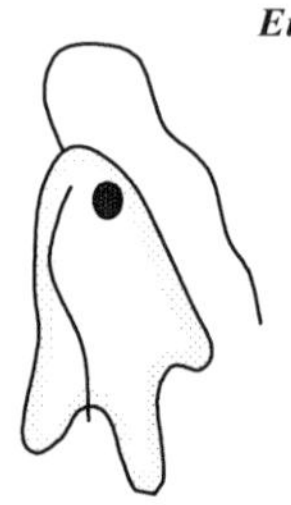

Cercomonas longicauda

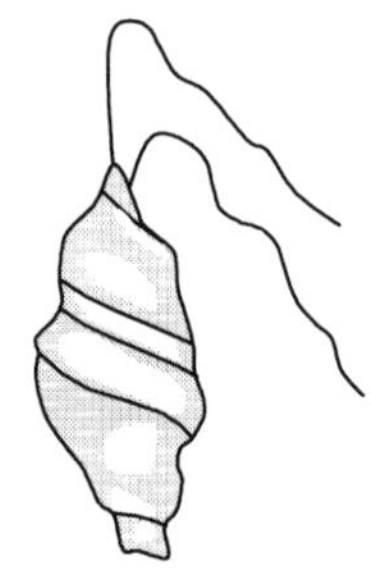

Heteronema acus

</td>
<td>

1. **Flagella:** These are long whip-like structures that function for the locomotion unicellular organisms. Each organism has one to several flagella.
2. **Pellicle:** It is an elastic layer present outside the cell membrane.
3. **Mouth:** A mouth is present anteriorly, which is indistinct.
4. **Chloroplast:** These are organelles containing chlorophyll pigments required for photosynthesis. Therefore, these are present in photosynthetic forms only.
5. **Eyespot:** It is a light-sensitive pigmented spot present anteriorly.
6. **Nucleus:** A spherical nucleus is present posteriorly.

</td>
</tr>
<tr>
<td>

Class Ciliophora

PARAMECIUM
STENTOR
VORTICELLA

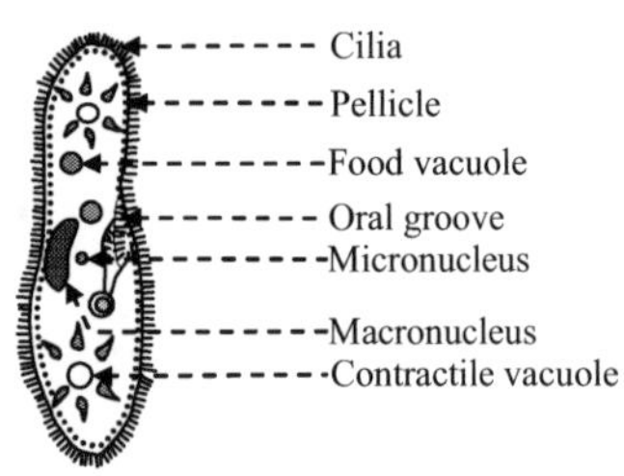

Paramecium caudatum

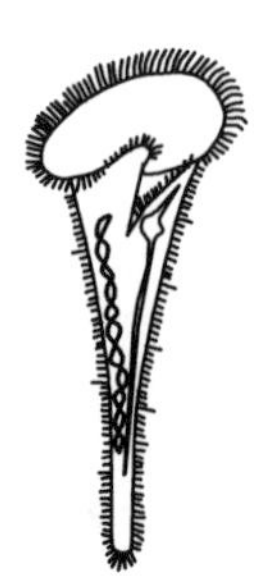

Stentor polymorpha

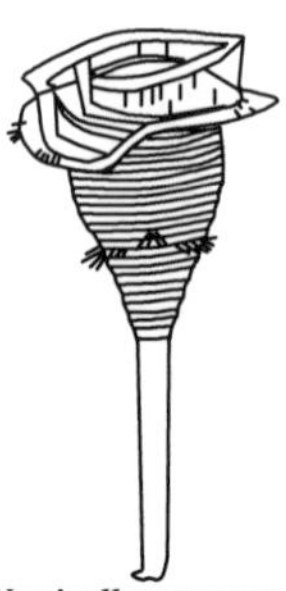

Vorticella campanula

</td>
<td>

1. **Cilia:** These are numerous short hair-like structures present on the cell surface of unicellular organisms that function for their locomotion.
2. **Pellicle:** It is an elastic layer present outside the cell membrane.
3. **Contractile vacuole:** These are large, clear circular membrane-bound organelles that regulate internal water pressure. They have radiating canals, which regulate osmotic pressure.
4. **Oral groove:** It is the indentation that leads to the mouth and gullet.
5. **Food vacuoles:** These are membrane-bound organelles, which contain engulfed food undergoing digestion.
6. **Macronucleus:** It is a large nucleus that functions to control the cell's activities. Its number in the cell varies from one to many.
7. **Micronucleus:** It is a small nucleus that functions during conjugation, which is a sexual mode of reproduction.

</td>
</tr>
</table>

Figure 9.1: Identifying characteristics of some free-living protozoa

Class Sarcodina

ENTAMOEBA HISTOLYTICA

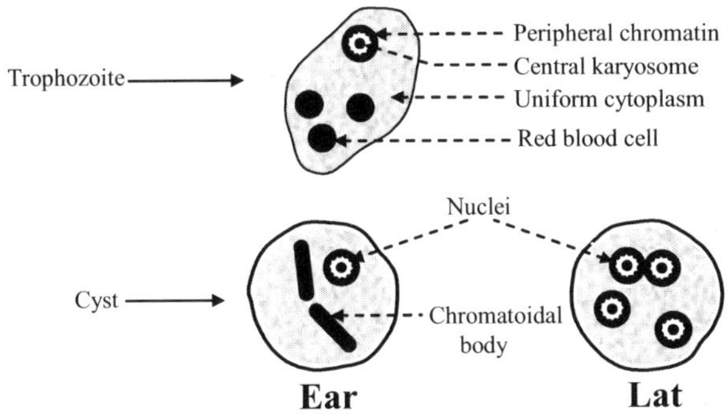

Entamoeba histolytica

TROPHOZOITE

1. **Shape:** The trophozoite has variable shape.
2. **Nucleus:** Nucleus has discrete nuclear membrane with central karyosome and peripheral chromatin granules.
3. **Cytoplasm:** Cytoplasm is uniform and clear. Red blood cells may be present in it.

CYST

1. **Shape:** The shape of the cyst is round to oval with thick wall.
2. **Nuclei:** Number of nuclei varies from one to four. The mature cyst is quadri-nucleated.
3. **Chromatoidal bodies:** Sausage-shaped chromatoidal bodies with rounded ends are present in young cysts only.

Class Mastigophora

TRYPANOSOMA GAMBIENSE

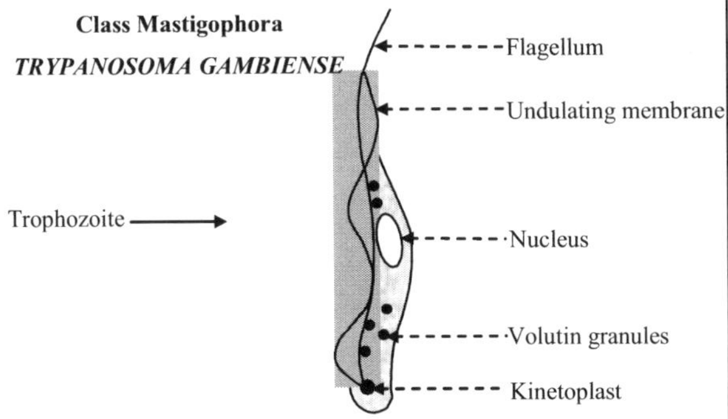

Trypanosoma gambiense

TROPHOZOITE

1. **Shape:** The trophozoite is crescent-shaped.
2. **Nucleus:** The nucleus is large and polymorphic located centrally.
3. **Cytoplasm:** The cytoplasm is granular with large number of volutin granules.
4. **Flagella:** A single flagella is present along undulating membrane having its root in the kinetoplast.

Class Mastigophora

GIARDIA LAMBLIA

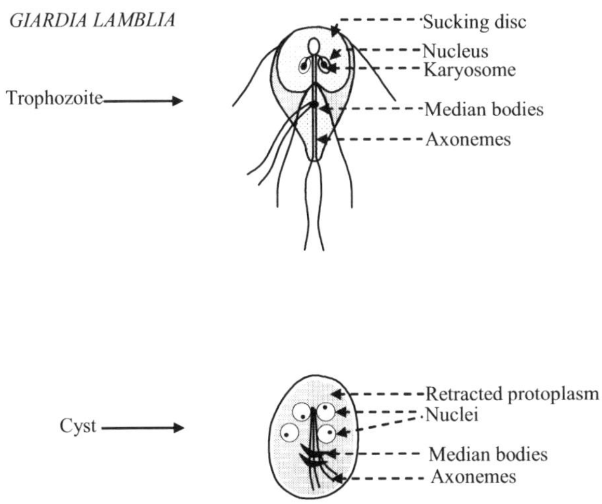

Giardia lamblia

TROPHOZOITE

1. **Shape:** The trophozoite is pear-shaped with two concave sucking discs.
2. **Nuclei:** Two nuclei are present located bilaterally. Each nucleus has central karyosome with no peripheral chromatin.
3. **Cytoplasm:** Cytoplasm is uniform and clear.
4. **Flagella:** Four pairs of flagella are present distributed with bilateral symmetry. The flagella are supported by the cytoskeleton called 'axonemes'.

CYST

1. **Shape:** The shape of the cysts is oval to ellipsoidal.
2. **Nuclei:** The number of nuclei varies from two to four.
3. **Cytoplasm:** The cytoplasm is uniform, clear and retracted from cyst wall.
4. **Flagella:** Each cyst has four pairs of flagella supported by axonemes.

Class Ciliophora

BALANTIDIUM COLI

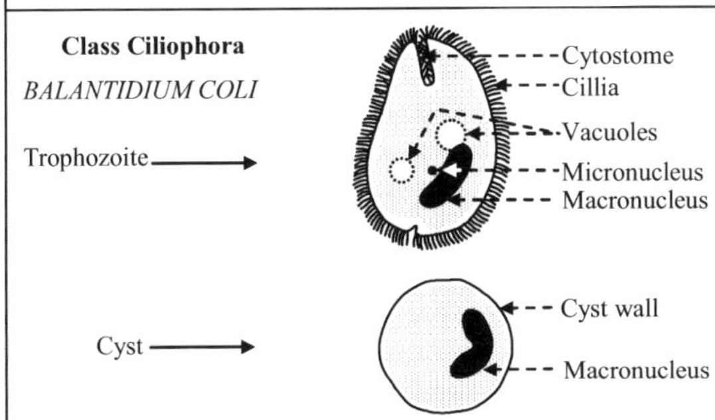

Balantidium coli

TROPHOZOITE

1. **Shape**: The shape of the trophozoite is oval.
2. **Nuclei:** A kidney-shaped macronucleus and a spherical micronucleus are present.
3. **Cytoplasm:** The cytoplasm is vacuolated.
4. **Cilia:** Cilia are present all over the cell surface.

CYST

1. **Shape:** The cyst is round and thick-walled.
2. **Nuclei:** One macronucleus and a micronucleus that is not visible are present.
3. **Cilia:** Cilia are present within the cyst.

Figure 9.2: Identifying characteristics of some parasitic protozoa

structural characteristics using available literature. The structural characteristics of some important parasitic protozoa have been given in Figure 9.2.

Materials Required

Prepared slides of the parasitic protozoa like *Entamoeba histolytica* (Trophozoite and cyst), *Trypanosoma gambiense, Giardia lamblia* (Trophozoite and cyst) and *Balantidium coli* (Trophozoite and cyst), compound microscope.

Procedure

1. The prepared slides of the parasitic protozoa like *Entamoeba histolytica* (Trophozoite and cyst), *Trypanosoma gambiense, Giardia lamblia* (Trophozoite and cyst) and *Balantidium coli* (Trophozoite and cyst) are taken.
2. The slides are examined under microscope using oil-immersion objective.
3. They are identified by comparing their structural characteristics with those available in literature (Figure 9.2).

Observations

Sketches of the parasitic protozoa are drawn as observed under the microscope. Their distinguishing structural characteristics are labeled.

10

Identification of Microscopic Fungi

A. Definition

Microscopic fungi are eukaryotic, heterotrophic microorganisms that fail to show any cellular differentiation into true tissues like root, stem or leaf and in which vascular system is absent.

B. Characteristics of Fungi

The major distinguishing characteristics of fungi are given below.

1. *Absence of Chlorophyll*: Due to absence of chlorophyll, they cannot synthesise their own food and depend upon food synthesised by others. Therefore, they have heterotrophic mode of nutrition. Depending on the source of food, they are of the following types.
   (*a*) *Saprophytic*: They use dead organic matter, such as wood and hay. Examples: Mucor, yeast, mushroom.
   (*b*) *Parasitic*: They live on other living plants or animals. Examples: Rusts, smuts.
2. *Thalloid Body*: The body of fungi consists of a thallus. A thallus is a plant body, which is not differentiated into true tissues like root, stem or leaf. The thallus of fungi is either a single cell or consists of branching filaments called 'hyphae'. The fungal hyphae are interwoven loosely or compactly to form the 'mycelium'. Thus, a fungus can be either unicellular or filamentous.

C. Classification of Fungi

The classification of fungi depends on their sexual mode of reproduction. They are subdivided into the following four classes. Species marked with asterisks (*) have been described in details with illustrations.

1. Phycomycetes (Alga-like Fungi)

Reproductive spores are external and uncovered. Examples: Water mold, terrestrial mold, bread mold (*Rhizopus stolonifer**, *Mucor* spp.*), downy mildew (*Albugo candida*), *Phytopthora infestans* (causative agent of 'late blight disease' in potato).

2. Ascomycetes (Sac Fungi)

Sexual spores, called ascospores, are produced in a sac-like structure called ascus. Examples: Yeasts (*Torula* spp.*, *Candida albicans**, *Saccharomyces cerevisiae*), molds (*Aspergillus flavus**, *Penicillium notatum**, *Cladosporium fulvum**, *Cephalosporium acremonium**).

3. Basidiomycetes (Club Fungi)

Reproductive spores, called basidiospores, separate from specialised stalks called basidia. Examples: Fleshy fungi, toadstools, puffballs, bracket fungi, mushrooms (edible mushroom: *Agaricus campestris*; poisonous mushroom: *Amanita muscaria*).

4. Deuteromycetes (Fungi Imperfecti)

No sexual reproductive phase exists. Therefore, it is also called fungi imperfecti. Examples: *Alternaria solani** (causative agent of 'early blight disease' in potato), *Fusarium solani**, *Colletotrichum falcatum* (causative agent of 'red rot disease' in sugarcane).

D. Types of Fungi

Based on structure, fungi are of the following two types.

1. *Unicellular fungi*: Example: Yeasts
2. *Filamentous fungi*: Example: Molds

Experiment 54

E. Cultivation and Identification of Fungi

***Aim*: To cultivate and identify a fungi.**

Principle

The structural components of most of the fungi, particularly of the filamentous molds, are very delicate. Simple handling with an inoculating loop may result in mechanical disruption of their structure. Therefore, a special micro-technique is used to cultivate them for identification. A sterilised nutrient medium with acidic pH such as Sabouraud agar medium, which is suitable for fungal growth is poured into the depression of a cavity slide and covered with a cover slip. Fungi from a stock culture is inoculated aseptically on the surface of the medium on the slide and incubated in a moist chamber at room temperature. After suitable incubation period, their colonial morphology is observed with naked eye or if required using a hand lens. To observe the microscopic appearance, wet mount of the grown fungi is prepared using lactophenol cotton blue solution and viewed under low power and high power magnification of a dissecting microscope (simple microscope). The fungi is then identified using its colonial morphology and microscopic appearance. The identifying characteristics of few fungi have been given in Figures 10.2 to 10.4.

Materials Required

Petri dish, circular piece of filter paper, U-shaped glass rod, cavity slide, cover slip, conical flask, beaker, pipette, ethanol (95%), forceps, bunsen burner, toothpick, petroleum jelly, cotton plugs, inoculating loop, Sabouraud agar (*See* Appendix I at page 247), autoclave, bunsen burner, stock culture of fungi to be cultivated and identified, laminar flow chamber, dispose jar, incubator, lactophenol cotton blue solution (*See* Appendix II at page 251), simple microscope.

Procedure

1. The ingredients of Sabouraud agar medium (*See* Appendix I at page 247) or its ready-made powder, required for 100 ml of the medium is weighed and dissolved in 100 ml of distilled water in a 250 ml conical flask by shaking and swirling (Figure 10.1)
2. Its pH is determined using a pH paper or pH meter and adjusted to 5.6 using 0.1N HCl if it is more or using 0.1 N NaOH if it is less.
3. The flask is heated to dissolve the agar in the medium completely.
4. The flask is cotton-plugged, covered with craft paper and tied with thread or rubber band.
5. It is sterilised at 121°C (15 psi pressure) for 15 minutes in an autoclave.

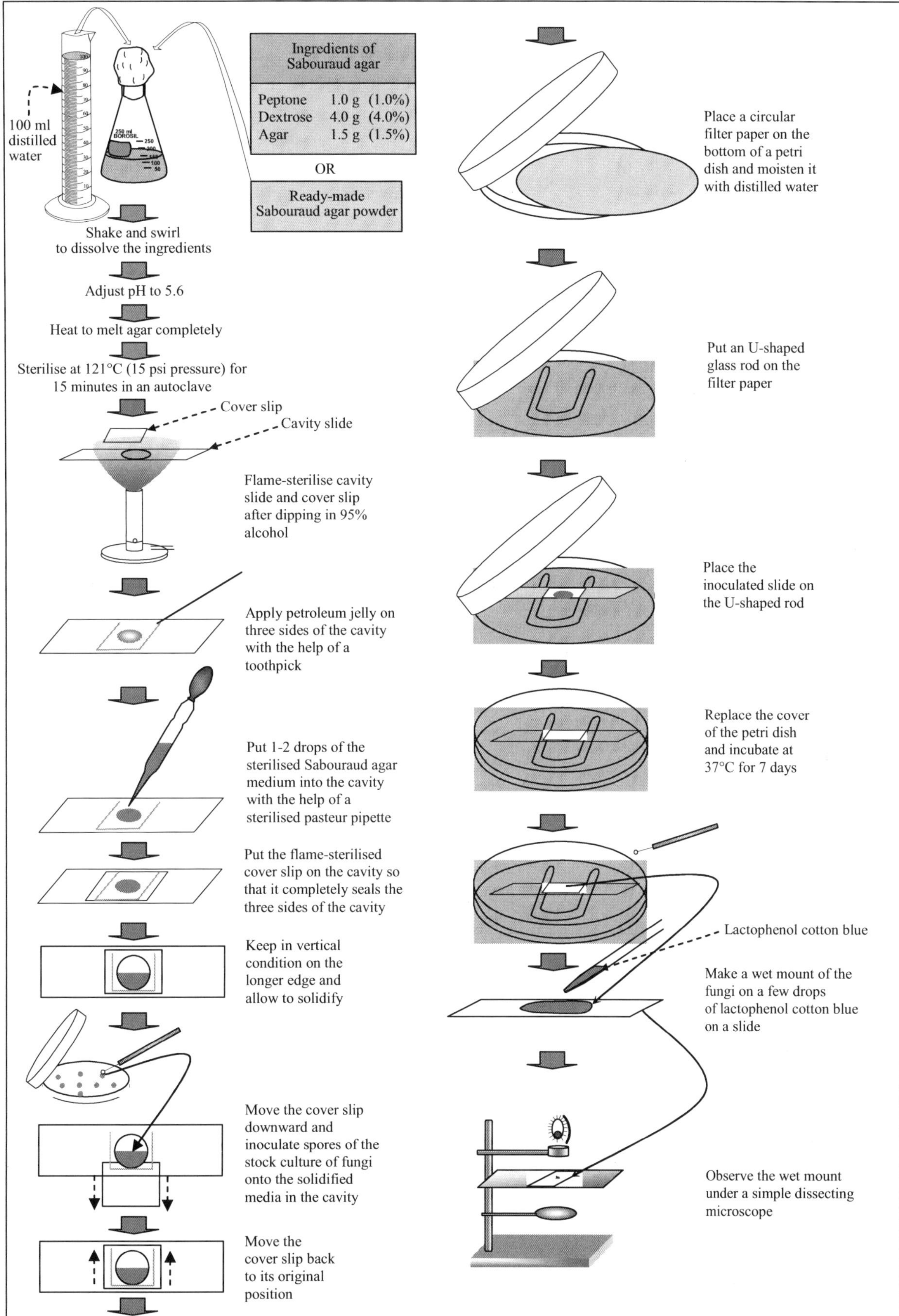

Figure 10.1: Cultivation and identification of microscopic fungi

6. After sterilisation, it is removed from the autoclave and allowed to cool for sometime, without allowing the medium to solidify. If the medium has already been prepared and solidified during storage, it has to be liquefied by heating carefully till it melts completely.
7. A cavity slide and a cover slip are flame-sterilised by dipping them, with the help of a forceps, in a beaker containing 95% ethanol and then passing them over the flame of a bunsen burner until all the ethanol has burnt off the slide and the cover slip.
8. With a toothpick, thin lines of petroleum jelly is applied on the three sides of the depression of the cavity slide so as to hold the cover slip, when placed on it. The fourth side, remaining towards the long side, of the slide serves as a vent for passage of air.
9. With the help of a sterile pasteur pipette, aseptically one to two drops of the sterilised cooled Sabouraud agar medium is put in the depression of the cavity slide.
10. The flame-sterilised cover slip is placed over the depression, so that it is completely sealed on the three sides.
11. The slide is kept in an upright position on the longer edge, so that the unsealed side remains to the top and the medium does not leak downwards. The medium is allowed to solidify in this position.
12. The cover slip is moved downwards and spores from test culture of fungi is inoculated on the solidified medium in the depression of the cavity slide with the help of a flame-sterilised loop aseptically, preferably in a laminar flow chamber.
13. The cover slip is pushed upward to the original position, thereby sealing off the cavity.
14. A circular piece of filter paper is placed on the bottom of a petri dish and moistened with sterile water to provide a moist atmosphere inside the petri dish.

Class Ascomycetes (Yeast)

TORULA

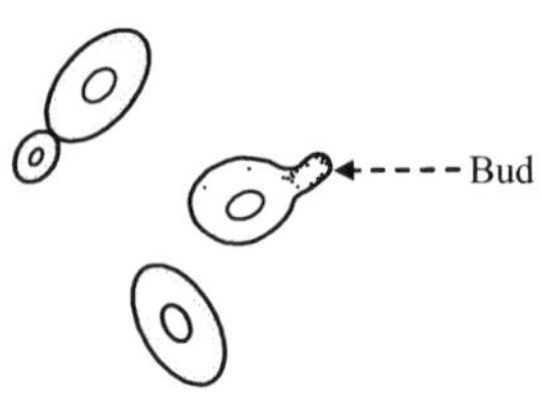

***Torula* spp.**

1. **Colonial morphology:** Colonies are pink, moist, with unbroken, even edges.
2. **Microscopic appearance:** Cells are oval, colourless and reproduce by budding.
3. **Importance:** Torula, in its inactive form (usually labeled as 'torula yeast'), is widely used as a flavouring in processed foods and pet foods. It is produced from wood sugar, as a by-product of paper production. It is pasteurised and spray-dried to produce a fine, light grayish-brown powder with a slightly yeasty odour and gentle, slightly meaty taste.

Class Ascomycetes (Yeast)

CANDIDA

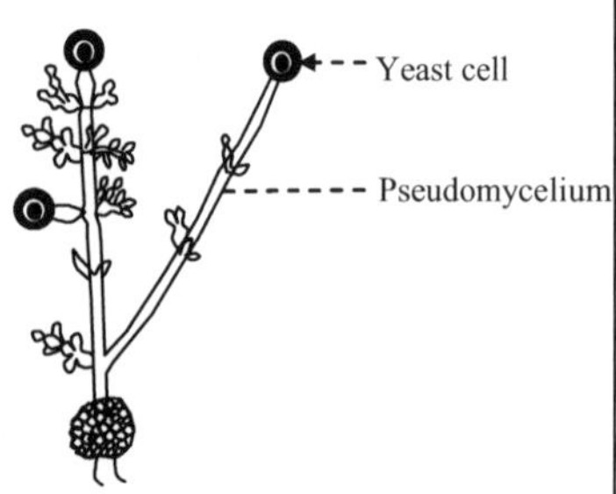

Candida albicans

1. **Colonial morphology:** Colonies are small, round, moist and colourless with unbroken, even edges.
2. **Microscopic appearance:** It is a yeast-like fungus, which produces pseudomycelium.
3. **Importance:** *Candida albicans* is a comensal and is among the gut flora. Under normal circumstances, it lives in 80% of the human population with no harmful effect, although overgrowth results in candidiasis. To infect host tissue, the usual unicellular yeast-like form reacts to environmental cues and changes into an invasive, multicellular filamentous form. It is a causative agent of oral and genital infections in human beings. Systemic infections (fungemias) are important causes of morbidity and mortality in immunocompromised patients (*e.g.*, AIDS, cancer chemotherapy, organ or bone marrow transplantation).

Figure 10.2: Identifying characteristics of some microscopic fungi *(Torula* and *Candida)*

Class Phycomycetes (Molds)

RHIZOPUS

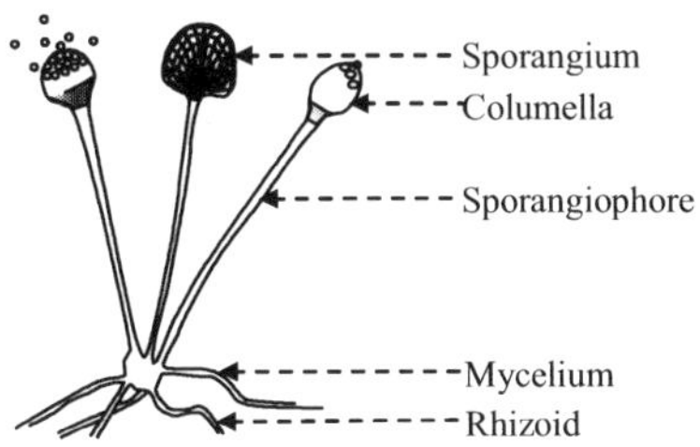

Rhizopus stolonifer

1. **Colonial morphology:** It is a rapidly growing white-coloured fungus, which swarms over the entire plate. The aerial mycelium is cottony and fuzzy.
2. **Microscopic appearance:** Its spores are oval, colorless or brown. The non-septate mycelium gives rise to straight sporangiophores that terminate with black sporangium, each containing a columella. The root-like hyphae (rhizoids) penetrate the medium.
3. **Importance:** It is a cosmopolitan filamentous fungus found in soil, animal faeces, old bread, decaying fruit and vegetables,. Some species are opportunistic agents of human zygomycosis. They may cause serious (and often fatal) infections in humans and animals because of their rapid growth rate and growth at relatively high temperatures. Rhizopus infection is an associated complication of diabetic ketoacidosis. Some species are plant pathogens. Two are used in food fermentation: (1) *Rhizopus oligosporus*, is used in the production of 'tempeh', a fermented food derived from soybeans and, 'oncom'. (2) *R. oryzae* is used in the production of alcoholic beverages in parts of Asia and Africa.

Class Phycomycetes (Molds)

MUCOR

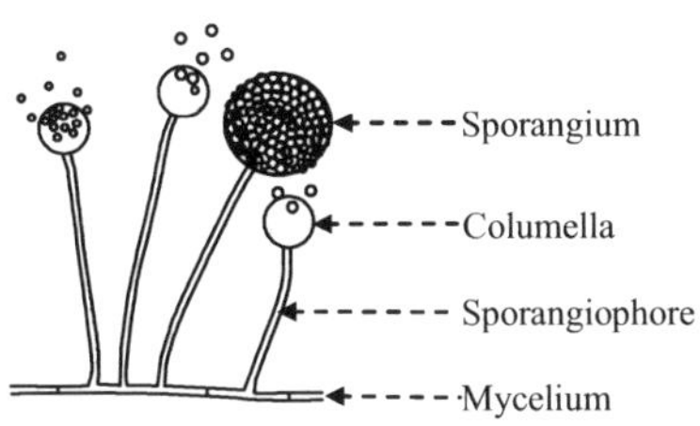

Mucor racemosus

1. **Colonial morphology:** Its colonies resemble those of *Rhizopus.*
2. **Microscopic appearance:** Its spores are oval. The non-septate mycelium gives rise to single sporangiophores with globular sporangium, each containing a columella. There are no rhizoids.
3. **Importance:** It has worldwide distribution and is primarily a soil fungus, but is also found in horse manure, plant remains, grains, vegetables and nuts. In the tropics, it is found at higher altitudes and often seen on soft fruits, fruit juice and marmalade. It is also the dominating mold in floor dust of houses.

Class Deuteromycetes (Molds)

ALTERNARIA

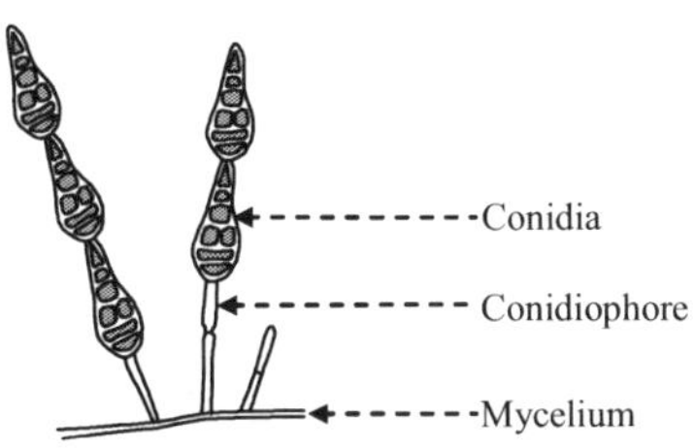

Alternaria solani

1. **Colonial morphology:** Its colonies are grayish-green or black with gray edges, which rapidly swarm over the entire plate. The aerial mycelium is not very dense and appears grayish to white.
2. **Microscopic appearance:** It has multicelled spores (conidia), which are pear-shaped and are attached to single conidiophores arising from a septate mycelium.
3. **Importance:** It is an outdoor mold, which appears when the weather is warm. It frequently grows in textiles, foodstuffs and soils. The black spots seen on tomatoes are usually of the *Alternaria* mold species. It is also found on condensed window frames. *Alternaria solani* is the causative agent of 'early blight disease' in potato.

Class Deuteromycetes (Molds)

FUSARIUM

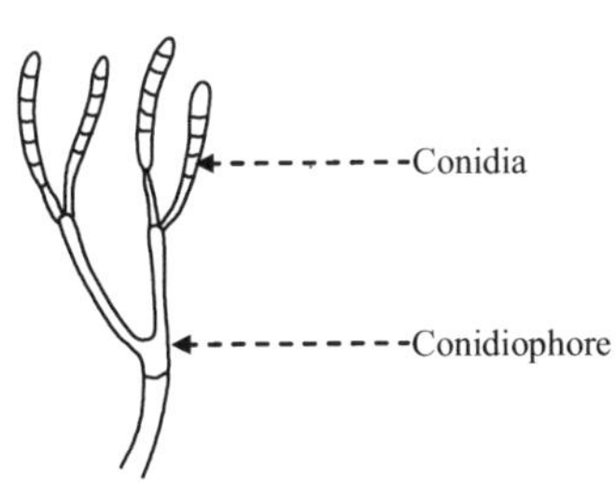

Fusarium solani

1. **Colonial morphology:** Its colonies are woolly, white, fuzzy changing color to pink, purple or yellow.
2. **Microscopic appearance:** It has multicelled spores (conidia), which are oval or crescent-shaped and are attached to conidiophores arising from a septate mycelium.
3. **Importance:** This mold is a common soil fungus and is widely found on numerous grasses and other plants. It can cause plant diseases and is a major parasite of rice, sugar cane, sorghum and especially maize grains. It is found regularly on banana roots and other fruits and vegetable, *e.g.*, tomato and watermelon. It sporulates in warm wet weathers and shares some of the same allergenic determinants as *Penicillium* and *Aspergillus*.

Figure 10.3: Identifying characteristics of some microscopic fungi *(Rhizopus, Mucor, Alternaria and Fusarium)*

Class Ascomycetes (Molds)

ASPERGILLUS

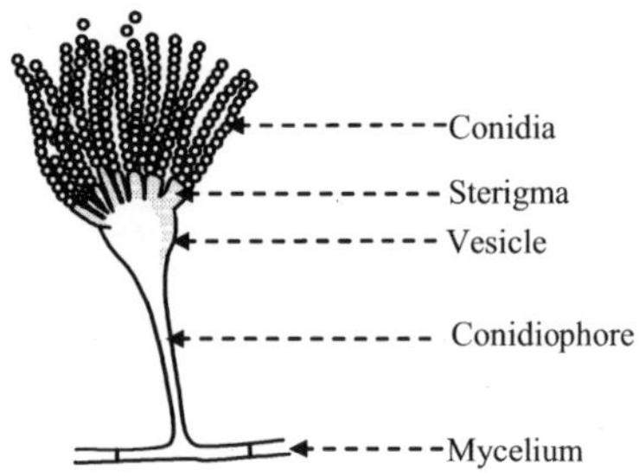

Aspergillus flavus

1. **Colonial morphology:** It shows white colonies, which become greenish-blue, black or brown as its cultures mature.
2. **Microscopic appearance:** Single-celled spores (conidia) in chains develop at the end of the sterigma arising from the terminal bulb of the conidiophore. The vesicle and the long conidiophores arise from a septate mycelium.
3. **Importance:** It is a mold found in damp conditions, both indoor and outdoor, where the temperature is approximately 40°C. It is found in soils, leaf, plant litter, decaying vegetables, roots, bird droppings, tobacco and stored sweet potatoes. Some diseases associated with the *Aspergillus* are farmers lung, bakers asthma and malt workers lung. Inhalation of conidia and mycelium of *Aspergillus* can lead to several diseases, the severity of which depends on the host's immune response. *Aspergillus flavus* produces the mycotoxin named aflatoxin.

Class Ascomycetes (Molds)

PENICILLIUM

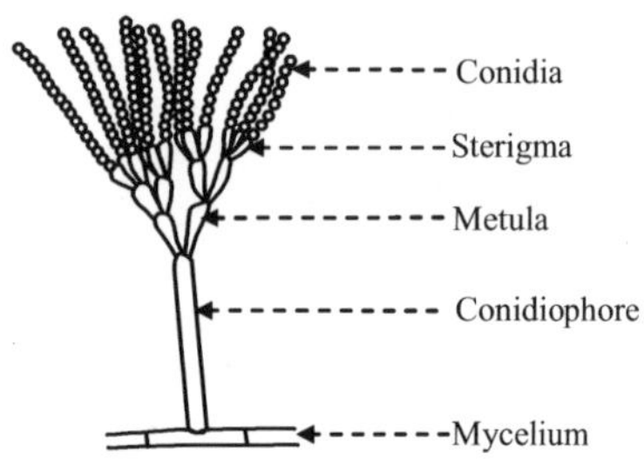

Penicillium notatum

1. **Colonial morphology:** Its mature cultures usually look greenish or blue-green.
2. **Microscopic appearance:** Single-celled spores (conidia) in chains develop at the end of the sterigma arising from the metula of the conidiophore. Branching conidiophores arise from a septate mycelium.
3. **Importance:** It is found in the soil of citrus plantations and has been isolated from decaying cabbage and barley plants, stored seeds of cereals, grapes, nuts, dried fruits and fruit juices. It is one of the most dominant and important house molds. The indoor mold can be readily seen on stale bread, citrus fruits and apples. It is frequently found in wine cellars.

Class Ascomycetes (Molds)

CLADOSPORIUM

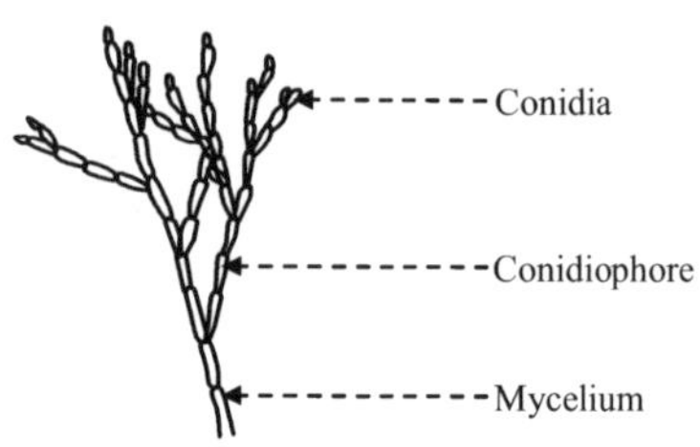

Cladosporium fulvum

1. **Colonial morphology:** Its colonies are small, heaped and powdery with greenish-black appearance.
2. **Microscopic appearance:** Spores (conidia) develop at the end of complex conidiophores arising from a septate mycelium that is usually brownish.
3. **Importance:** It is the most frequent of all the molds encountered in the air. It is found most commonly on dying and dead plant substrates, especially on leaves and stems of ferns, mosses as well as on desert and aquatic plants. It is found in various soil types and on food items such as cereals, cucumbers, tomatoes and peaches. It is also found in fuel tanks, face creams, paints and textiles. It is the causative agent of leaf mold disease in tomato.

Class Ascomycetes (Molds)

CEPHALOSPORIUM

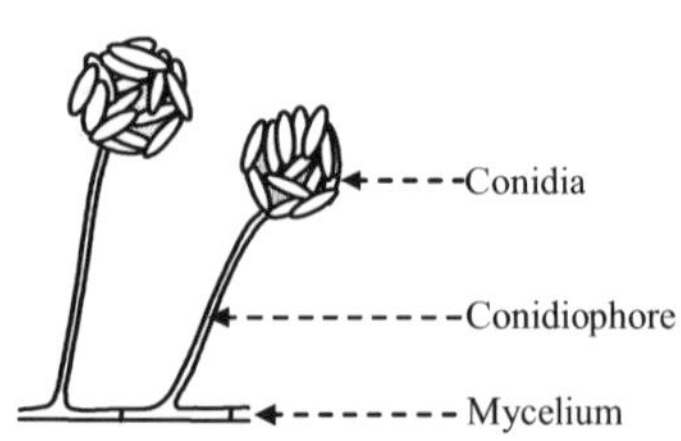

Cephalosporium acremonium

1. **Colonial morphology:** It has rapidly growing compact and moist colonies, which become cottony with aerial hyphae that are gray or pink.
2. **Microscopic appearance:** Single-celled conical or elliptical spores (conidia) are held together in clusters at the tips of the conidiophores by a mucoid substance. Erect, unbranched conidiophores arise from a septate mycelium.
3. **Importance:** It is found in decomposing vegetation, and is a soil inhabitant. It is also found in dust from textile plants, soil when gardening, bathrooms and damp old houses. It is also occasionally found in patients sensitive to *Candida albicans*.

Figure 10.4: Identifying characteristics of some microscopic fungi (*Aspergillus, Penicillium, Cladosporium and Cephalosporium*)

15. A U-shaped glass rod is put on the filter paper.
16. The inoculated slide is placed on the U-shaped rod.
17. The cover of the petri dish is replaced and the petri dish is incubated at 37°C for seven days in an incubator. The filter paper is remoistened, whenever necessary.
18. For microscopic observation, a wet mount of the cultured fungi is prepared by suspending some of the culture in a few drops of lactophenol cotton blue solution on a slide. Care is taken to avoid damaging the fungal structures.
19. The wet mount preparation is observed under low power and high power magnification with the aid of a dissecting microscope (simple microscope).

Observations

1. The colonial morphology of the cultured fungi is noted.
2. The microscopic appearance of the fungi under simple microscope is noted.
3. The fungi is then identified by comparing its colonial morphology and microscopic appearance with the identifying characteristics of different fungi. The identifying characteristics of few fungi have been given in Figures 10.2 to 10.4.

11

Identification of Microscopic Algae

A. Definition

Microscopic algae are eukaryotic, autotrophic microorganisms that fail to show any cellular differentiation into true tissues like root, stem or leaf and in which vascular system is absent.

B. Characteristics of Algae

The major distinguishing characteristics of algae are given below.

1. *Presence of Chlorophyll*: Algae are chlorophyll-bearing organisms; specifically 'chlorophyll a' is present in all types of algae. Other pigments are also present. The pigments in algae are of three types as follows:
   (*a*) *Chlorophyll*: Examples: Chlorophyll a, b, c, d and e.
   (*b*) *Carotenoids*: It includes the following two groups.
      (*i*) *Xanthophyll*: Examples: Zeaxanthine, astaxanthine, cryptoxanthine, lycopene and fucoxanthine.
      (*ii*) *Carotene*: Examples: α-, β-, γ- and e-carotene.
   (*c*) *Phycobilins*: Phycocyanin and phycoerythrin.

   Chlorophyll and carotenoids are fat-soluble, while phycobilins are water-soluble.
2. *Holophytic Mode of Nutrition*: Due to presence of the photosynthetic pigment, chlorophyll, they can synthesise their own food by photosynthesis. Therefore, they have autotrophic mode of nutrition. As their mode of nutrition is similar to that of higher plants (= phyta), such type of nutrition is also called holophytic mode of nutrition.
3. *Thalloid Body*: The body of algae consists of a thallus. A thallus is a plant body, which is not differentiated into true tissues like root, stem or leaf. Some algae show little differentiation of their tissues. However, even the complex thallus lacks vascular system and epidermis with stomata. The thallus of algae is either a single cell or consists of branching filaments, in which the cells are attached end to end. Thus, the size of algae varies from microscopic unicellular forms like *Microcystis* to large macrophytes like various seaweeds.
4. *True Parenchyma Cells*: The cells of algae are true parenchyma cells. Parenchyma cells are simple thin-walled plant cells, which are isodiametric in that they expand equally in all sides.
5. *Starch as Reserve Food*: In the cells of algae, the reserve food material is stored in the form of starch.

6. *Cellulose Cell Wall*: The cell wall of all algae is made of cellulose, except those of the blue green algae (Class Cyanophyceae), in which it is made of peptidoglycan similar to the cell wall of bacteria.
7. *Aquatic Habitat*: Most of the algae remain in freshwater, brackishwater or marine ecosystems. However, algae are ubiquitous and are found in all habitats.

C. Classification of Algae

The classification of algae depends on the structure of the thallus and the mode of reproduction. They are subdivided into the following eleven classes. Genera, marked with asterisks (*) have been described in details with illustrations.

1. Cyanophyceae

The members of this class are photosynthetic gram-negative prokaryotes, generally grouped as 'blue green algae (BGA)'. They are the only prokaryotic algae, as they do not contain membrane-bound nucleus in the cells. Algae of all the other ten classes are eukaryotic in that their cells contain nuclear material confined in membrane-bound nucleus. They are different from photosynthetic bacteria. The photosynthetic pigment in BGA is 'chlorophyll a' similar to the pigments in eukaryotic algae and higher plants, while that in the photosynthetic bacteria is bacteriochlorophyll. BGA also contain other pigments like carotenoids and phycobilins, which impart different shades of colours. Their chlorophyll pigments are not confined in chloroplast, as it is in eukaryotic algae and higher plants; rather are found in thin layers of membranes called thyllakoids. BGA are important due to their ability to fix atmospheric nitrogen. Most of the BGA are aquatic. They lack flagella. Examples: *Microcystis**, *Oscillatoria**, *Nostoc**, *Anabaena**, *Spirulina**, *Scytonema*, *Rivularia*.

2. Chlorophyceae

This class includes the 'green algae'. They are eukaryotic. Their colour is green due to the abundance of the green pigments 'chlorophyll a' and 'chlorophyll b' over other pigments in the plastids called chloroplasts. Chloroplasts usually contain proteinaceous bodies called 'pyrenoids'. Motile cells of primitive forms contain eyespot or 'stigma'. Examples: *Chlamydomonas**, *Chlorella**, *Spirogyra**, *Zygnema**, *Ulothrix**, *Oedogonium**, *Volvox**, *Hydrodictyon**, *Pediastrum**, *Gonium**, *Pandorina**, *Eudorina**, *Closterium**, *Cosmarium**, *Ulva*, *Enteromorpha*, *Cladophora*, *Pithophora*, *Caulerpa*, *Scenedesmus*, *Acetabularia*, *Monostroma*. One group of algae belonging to Chlorophyceae does not have flagella in any stage of the life and reproduces by conjugation, in which the gamete of one cell moves into another cell by amoeboid action and fuses with its gamete to produce the zygote. This group is called 'conjugales'. Conjugales are of two types; filamentous (*Spirogyra, Zygnema*) and unicellular. The unicellular conjugales are called 'desmids'. They are of two types; 'sacoderm desmids', in which the cell wall is a single piece and has no pores (*Mesotaenium, Cylindrocystis, Netrium, Roya*) and 'placoderm desmids', in which the cell wall has more than one piece and has pores on it (*Closterium, Cosmarium*).

3. Bacillariophyceae

Algae belonging to this class are called 'diatoms'. Their highly sculptured and symmetrically ornamented cell wall separates them from rest of the algae. The diatom cell, often called 'frustule' has a wall of usually two equal halves. Like a pair of petri dishes, the older half 'epitheca' fits closely over the younger half 'hypotheca'. In each half, the main surface is called valves and the circular projection at the margin of the surface is called 'connecting band'. The connecting band of epitheca overlaps that of the hypotheca. The overlapping region is called 'girdle', which remains united by some cementing organic substance. The common constituent of the cell wall is hydrated amorphous silica. Examples: *Pinnularia**, *Navicula**, *Nitzschia**, *Pleurosigma**, *Gyrosigma**, *Asterionella**, *Tabellaria**, *Diatoma**, *Fragilaria**, *Synedra**, *Rhabdonema**, *Surirella**, *Cyclotella**, *Biddulphia**, *Coscinodiscus**, *Melosira**, *Sceletonema**, *Thalassiosira**, *Rhizosolenia**, *Chaetoceros**, *Isocrysis*. Diatoms are of two types; the pennate diatoms (pennales), which are bilaterally symmetrical and the centric diatoms (centrales), which are radially symmetrical. Centric diatoms are far more abundant in the sea than in freshwater and the marine forms, moreover, attain a much larger size than the freshwater ones.

4. Rhodophyceae

This class includes the 'red algae', which are mostly macroscopic and constitute the majority of seaweeds. The characteristic red colour of these algae is due to the presence of two red phycobilin pigments (phycoerythrin and phycocyanin). The red pigments mask the presence of other pigments. Examples: *Porphyridium, Porphyra, Batrachospermum, Polysiphonia, Gonitrichum, Lemanea, Gelidium, Gracillaria, Gelidiella, Acanthophora.*

5. Phaeophyceae

This class includes the 'brown algae'. Most of them are macroscopic and some are seaweeds. The characteristic brown colour of these algae is due to the presence of golden brown xanthophyll pigment, 'fucoxanthine'. The reserve food material is usually 'laminarin'. Their thalli are very big and show some tissue differentiation, due to which most of the members look like other angiospermic plants. Examples: *Ectocarpus, Laminaria, Dictyota, Fucus, Sargassum, Macrocystis, Lessonia, Postelsia, Ascophyllum, Turbinaria, Undaria, Cystophyllum, Hormophysa, Padina.*

6. Xanthophyceae

This class includes the 'yellow-green algae'. Most of them are macroscopic. The characteristic yellow green colour of these algae is due to the presence of chlorophyll a, chlorophyll e, β-carotene and several xanthophylls. Flagella, if present, are two and are of unequal length. Reserve food material is fat. Examples: *Botrycoccus, Botrydium, Vaucheria.*

7. Charophyceae

This class includes a group of macroscopic green algae, which are called 'stoneworts' or 'brittleworts'. They are a unique group of algae with resemblance to Chlorophyceae in morphology (presence of chlorophyll a and b, storage of starch in their plastids and their total aquatic habitat) and with Bryophytes in reproduction (the structure of sex organs, sperm and germination of zygote). They are all aquatic, mostly found in freshwaters, but some have also been reported from saline waters. Many members are heavily calcified with growths on the bottom of lakes, leading to the formation of marl ($CaCO_3$ and $MgCO_3$ deposits) and hence the common name, the stoneworts. They are anchored to sandy or muddy substratum with the help of well-developed rhizoids. This class is so similar to the class Chlorophyceae that, sometimes it is kept under the class Chlorophyceae instead of having a separate class. However, this class is different from the class Chlorophyceae in that the plant body of its members consists of an erect axis differentiated into nodes and internodes with laterals of limited growth at the nodes. Examples: *Chara, Nitella, Nitellopsis, Tolypella.*

8. Euglenophyceae

The members of this class are motile flagellated algae. Each cell has flagella, may be one or two, arising from the base of a canal like invagination at the front end. The cell has complex vacuolar system and a large, prominent nucleus. Each cell has several plastids (chromatophores). Plastids are pure green in colour. These algae are found only in freshwater bodies. Sometimes, they are put under protozoa as all members are unicellular. Example: *Euglena**, *Cercomonas**, *Heteronema**, *Paranema* (*See* page 208).

9. Chrysophyceae

This class includes the 'golden-brown algae'. The plastids (chromatophores) of these algae are brown or orange coloured. Cells commonly contain one or two parietal (lying along the inner wall of the cell) chromatophores. Phycochrysin serves as the chief accessory pigment. The reserve food material is fat and leucosin. They are unicellular to branched filamentous. Flagella are unequal, attached at the front end. Most of the members are found in cold freshwater, but few are marine. Examples: *Ochromonas, Mallomonas, Chrysochromulina, Phaeothamnion.*

10. Cryptophyceae

The cells of the members of this class have chromatophores, which show diverse pigmentation and are usually parietal. There may be some shade of brown. Reserve food material is solid carbohydrates or in some cases starch. Plants are largely represented by motile cells, but most advanced forms are coccoid[1]. Flagella are slightly unequal. They are equally distributed both in marine and freshwater habitats. Examples: *Cryptomonas, Rhabdomonas, Protochrysis, Zooxanthella.*

11. Dinophyceae (Pyrrophyceae)

The chromatophores of the members of this class are dark yellow or brown, which contains a number of special pigments. Chromatophores are numerous in the cells. Reserve food material is starch or oil. They are unicellular to branched filamentous. The bodies of motile cells have two furrows, a transverse furrow having a transverse flagellum, which encircles the body and a longitudinal furrow with backwardly directed longitudinal flagellum. They are mostly marine, but few are found in freshwaters. Examples: *Gymnodinium*, Gonyaulax*, Ceratium*, Noctiluca*, Peridinium.*

D. Types of Algae

Algae are grouped into the following types.

I. Based on Type of Cell

Based on the type of cell, algae are grouped into two categories as follows.

1. Prokaryotic Algae

It includes the blue green algae (BGA), which have been classified as Class Cyanophyceae. These algae are made of prokaryotic cells similar to the bacteria cells, which are also prokaryotic. Prokaryotic cells are those primitive types of cells, in which the nucleus is absent and the nuclear material remains in the protoplasm concentrated mostly at the center of the cells. In other words, the nuclear membrane is absent. The cell wall is made of peptidoglycan, similar to the cell wall of bacteria. Like bacteria cells, the cells of prokaryotic algae lack membrane-bound organelles like plastids, mitochondria, golgi bodies and endoplasmic reticulum, but possess ribosomes scattered in the protoplasm. The chlorophyll pigments are bound to photosynthetic lamellae or thyllakoids, which are arranged parallel and not superimposed to from grana. Due to their similarity with bacteria, blue green algae are sometimes called cyanobacteria.

2. Eukaryotic Algae

It includes the algae of all the other 10 classes. Their cells resemble the eukaryotic cells of higher plants and animals. The eukaryotic cells are those cells, in which the nucleus is present. In other words, the nuclear material is confined in the protoplasm within a membrane-bound body called nucleus. The cell wall is made of cellulose as in the cells of higher plants. Membrane-bound organelles like plastids, mitochondria, golgi bodies and endoplasmic reticulum are present. Ribosomes are either scattered in the cytoplasm or attached to the endoplasmic reticulum. The chlorophyll pigments are bound to photosynthetic lamellae or thyllakoids, which do not remain in superimposed manner to from grana, rather remain suspended in the fluid stroma enclosed within the chloroplast.

II. Based on Size and Structure

Based on the size and structure, algae are of the following two types.

1. Microscopic Algae

Their structural details can be seen only under a microscope. These algae come under the purview of microbiology. Therefore, their identification has been described below. They are of two types as follows.

---

1 Coccoid is a resting, motionless state found in few motile unicellular algae, during which the flagella are drawn in before division of the protoplast to form a new generation of free-moving individual cells.

(*a*) *Unicellular Algae*: Made of single cell. Example: *Chlamydomonas.*

(*b*) *Filamentous Algae*: Cells joined end to end to form filaments. Example: *Spirulina.*

2. Macrophytic Algae

They include large algae, looking like other angiospermic plants. Examples: *Chara, Nitella*. They are not dealt with under microbiology.

Experiment 55

E. Identification of Microscopic Algae

***Aim*: To identify an unknown microscopic algae.**

Principle

There are more than 30,000 known species of microscopic algae. They are identified with the help of their structural characteristics observed under microscope. The structural characteristics of few of the microscopic algae and meaning of these structures have been given in Figures 11.1 to 11.21.

Materials Required

Water sample, sampling bottle, dropper, glass slide, methylcellulose, cover slip, compound microscope

Procedure

1. Water sample is collected in a sampling bottle from the water body (sea, lagoon, lake, river pond, ditch etc.).
2. A drop of the water is placed in the center of a clean slide.
3. One edge of a cover slip is placed against the outer edge of the drop of the water.
4. After the drop of water spreads along the inner edge of the cover slip, the cover slip is gently lowered onto the slide.
5. The slide preparation is observed under low power and high power objectives of a compound microscope with diminished light.

Observations

Microscopic algae can be seen in the water. They are identified by comparing their physical structures with the literature available on the structure of different algae (Figures 11.1 to 11.21).

Class Cyanophyceae

MICROCYSTIS

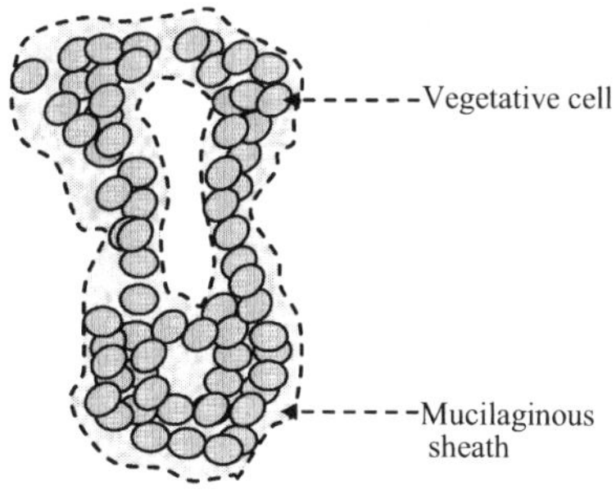

Colony

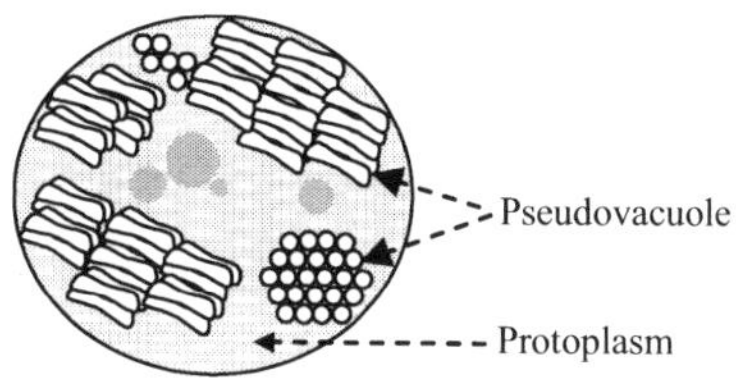

A single vegetative cell
Microcystis aeruginosa

1. **Habitat:** It is a freshwater planktonic colonial form. Some important species are *Microcystis aeruginosa, M. flosaquae, M. viridis, M. parasitica* and *M. densa*.
2. **Colony:** Cells have thick mucilaginous membrane, for which they remain in colony. The colony may be shapeless, spherical, ellipsoidal, irregularly elongated or clathrate.
3. **Thallus:** Unicellular, non-motile.
4. **Cells:** The cells are spherical in shape. They have vacuole-like structures present in the protoplasm, which are not actually vacuoles; rather they are pseudovacuoles (cylindrical gas vesicles) observable in both longitudinal and cross-section.
5. **Reproduction:** Reproduction is only by binary fission.

Class Cyanophyceae

OSCILLATORIA

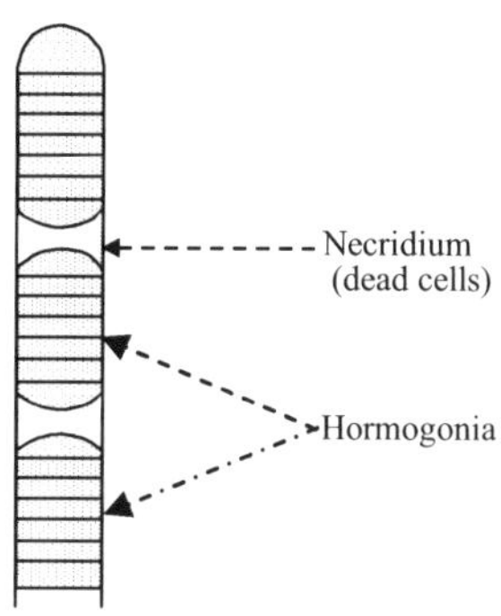

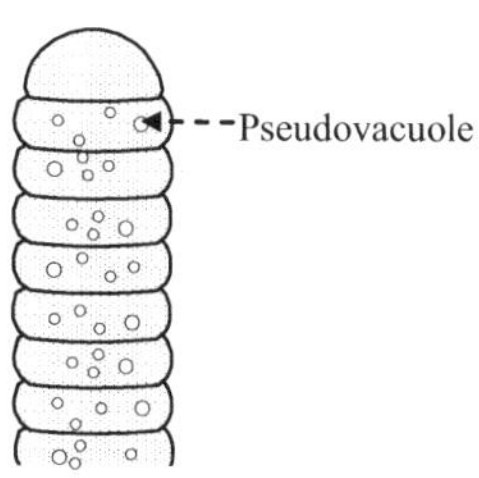

Oscillatoria annae

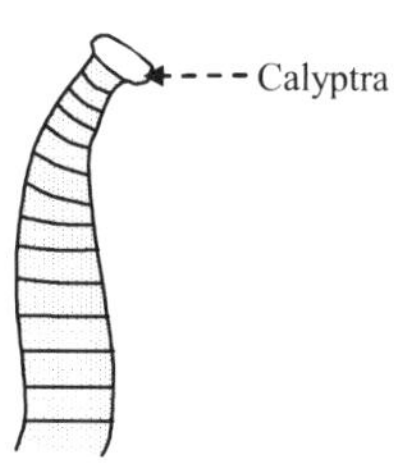

O. proboscidea

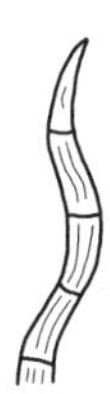

O. acuminata

1. **Habitat:** It is a freshwater planktonic form usually found in algal blooms in fish ponds. Marine species are also found. Some important species are *Oscillatoria annae, O. proboscidea, O. acuminata, O. princeps, O. curviceps, O. irrigua* and *O. nigra*.
2. **Thallus:** Thallus is filamentous. The cells are discoid, which join end-to-end forming the trichome. A trichome is a row of cells without any sheath. (When sheath surrounds individual trichome, it is called filament)
3. **Cells:** The cells are discoid in shape. In some forms like *O.proboscidae*, the apical cell is tipped with a thickened membrane called calyptra. Floating species often possess pseudovacuoles, which appear like shining granules.
4. **Reproduction:** Reproduction is by vegetative means through formation of hormogonia. Hormogonia are short sections of trichome separated from each other by dead cells called necridium. Each hormogonium develops into a new filament.

Figure 11.1: Identifying characteristics of some microscopic algae (*Microcystis* and *Oscillatoria*)

Class Cyanophyceae

NOSTOC

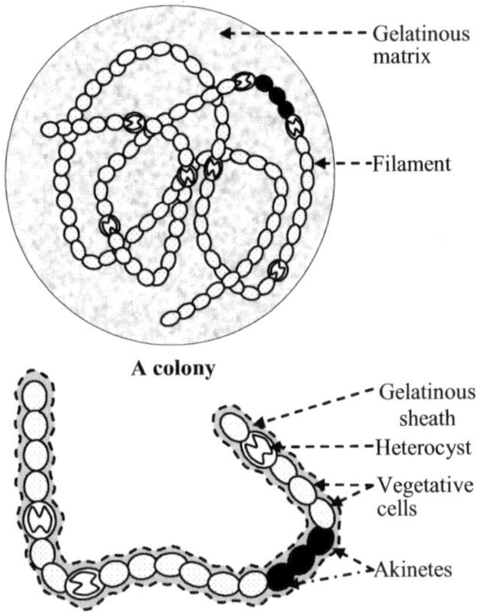

Nostoc sphaericum

1. **Habitat:** It is found both in terrestrial and aquatic habitats. Aquatic forma may be free-floating, lying on the floor or attached to submerged vegetation of freshwater ponds. Some prefer swift running water. Some important species are *Nostoc sphaericum, N. azollae, N. carneum* and *N. punctiforme.*
2. **Thallus:** Thallus consists of unbranched filamentous trichome embedded within a gelatinous sheath. Trichomes of varying lengths are contorted in a gelatinous matrix to form ball-shaped colonies. Colonies may be microscopic to a diameter of 30 cm.
3. **Cells:** Vegetative cells are generally oval, for which the trichome appears beaded. Intercalary heterocysts and akinetes are usually present. Heterocysts are specialised enlarged vegetative cells with thick wall. They are the sites of nitrogen fixation. Akinetes are thick-walled spores.
4. **Reproduction:** Reproduction is either by vegetative means through formation of hormogonia or by means of heterocysts or akinetes.

Class Cyanophyceae

ANABAENA

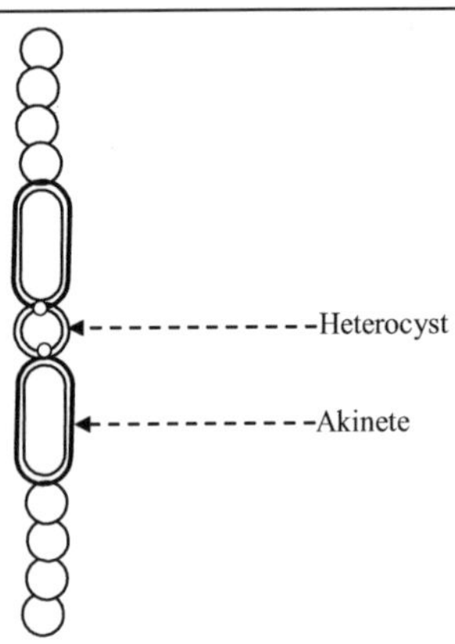

Anabaena levanderi

1. **Habitat:** It is a freshwater planktonic form, usually found in algal blooms in fish ponds. Some are symbiotic. Some important species are *Anabaena levanderi, A. azollae, A. aequalis* and *A. affinis.*
2. **Thallus:** Thallus consists of unbranched filamentous trichome embedded within a watery sheath. It is different from *Nostoc* in that trichomes are not contorted and do not form colonies.
3. **Cells:** Vegetative cells are generally barrel-shaped or oval, for which the trichome appears beaded. Intercalary heterocysts and akinetes are usually present.
4. **Reproduction:** Reproduction is either through hormogonia, heterocysts or akinetes like that of *Nostoc.*

Class Cyanophyceae

SPIRULINA

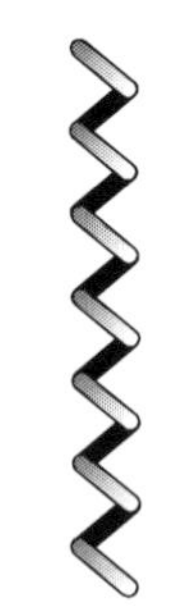

Spirulina platensis

1. **Habitat:** It is a free-floating freshwater algae. Some important species are *Spirulina (Arthrospira) platensis, S. maxima* and *S. fusiforms.*
2. **Thallus:** Thallus consists of filamentous trichome loosely or tightly coiled into more or less regular left-handed helix. Cross walls are not distinct.
3. **Apical cell:** The apical cells are widely rounded and usually with thickened outer cell wall without calyptra.
4. **Reproduction:** Cell division takes place perpendicularly to the long axis of the trichome. The daughter cells grow more or less to the original size before the next division. All cells are capable to divide with the exception of apical ones. Reproduction is by fragmentation of trichomes into motile hormogonia, which separate by help of necridium cells (*See* page 223).
5. **Nutritional value:** It is a rich source of protein, containing about 40-50% crude protein, for which it is being used as human food. Spirulina tablets are available in market to be used against protein deficiency.

Figure 11.2: Identifying characteristics of some microscopic algae (*Nostoc, Anabaena* and *Spirulina*)

Class Chlorophyceae

CHLAMYDOMONAS

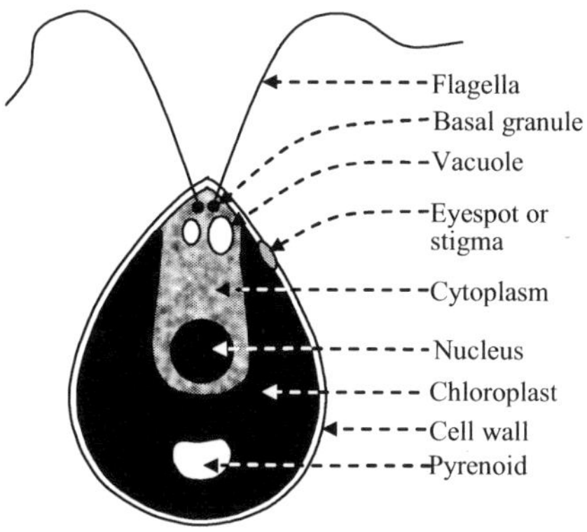

Chlamydomonas eugametos

1. **Habitat:** It is a freshwater planktonic form, which grows in stagnant water bodies and imparts green colour to them. It forms algal blooms. Few members are marine. Some important species are *Chlamydomonas augametos, C. alpina, C. angulosa, C. nivalis, C. elegans* and *C. caudate.*
2. **Thallus:** Unicellular, motile.
3. **Cell:** Cell is oval, spherical, pear-shaped or elongated. Anterior end is pointed. From the basal granules at the anterior end arise two flagella of equal length. Flagella help in motility of the algae. A cup-shaped chloroplast almost fills the cell. Nucleus is present in the cup-shaped cavity of the chloroplast. Towards the anterior end of the chloroplast is present a light sensitive stigma or eyespot. A pyrenoid is founded embedded in the mid basal part of the chloroplast. A pyrenoid is a proteinaceous area of the chloroplast associated with the formation of storage products. Vacuoles are present in cytoplasm.
4. **Reproduction:** Reproduction is either asexual through spore formation or sexual through isogamy, anisogamy or oogamy.

Class Chlorophyceae

CHLORELLA

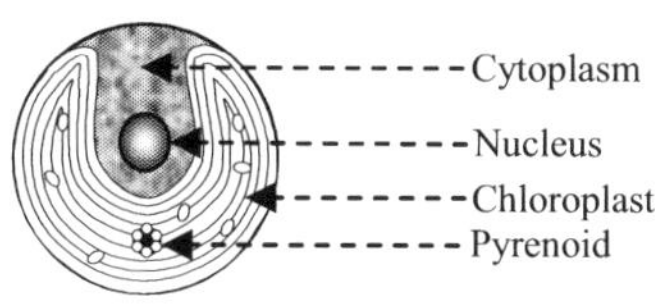

A single *Chlorella* cell

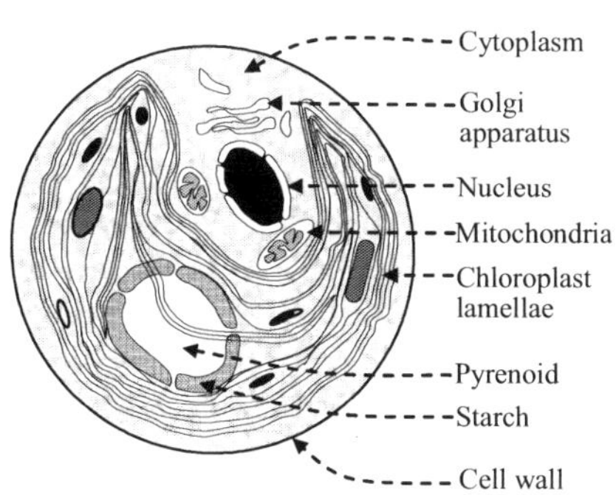

An enlarged *Chlorella* cell

Chlorella vulgaris

1. **Habitat:** It is a freshwater planktonic form, which grows in stagnant water bodies and imparts green colour to them. It forms algal blooms. Few members are symbiotic. Some important species are *Chlorella vulgaris, C. minutissa* and *C. pyrenoidosa.*
2. **Thallus:** Unicellular, small (5-10μ diameter), non-motile, often occurs singly, but occasionally in groups.
3. **Cell:** Cell is spherical to ellipsoidal. A cup-shaped chloroplast almost fills the cell. The chloroplast lamellae are visible. An indistinct pyrenoid is founded embedded in the mid basal part of the chloroplast. Starch produced by the pyrenoid can be seen in its periphery. Nucleus is present in the cup-shaped cavity of the chloroplast. Golgi apparatus and mitochondria are present in the cytoplasm.
4. **Reproduction:** Reproduction is asexual through autospore formation.
5. **Nutritional value:** Due to its high content of proteins, fats, carbohydrates and vitamins, it has potential use as human food.

Figure 11.3: Identifying characteristics of some microscopic algae (*Chlamydomonas* and *Chlorella*)

Class Chlorophyceae

SPIROGYRA

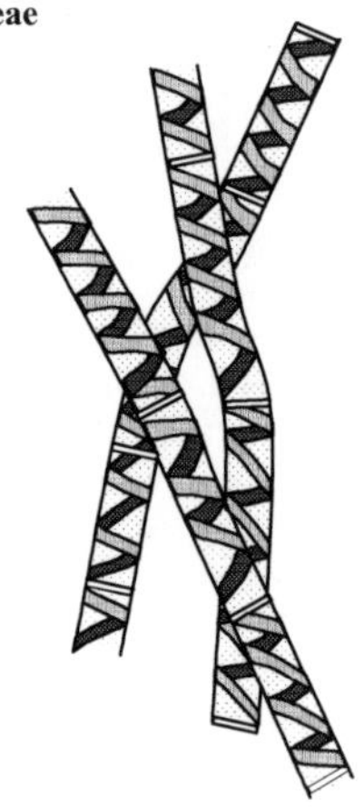

Filaments

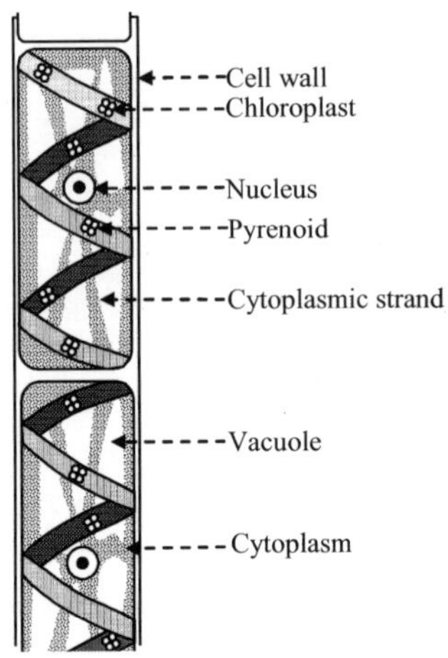

Enlarged portion of a filament

Spirogyra indica

1. **Habitat:** It is a freshwater free-floating algae, which grows as extensive masses, called 'pond scum', in stagnant water bodies. It looks like a mass of shining silky long filaments and hence is popularly known as 'pond silk'. Few members grow in slow-running water. Some important species are *Spirogyra indica, S. affinis. S. adnata, S. maxima* and *S. mirabisis*.
2. **Thallus:** Thallus consists of unbranched filaments. Young ones are attached to some substratum by a modified basal cell called hapteron or holdfast, while adults are always free-floating. Each filament consists of a single row of cells.
3. **Cells:** Cells are cylindrical. Each cell consists of a firm cell wall enclosing a mass of protoplast. Cell wall is commonly two-layered; the inner is made of cellulose, while the outer is made of pectic substances. These pectic substances gelatinise in presence of water and renders the plant slimy to touch. Cytoplasm is peripheral with a large central vacuole, which is traversed by several cytoplasmic strands. A single nucleus is found centrally suspended by these cytoplasmic strands. Chloroplast is flat ribbon-shaped present as a spiral, which is twisted anticlockwise. Each chloroplast has pyrenoids at intervals.
4. **Reproduction:** Reproduction is either by vegetative means through fragmentation or by sexual means through isogamous conjugation.

Class Chlorophyceae

ZYGNEMA

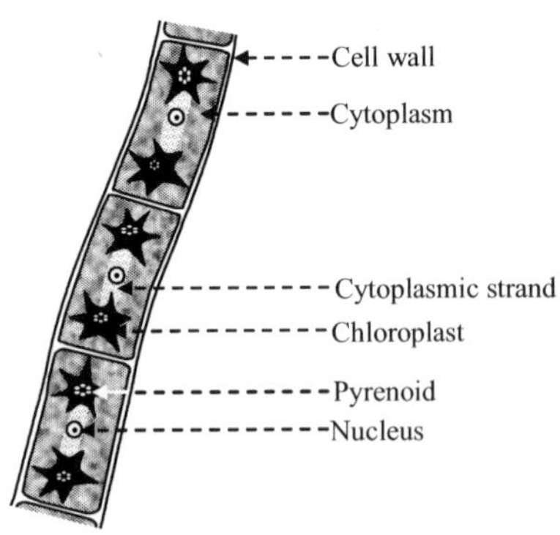

Zygnema pectinatum

1. **Habitat:** It is a freshwater free-floating algae, which grows in ponds, pools and streams to form yellowish-green scum. All members are aquatic except *Zygnema terrestre*. Some important species are *Zygnema pectinatum, Z. reticulatum* and *Z. spontaneum*.
2. **Thallus:** Thallus consists of unbranched filaments. The filament remains covered with mucilage. Young ones are attached to substratum by holdfast, while adults are always free-floating. Each filament consists of a single row of cells.
3. **Cells:** Cells are cylindrical. Each cell consists of a two-layered cell wall enclosing a mass of protoplast. Cytoplasm is peripheral. A single nucleus remains centrally suspended by cytoplasmic strands connecting the two chloroplasts. Two star-shaped chloroplasts are present in each cell, each with a prominent centrally located pyrenoid.
4. **Reproduction:** Reproduction is asexual (fragmentation or sporulation) or sexual (isogamous conjugation)

Figure 11.4: Identifying characteristics of some microscopic algae (*Spirogyra* and *Zygnema*)

Class Chlorophyceae

ULOTHRIX

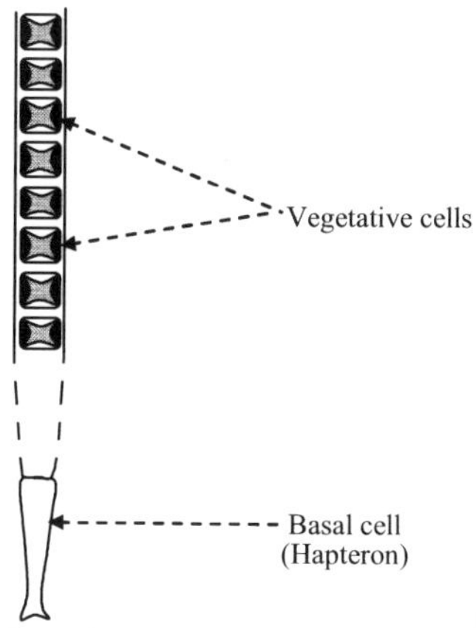

Filament

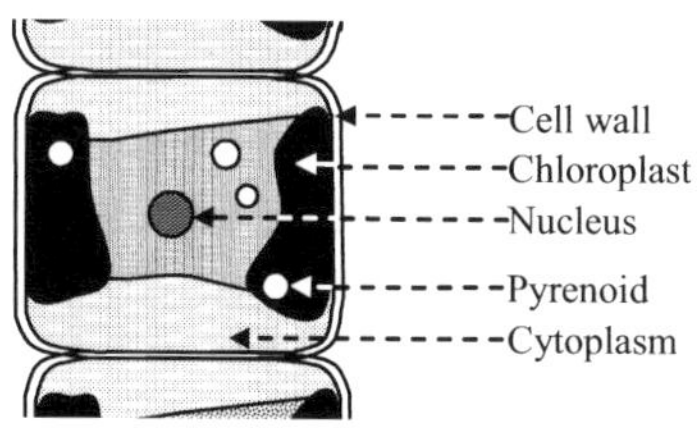

Enlarged portion of a filament

Ulothrix zonata

1. **Habitat:** It is a freshwater free-floating algae, which grows in ponds, pools and streams. Few are found attached to rocks and submerged grasses. A few forms are marine. Some important species are *Ulothrix zonata, U. flacca* and *U. tenuissima.*
2. **Thallus:** Thallus consists of unbranched filaments. Young ones are attached to substratum by holdfast (hapteron), while adults are always free-floating found as tangled masses on the surface of water. Each filament consists of a single row of cells.
3. **Cells:** All cells are broader than long except the basal cell, holdfast, which is colourless and sometimes slightly ramified and rhizoid-like. Each cell consists of a two-layered cell wall enclosing a mass of protoplast. Cytoplasm is peripheral. A single nucleus is present in the center of the cell. Each cell has a girdle-shaped chloroplast with one or more pyrenoids. Shape of chloroplast varies from species to species.
4. **Reproduction:** Reproduction is either asexual (fragmentation or sporulation) or sexual (isogamous conjugation).

Class Chlorophyceae

OEDOGONIUM

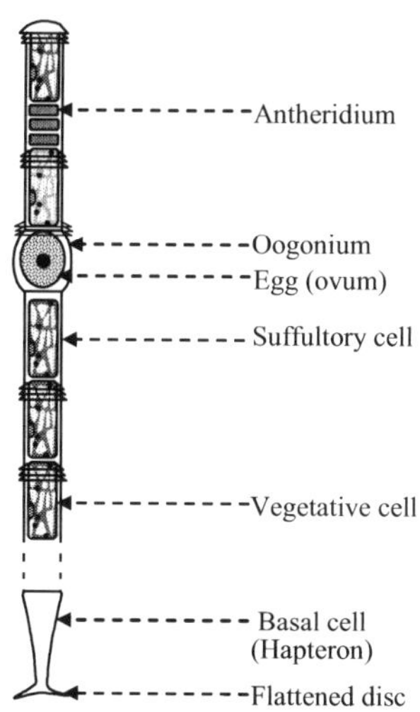

Filament

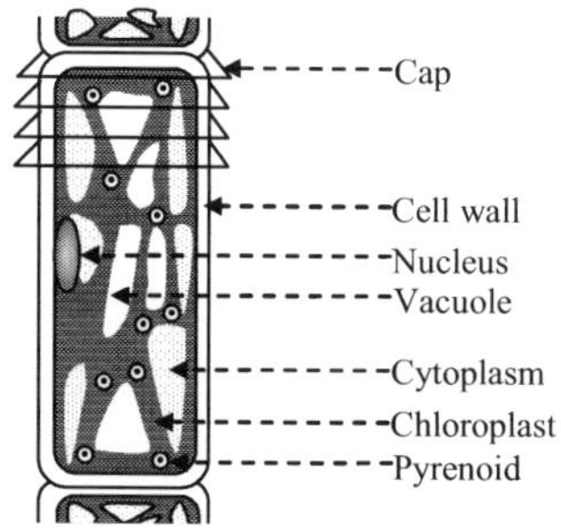

Enlarged vegetative cell

Oedogonium borisianum

1. **Habitat:** It is a freshwater algae, which grows in ponds, pools and streams. Few are found attached to rocks and submerged grasses. It is invariably aquatic except a few terrestrial species. Some important species are *Oedogonium borisianum, O. macrandrous*, *O. americanum* and *O. foveolatum.*
2. **Thallus:** Thallus consists of unbranched filaments. Young ones are attached to some substratum by a modified basal cell called hapteron or holdfast, while adults are always free-floating. The base of the holdfast is formed into a flattened disc, with which the algae attaches to the substratum. Each filament consists of a single row of cells. There is generally no slime around the filament.
3. **Cells:** Its thallus is like that of *Ulothrix*, but shows more marked specialisation of cells with greater interdependence. Besides the vegetative cells, there are specialised cells like a basal cell, suffultory cells, oogonium and antheridium. Vegetative cells are cylindrical. Each cell consists of a firm three-layered cell wall enclosing a mass of protoplast. The outermost layer of the cell wall is made of chitin, the middle layer, of pectin and the innermost layer, of cellulose. Each cell has a perietal large single flat circular nucleus and a peripheral network of chloroplast around a central vacuole. The chloroplast extends from end to end and bears many pyrenoids with starch sheaths, each situated at the interstices of network. Certain cells in every filament possess one or more ring-like markings of hemicellulose at their distal ends. Such structures are called apical caps. Cells with apical caps are called cap cells. These cells are found at variable intervals in the filament.
4. **Reproduction:** Reproduction is either by vegetative means through fragmentation or by sexual means through isogamous conjugation.

Figure 11.5: Identifying characteristics of some microscopic algae (*Ulothrix* and *Oedogonium*)

Class Chlorophyceae

VOLVOX

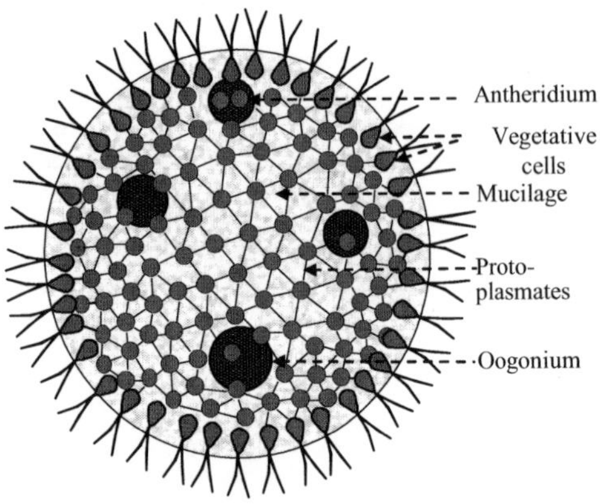

A colony

Volvox globator

1. **Habitat:** It is a freshwater algae, which grows in ponds, pools and lakes imparting green colour to the water. Important species are *Volvox globator*, *V. aureus* and *V. carteri*.
2. **Thallus:** Thallus consists of a coenobium. A coenobium is a colony of algal cells in a specific arrangement and number that does not increase once mature. The *Volvox* coenobium is a hollow sphere of mucilage with numerous vegetative cells arranged in a single layer near the surface. The extracellular matrix of the coenobium is made of a gelatinous glycoprotein. The individual cells are connected by thin strands of cytoplasm called protoplasmates. The cells swim in a coordinated fashion, with distinct anterior and posterior poles.The cells have eyespots, more developed near the anterior, which enable the colony to swim towards light.
3. **Cells:** The vegetative cells in the *Volvox* colony resemble *Chlamydomonas* cells.
4. **Reproduction:** Reproduction is asexual or sexual. For asexual reproduction, few specialised cells of the coenobium differentiate to gonidium by growing larger with the disappearance of flagella and gradual thickening. The gonidium escapes from the mother colony and increases in number by binary fission to produce a new *Volvox* colony. For sexual reproduction, some cells of the colony become oogonium and each oogonium develops into an ovum (egg). Some other cells become antheridium and each antheridium divides to become a large number of spindle-shaped male gametes (sperm). One of the several sperm cells fertilises an ovum and produces the zygote. The zygote develops to a new coenobium of *Volvox*.

Class Chlorophyceae

HYDRODICTYON

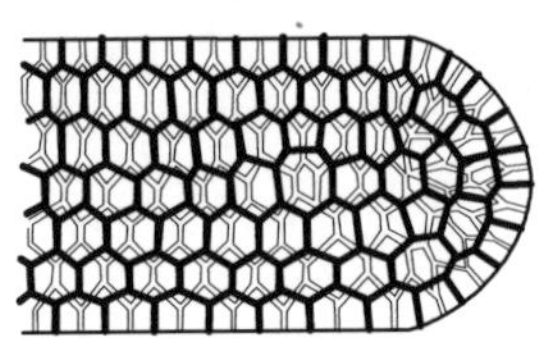

Net-like colony with hexagonal mesh

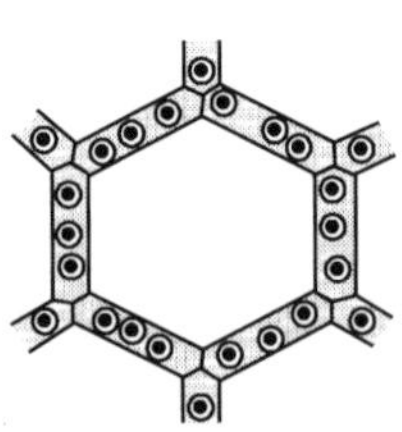

A single mesh formed by six cells

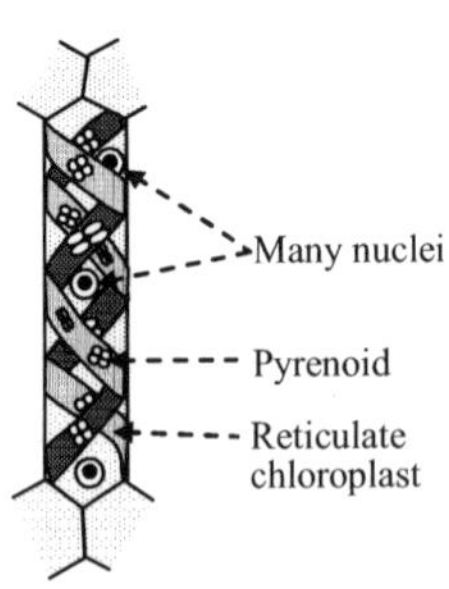

A single cell

Hydrodictyon indicum

1. **Habitat:** It is a beautiful freshwater algae of ponds and pools. It is commonly called 'water net' because of its net-like appearance. Important species are *Hydrodictyon indicum*, *H. africanum*, *H. patenaeforme* and *H. reticulatum*.
2. **Thallus:** Thallus is a coenobium consisting of a net-like colony with hexagonal or pentagonal meshes. The net may be either a flat net or a single-layered network of cells arranged in a hollow cylinder closed at both ends.
3. **Cells:** The cells in the colony form the sides of a hexagon or that of a pentagon. Each cell is cylindrical. At each corner, the triangular ends of three cells are in contact. Each cell has large number of nuclei (coenocytic). Chloroplast is reticulate with large number of pyrenoids. Cytoplasm occupies a peripheral position enclosing a large central vacuole, which contains a watery cell-sap.
4. **Reproduction:** Reproduction is both asexual through zoospore formation and sexual through isogamy.

Figure 11.6: Identifying characteristics of some microscopic algae (*Volvox* and *Hydrodictyon*)

Class Chlorophyceae

PEDIASTRUM

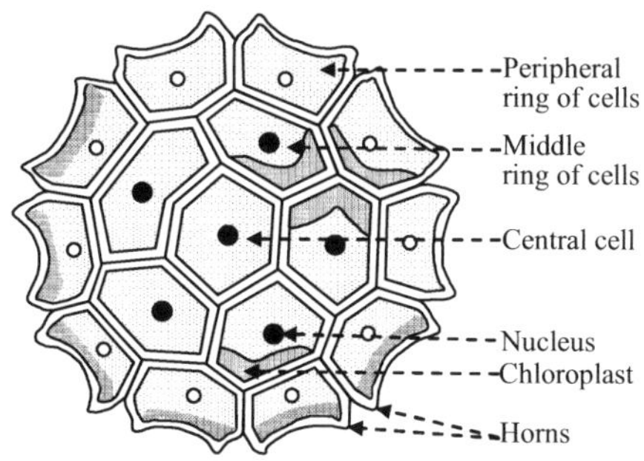

A young colony (16 cells)

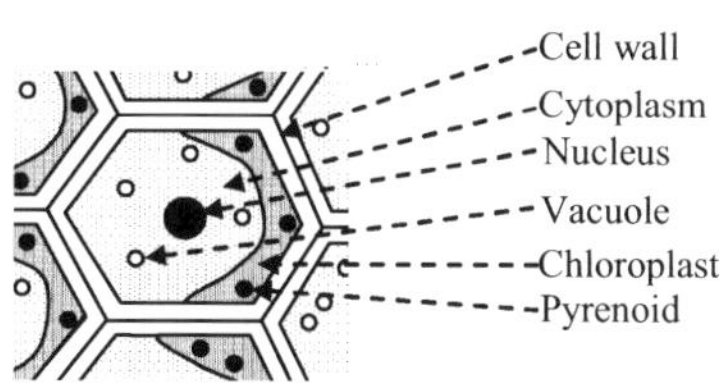

An enlarged individual cell

Pediastrum boryanum

1. **Habitat:** It is a freshwater algae found in ponds, pools, ditches and lakes amongst other aquatic plants. Common species are *Pediastrum boryanum*, *P. simplex* and *P. tetras*.
2. **Thallus:** Thallus consists of a coenobium containing a colony of 2 to 128 cells depending on the species. The number of cells is some power of 2 (*e.g.* 2^1, 2^2, 2^3, 2^4, 2^5, 2^6, 2^7 etc.). Each species has a fixed number of cells. *P. tetras* has 4 to 8 cells, while *P. boryanum* has upto 128 cells. The cells are arranged in a single layer forming a round plate. They are arranged in concentric rings in the plate. Each ring has a definite number of cells. An 8-celled coenobium has one central cell surrounded by a peripheral ring of 7 cells. Similar arrangement is also there for 16-celled (1+5+10) and 32-celled (1+5+10+16) coenobium.
3. **Cells:** Individual cells are polygonal in shape, which are arranged compactly. They are non-motile and lack eyespot and flagella. Each young cell has a single nucleus and a perietal chloroplast containing one pyrenoid. Older cells have more nuclei (1-8) and diffused perforated chloroplast containing more pyrenoids (1-4). Cell wall is smooth or granular. The cells of the peripheral ring of cells usually have outwardly projecting processes called 'horns' (1-3 on each cell). The horns are the extensions of the cell wall, which become gelatinised.
4. **Reproduction:** Reproduction is both asexual through zoospore formation and sexual through isogamy.

Class Chlorophyceae

GONIUM

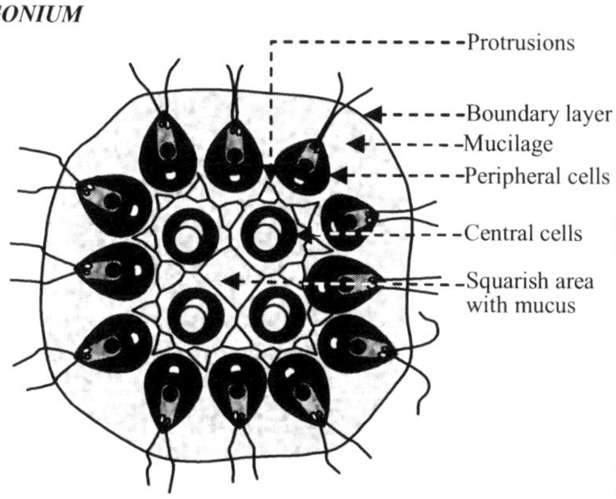

A colony

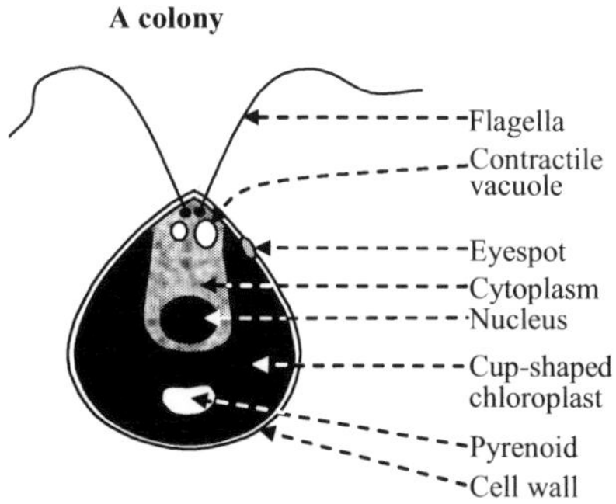

An enlarged individual cell

Gonium pectorale

1. **Habitat:** It is usually found intermingled with other algae of freshwater ponds, pools and ditches.
2. **Thallus:** Thallus consists of a coenobium containing a colony of 4, 16 or 32 cells arranged in a rectangular plate. In a 16-celled coenobium, there are four central cells and 12 peripheral cells, three on each side. The cells remain embedded in mucilage with a firm boundary layer. The cells are connected by slight protrusions, so that there are small triangular spaces between them, while in the center of the whole coenobium, there is a large squarish area occupied by mucus.
3. **Cells:** Individual cells are ovoid to pyriform in shape. Two flagella are present at the anterior end. Two contractile vacuoles are present at the base of the flagella. A single eyespot is present in the anterior end of the cell. Chloroplast is cup shaped with one pyrenoid.
4. **Reproduction:** Reproduction is either by vegetative means through fragmentation or by sexual means through isogamy.

Figure 11.7: Identifying characteristics of some microscopic algae (*Pediastrum* and *Gonium*)

Class Chlorophyceae ***PANDORINA*** 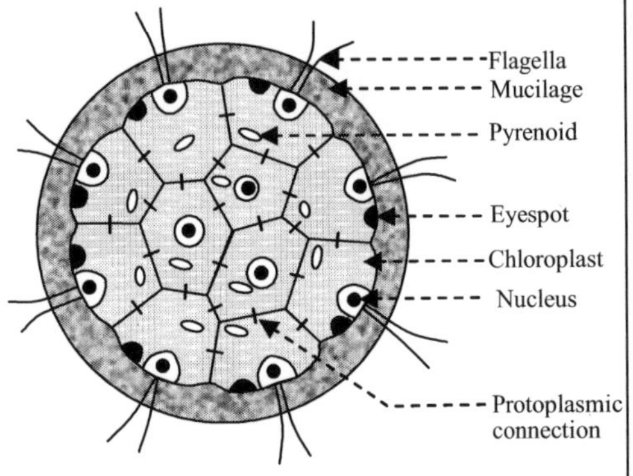 ***Pandorina morum***	1. **Habitat:** It is a freshwater algae, which grows in ponds and pools. Some important species are *Pandorina morum, P. unicocca* and *P. charkowiensis.* 2. **Thallus:** Thallus consists of a coenobium containing a colony of 4, 8, 16 or 32 cells, which remain embedded in a common gelatinous matrix. *Pandorina morum,* which occurs in India has a 16-celled coenobium. In the coenobium, the neighbouring cells are connected by protoplasmic connections. The coenobium is spherical or ellipsoidal. A well-defined envelope of mucilage surrounds the whole colony. It is different from *Gonium* in that (a) Its coenobium is spherical or ellipsoidal while that of *Gonium* is rectangular, (b) The individual cells in *Pandorina* are more tightly packed than those in *Gonium* and (c) In *Pandorina,* the broader ends of individual cells remain outwards while in *Gonium* they remain inwards. 3. **Cells:** Individual cells are originally pyriform in shape, but are so tightly packed that owing to their mutual pressure, they become laterally flattened with the broad ends outward. Two flagella are present at the middle of the broader end. Each cell has a single eyespot and a contractile vacuole at the flagellated end. Chloroplast is cup-shaped, which almost completely fills the cell. Each chloroplast may contain one or more pyrenoids. 4. **Reproduction:** Reproduction is both asexual and sexual.
Class Chlorophyceae ***EUDORINA*** 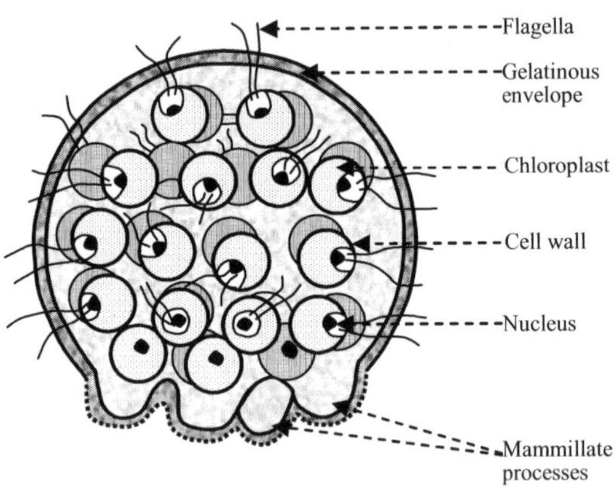 ***Eudorina illinoiensis***	1. **Habitat:** It is a freshwater algae of ponds and pools. Some important species are *Eudorina illinoiensis* and *E. elegans.* The Indian species is *E. indica.* 2. **Thallus:** Thallus consists of a hollow spherical or ellipsoidal coenobium containing 16, 32 or 64 cells inside a gelatinous envelope. It is different from *Pandorina* in that, the individual cells are loosely arranged forming a single layer in the peripheral mucilage, which surrounds a hollow space. The posterior end of the coenobium bears few mammillate processes. The cells are arranged in tiers, each tier having a ring of cells surrounding a hollow space. In a 32-celled coenobium, there are 5 tiers of rings; the 3 middle tiers have larger rings of 8 cells each while the 2 polar rings have only 4 cells each (4+8+8+8+4=32). 3. **Cells:** The individual cells are pyriform or spherical in shape, each with two flagella, a cup-shaped chloroplast having one or more pyrenoids, two contractile vacuoles at the base of the flagella and an eyespot at the same end. Each cell has a nucleus present in the cup-shaped cavity of the chloroplast. Cells are connected to neighbouring cells by protoplasmic connections. 4. **Reproduction:** Reproduction is both asexual and sexual.

Figure 11.8: Identifying characteristics of some microscopic algae (*Pandorina* and *Eudorina*)

Class Chlorophyceae

CLOSTERIUM

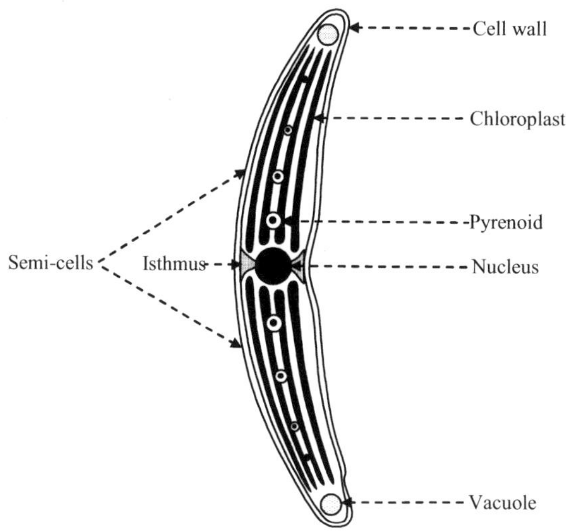

Closterium moniliforme

1. **Habitat:** It is an unconstricted placoderm desmid (*See* page 219). It is found solitarily at the bottom of freshwater ponds and drains. Common species are *Closterium moniliforme*, *C. acerosum*, *C. lanceolatum*, *C. lineatum* and *C. striolatum*.
2. **Thallus:** Unicellular, non-motile.
3. **Cell:** Cell is elongated, tapering from the middle towards both the ends. It usually has crescent shape like a curved moon and is circular in cross section. The cell consists of two symmetrical halves known as the semi-cells joined together by a connecting zone called isthmus. The cell is not constricted at the isthmus zone so that the thallus is distinctly a single cell. Nucleus is embedded in a small median mass of cytoplasm in the region of the isthmus. Each semi-cell has an axial elongated chloroplast in the form of a curved cone, which bears several longitudinal ridges. In the chloroplasts, the pyrenoids are located in the central portion in a row. Both the tips of the cell contain hyaline cytoplasmic regions, each tip containing a small spherical polar vacuole. Cell wall is made of two halves; one older than the other. The two halves have beveled edges and fit so closely that they are not easily recognisable. The wall is further composed of two well-differentiated layers. The cell wall has several pores arranged in longitudinal rows in the narrow grooves between the fine ridges. A layer of mucilage secreted through the pores surrounds the cell wall.
4. **Reproduction:** Reproduction is both asexual through transverse cell division and sexual through conjugation.

Class Chlorophyceae

COSMARIUM

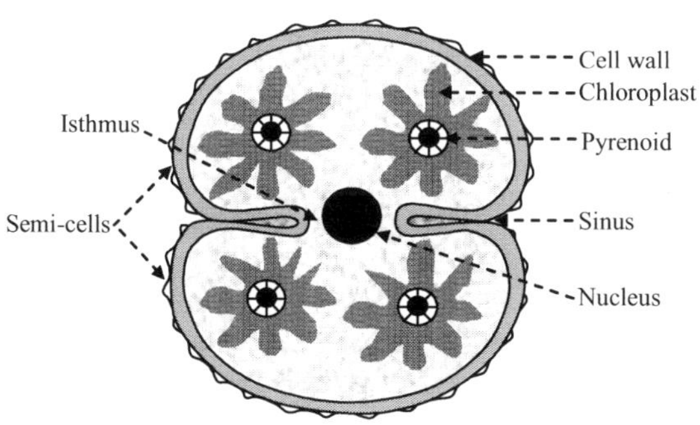

Cosmarium reniforme

1. **Habitat:** It is a constricted placoderm desmid (*See* page 219). It is found as a solitarily free-floating desmid in freshwater ponds intermingled with other algae. Common species are *Cosmarium reniforme, C. angulosum, C. costatum, C. granatum, C. rectangulare, C. sexangulare* and *C. undulatum.*
2. **Thallus:** Unicellular, non-motile.
3. **Cell:** Cell is flattened and exhibits distinct constriction, which divides it into two perfectly symmetrical halves called semi-cells. The narrower part connecting the two semi-cells is known as isthmus. The constricted portion is known as sinus. Nucleus is embedded in a small median mass of cytoplasm in the region of the isthmus. Each semi-cell has two chloroplasts, which are richly lobed. The lobes spread towards the periphery of the cell. Each chloroplast contains a pyrenoid. In the chloroplasts, the pyrenoids are located in the central portion in a row. Cell wall is similar to *Closterium* and has pores, through which mucilage is secreted to the surrounding.
4. **Reproduction:** Reproduction is both asexual through transverse cell division and sexual through conjugation.

Figure 11.9: Identifying characteristics of some microscopic algae (*Closterium* and *Cosmarium*)

Class Bacillariophyceae (Diatoms)

PINNULARIA

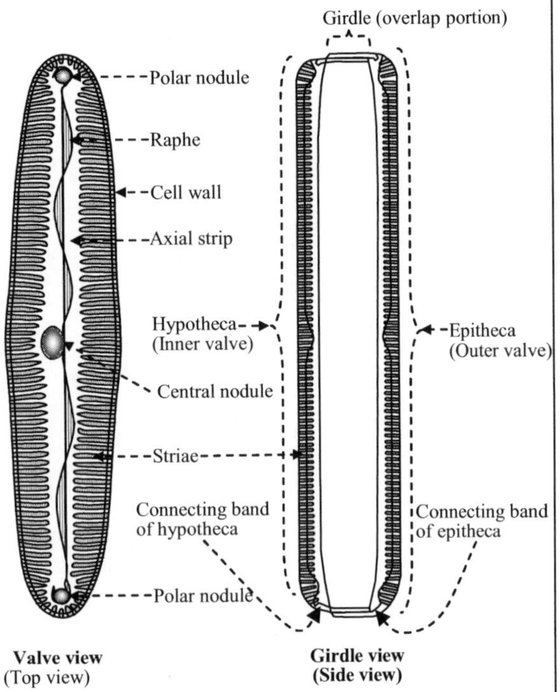

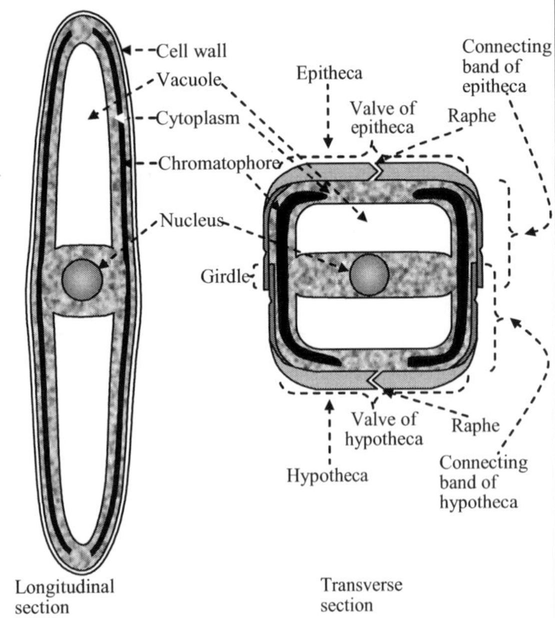

Pinnularia viridis

1. **Habitat:** It is freshwater pennate diatom (pennale) (*See* page 219) found in ponds, pools, ditches and lakes. Common species are *Pinnularia viridis, P. debesii, P. major, P. socialis* and *P. streptoraphe*.
2. **Thallus:** Unicellular, motile.
3. **Cells:** The diatom cell, often called 'frustule' is oblong elliptical with blunt ends in case of *Pinnularia*. As the cell is bilaterally symmetrical, it is a pinnate diatom. The cell wall has two layers, the inner thin continuous membranous wall made of pectin that encloses the protoplast and the outer thick armorous wall. The outer wall is made of two equal halves. The older half 'epitheca' fits closely over the younger half 'hypotheca', just like a pair of petri dishes. Each half consists of the main surface called 'valve' and the circular projection at the margin of the surface called 'connecting band'. The connecting band of epitheca overlaps that of the hypotheca. The overlapping region is called 'girdle', which remains united by some cementing organic substance. On the valve surface, there are two rows of ridges called striae arranged on both the side of an axial strip to produce beautiful ornamentation. The connecting bands are smooth and lack such ornamentation. A longitudinal slot called raphe extends from one end of the valve to the other along the middle of the axial strip. Raphe helps diatoms for their movement. Therefore, all diatoms possessing raphe are motile and those, which do not have raphe are non-motile. The *Pinnularia* frustule has two polar nodules at the ends and a central nodule in the middle of the cell wall. The nodules are modifications of the cell wall. The common constituent of the cell wall is hydrated amorphous silica. The cell can be seen in two views; the valve view, when seen from the top and the girdle view, when seen from the side. Longitudinal and transverse sections through the cell show that, the cytoplasm forms a thick layer just below the cell wall. There is a large central vacuole. A cytoplasmic band runs across the middle of the central vacuole. A large nucleus is embedded in the center of the cytoplasmic band. There are two perietal chromatophores, which extend through the whole length of the cell and contain pyrenoids.
4. **Reproduction:** Reproduction is mainly asexual through cell division or fission. During each cell division, the overlapping theca (epitheca and hypotheca) loosen their hold from each other and slightly separate at the girdle. The protoplast divides into two equal halves longitudinally in a plane parallel to the valve face, producing two daughter cells. One of the daughter cells remains in the epitheca and the other in the hypotheca of the mother cell. Their opposite sides are naked. Now, the protoplast of each daughter cell covers its naked face by secreting a new theca fitting inside the old theca. Thus, the two new theca always become the hypotheca of the daughter cells. The daughter cell, which carries the epitheca of the mother cell, remains same in size as that of the mother cell, while the one, which carries the hypotheca of the mother cell, is slightly smaller. This results in a gradual reduction of the size of one of the daughter cells after each division. Before a daughter cells reaches its lower limit of size, it goes for sexual reproduction to restore back the normal size. Sexual reproduction takes place through formation of auxospores (*auxo* : grow).

Figure 11.10: Identifying characteristics of some microscopic algae (*Pinnularia*)

Class Bacillariophyceae (Diatoms)

NAVICULA

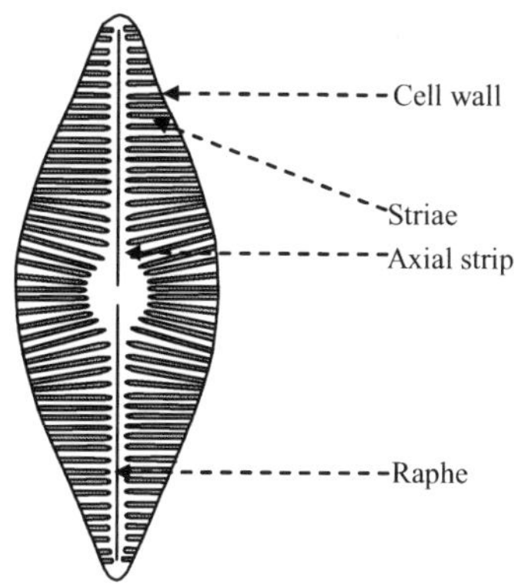

Navicula cuspidata

1. **Habitat:** It is a pennate diatom (pennale) (*See* page 219). A large number of species of this genus are found in freshwater. Some are also marine. Common species are *Navicula cuspidata*, *N. mutica*, *N. oblonga*, *N. ostrearia*, *N. seminulum*, *N. amphisbaena* and *N. grevillei*.
2. **Thallus:** Unicellular, motile.
3. **Cell:** The diatom frustule is oblong and boat-shaped with pointed or capitate ends. It is different from *Pinnularia* in that the cell has a single chromatophore opposed to one of the valves, which spreads onto the girdle. Pyrenoids are absent. Other structures are similar to *Pinnularia*.
4. **Reproduction:** Reproduction is mainly asexual through cell division or fission. Sexual reproduction takes place through formation of auxospores (*auxo* : grow) similar to *Pinnularia*.

Class Bacillariophyceae (Diatoms)

NITZSCHIA

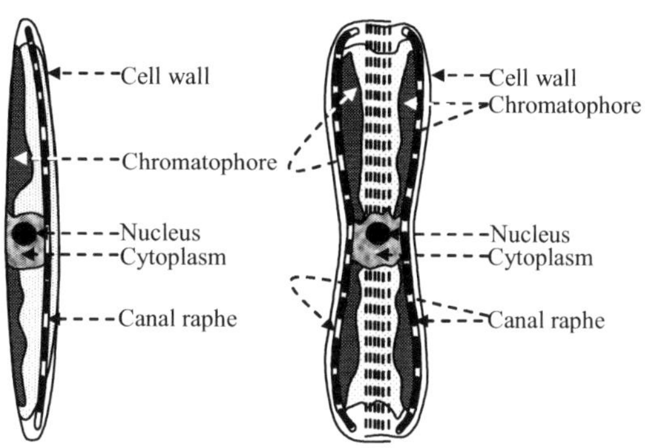

Valve view **Girdle view**

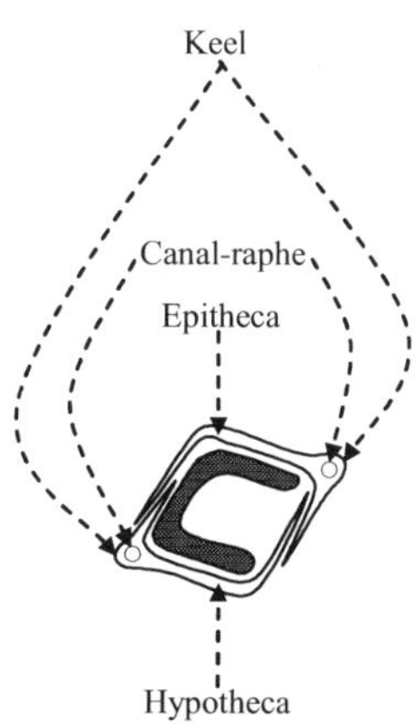

Transverse section

Nitzschia commutata

1. **Habitat:** It is a pennate diatom (pennale) (*See* page 219) found in both freshwater and marine environments. Common species are *Nitzschia commutata*, *N. closterium*, *N. fonticola*, *N. granulata*, *N. leucosigma*, *N. linearis*, *N. longissima*, *N. obtusa*, *N. palea*, *N. putrida*, *N. scalaris*, *N. sigma*, *N. sigmoidea*, *N. subtilis*, *N. tryblionella* and *N. vitrea*.
2. **Thallus:** Unicellular, motile.
3. **Cells:** The 'frustule' is oblong elliptical and is depressed in the middle. Each valve has a projecting keel, which runs along the whole length and is marked with evenly spaced carinal dots. Keel is displaced towards one margin of the valve. Cross section of the frustule is rhomboidal, the epitheca and hypotheca meet at an acute angle in the keel. Raphe is present as a longitudinal cylindrical canal (canal-raphe) without nodules and is located in the keel. Longitudinal section through the cell shows that the cytoplasm forms a thick layer just below the cell wall. There is a large central vacuole. A cytoplasmic band runs across the middle of the central vacuole. A large nucleus is embedded in the center of the cytoplasmic band. There are two perietal chromatophores, which extend through the whole length of the cell and contain pyrenoids.
4. **Reproduction:** Reproduction is mainly asexual through cell division or fission. Sexual reproduction takes place through formation of auxospores.

Figure 11.11: Identifying characteristics of some microscopic algae (*Navicula* and *Nitzschia*)

Class Bacillariophyceae (Diatoms)

PLEUROSIGMA

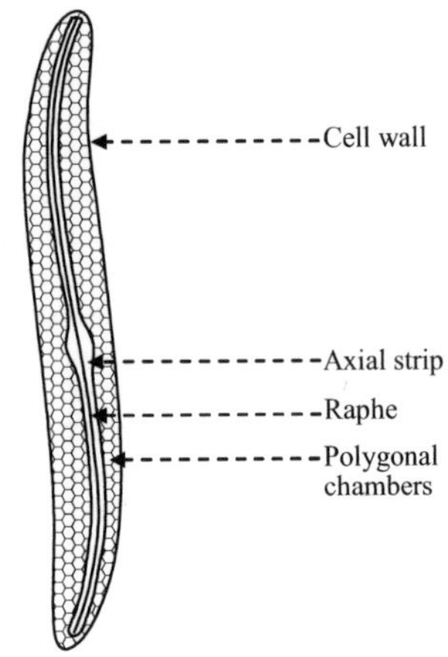

Valve view

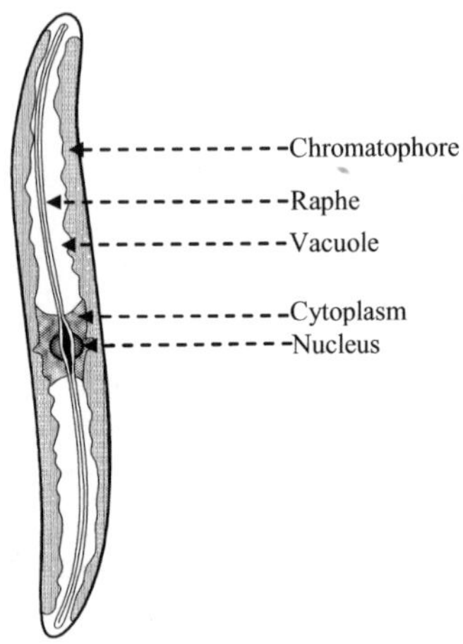

Longitudinal section

Pleurosigma spenceri

1. **Habitat:** It is a fresh water pennate diatom (pennale) (*See* page 219) found in ponds, pools ditches and lakes. Common species are *Pleurosigma spenceri, P. balticum* and *P. gigantium*.
2. **Thallus:** Unicellular, motile.
3. **Cells:** The 'frustule' is oblong and sigmoid in shape (S-shaped). The wall of the valve is occupied by innumerable minute polygonal chambers. Raphe and axial strip extend from one end of the valve to the other along the middle in the form of a sigmoid curve. Longitudinal section through the cell shows that the cytoplasm forms a thick layer just below the cell wall. There is a large central vacuole. A cytoplasmic band runs across the middle of the central vacuole. A large nucleus is embedded in the center of the cytoplasmic band. There are two perietal chromatophores, which extend through the whole length of the cell and contain pyrenoids.
4. **Reproduction:** Reproduction is mainly asexual through cell division or fission. Sexual reproduction takes place through formation of auxospores.

Class Bacillariophyceae (Diatoms)

GYROSIGMA

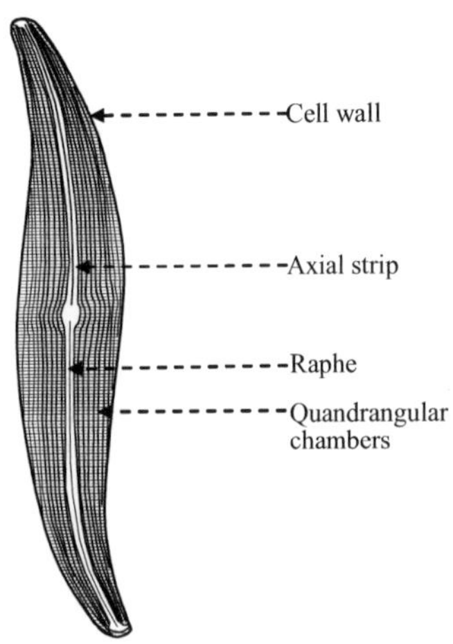

Girdle view

Gyrosigma attenuatum

1. **Habitat:** It is a pennate diatom (pennale) (*See* page 219) found in marine environment. Common species are *Gyrosigma attenuatum* and *G. acuminatum.*
2. **Thallus:** Unicellular, motile.
3. **Cells:** The 'frustule' is oblong and sigmoid in shape (S-shaped). It is different from *Pleurosigma* in that, the wall of its valve is occupied by innumerable minute quadrangular chambers. Raphe and axial strip extend from one end of the valve to the other along the middle in the form of a sigmoid curve. Longitudinal section through the cell shows that the cytoplasm forms a thick layer just below the cell wall. There is a large central vacuole. A cytoplasmic band runs across the middle of the central vacuole. A large nucleus is embedded in the center of the cytoplasmic band. There are two perietal chromatophores, which extend through the whole length of the cell and contain pyrenoids.
4. **Reproduction:** Reproduction is mainly asexual through cell division or fission. Sexual reproduction takes place through formation of auxospores.

Figure 11.12: Identifying characteristics of some microscopic algae (*Pleurosigma* and *Gyrosigma*)

Class Bacillariophyceae (Diatoms)

ASTERIONELLA

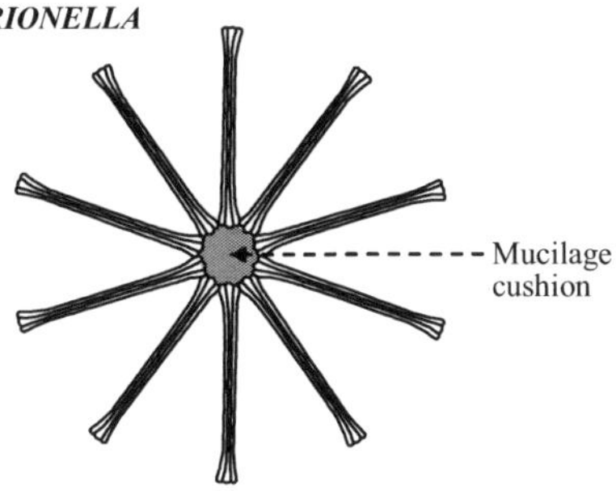

A colony

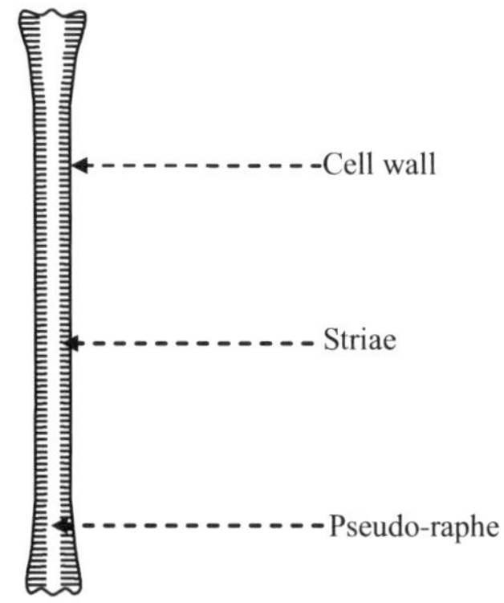

An individual cell

Asterionella gracillima

1. **Habitat:** It is a pennate diatom (pennale) (*See* page 219) found in freshwater and marine environments as free-floating plankton. Some important species are *Asterionella gracillima, A. formosa, A. glacialis, A. japonica* and *A. kariana*.
2. **Thallus:** Thallus consists of a star-shaped colony of non-motile cells arranged radially. Cells are united by a basal mucilage cushion to form characteristic stellate (star-shaped) groups.
3. **Cells:** The 'frustule' is straight, rod-shaped. Raphe is absent, for which it is non-motile. Only a pseudo-raphe is present. A pseudo-raphe is a narrow linear smooth area separating the two systems of striae. It is devoid of markings (striae) and extends from one end of the valve to the other end. This smooth area looks like a true raphe and is therefore called pseudo-raphe.
4. **Reproduction:** Reproduction is mainly asexual through cell division or fission. Sexual reproduction takes place through formation of auxospores.

Class Bacillariophyceae (Diatoms)

TABELLARIA

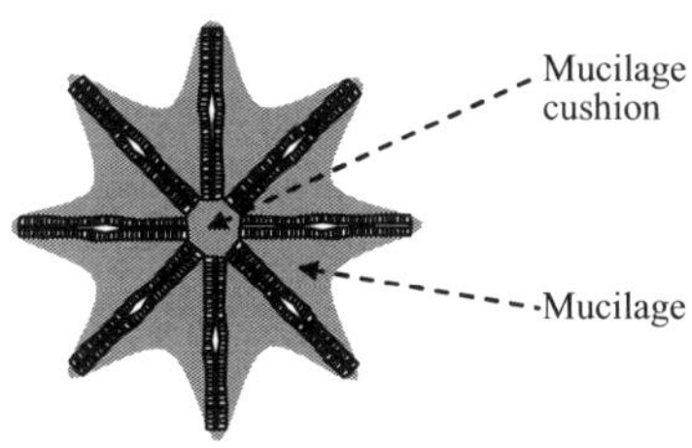

A colony

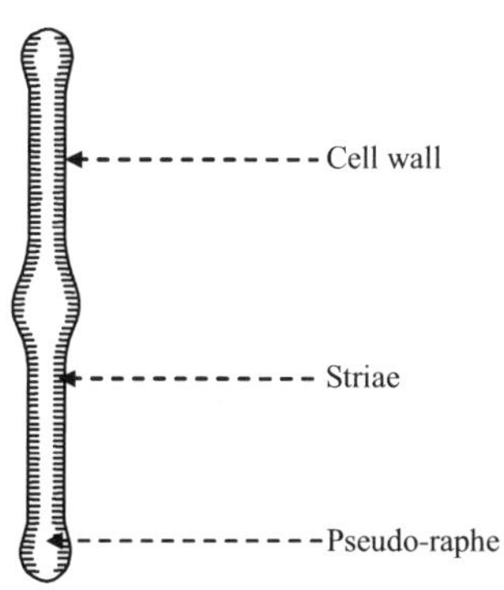

An individual cell

Tabellaria flocculosa

1. **Habitat:** It is a pennate diatom (pennale) (*See* page 219) found in freshwater as free-floating plankton. Some important species are *Tabellaria flocculosa, T. fenestrata* and *T. ventricosa*.
2. **Thallus:** Thallus consists of a star-shaped colony of non-motile cells arranged radially. Cells are united by a basal mucilage cushion to form characteristic stellate (star-shaped) groups. The cells also spread out between them, a delicate layer of mucilage, so that the whole has the character of a parachute. Sometimes cells may remain attached to each other at their ends with acute angles, so as to form zig-zag colonies.
3. **Cells:** The 'frustule' is straight, rod-shaped. Raphe is absent, for which it is non-motile. Only a pseudo-raphe is present, which extends from one end of the valve to the other end (*See Asterionella* described above).
4. **Reproduction:** Reproduction is mainly asexual through cell division or fission. Sexual reproduction takes place through formation of auxospores.

Figure 11.13: Identifying characteristics of some microscopic algae (*Asterionella* and *Tabellaria*)

Class Bacillariophyceae (Diatoms)

DIATOMA

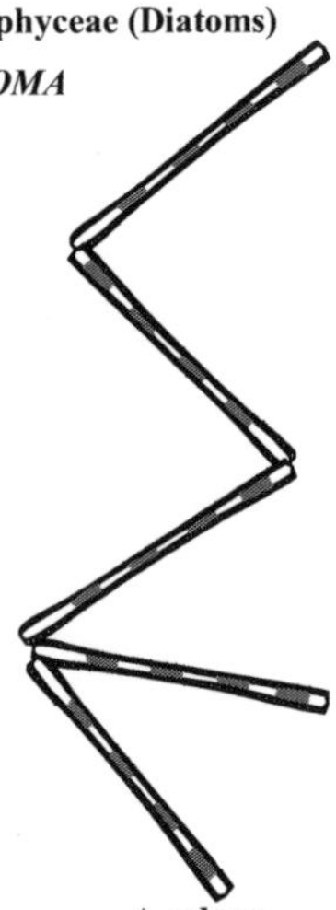

A colony

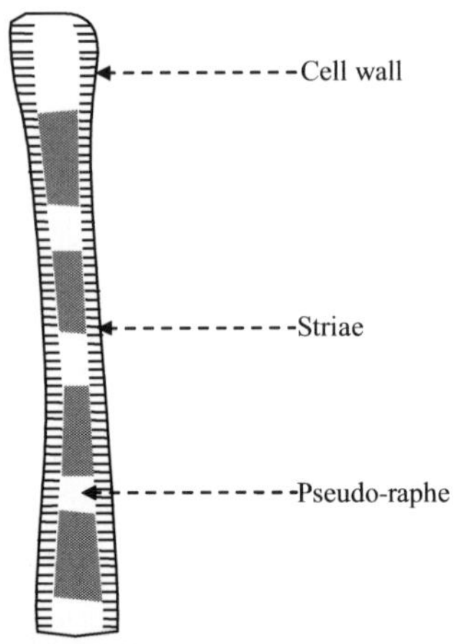

An individual cell

Diatoma elongatum

1. **Habitat:** It is a pennate diatom (pennale) (*See* page 219) found in freshwater as free-floating plankton. Common species are *Diatoma elongatum*, *D. hiemale* and *D. vulgare*.
2. **Thallus:** Thallus consists of a colony of non-motile cells arranged in a zigzag manner. Cells are connected to each other by mucilage secreted locally. Sometimes, the colony may be stellate (star-shaped).
3. **Cells:** The 'frustule' is straight, rod-shaped. Raphe is absent for which it is non-motile. Only a pseudo-raphe is present which extends from one end of the valve to the other end (*See* page 235).
4. **Reproduction:** Reproduction is mainly asexual through cell division or fission. Sexual reproduction takes place through formation of auxospores.

Class Bacillariophyceae (Diatoms)

FRAGILARIA

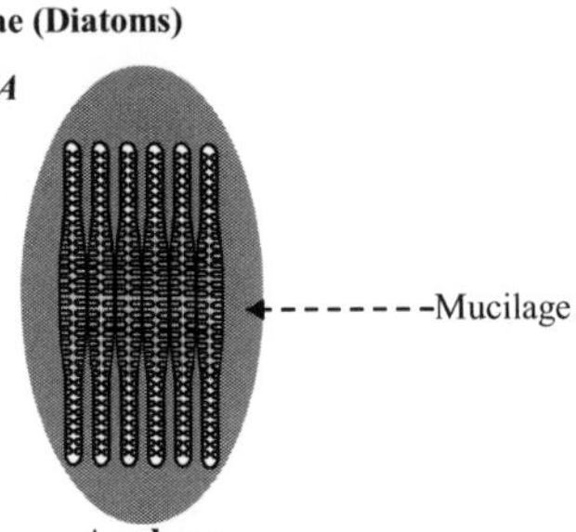

A colony

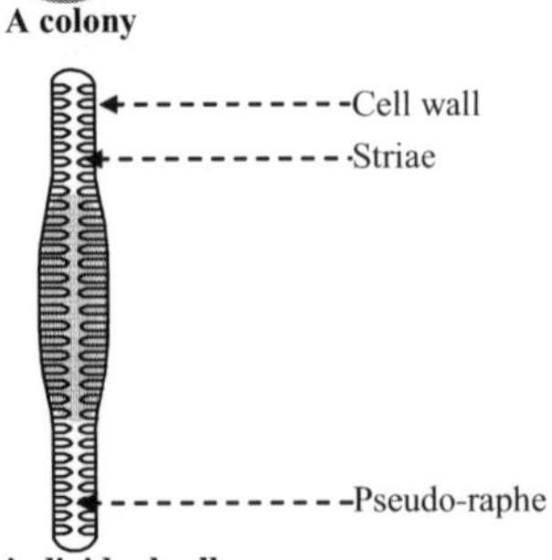

An individual cell

Fragilaria linearis

1. **Habitat:** : It is a pennate diatom (pennale) (*See* page 219) found in freshwater and marine environments as free-floating plankton. Common species are *Fragilaria linearis, F. pinnata, F. polygonata, F. sublinearis, F. voucheriae, F. virescens* and *F. oceanica*.
2. **Thallus:** Thallus consists of a colony of non-motile cells arranged side-by-side. Cells remain in mucilage.
3. **Cells:** The 'frustule' is straight, rod-shaped, wide in the middle portion and narrowed down towards the ends. Raphe is absent. A pseudo-raphe extends from one end of the valve to the other end (*See* page 235).
4. **Reproduction:** Reproduction is mainly asexual through cell division or fission. Sexual reproduction takes place through formation of auxospores.

Figure 11.14: Identifying characteristics of some microscopic algae (*Diatoma* and *Fragilaria*)

Class Bacillariophyceae (Diatoms)

SYNEDRA

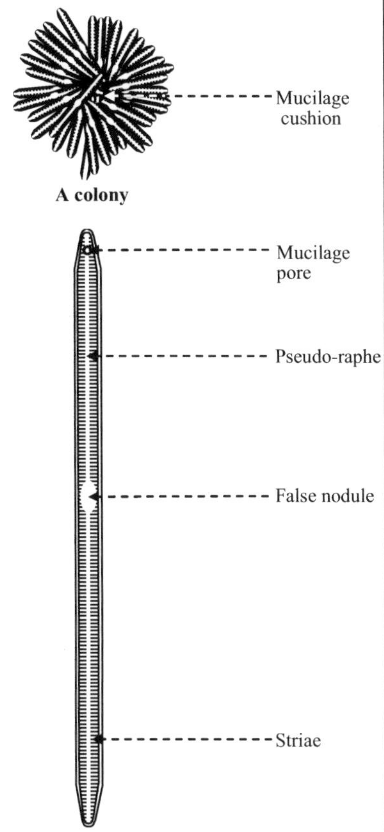

An individual cell
Synedra ulna

1. **Habitat:** It is a pennate diatom (pennale) (*See* page 219) found in freshwater and marine environments as free-floating plankton. Important species are *Synedra ulna, S. affinis, S. hyaline, S. splendens* and *S. thalassothrix*.
2. **Thallus:** Thallus consists of a colony of non-motile cells arranged radially. A number of individual cells occur attached in tufts by means of mucilage-cushion. Few species are unicellular which attach to some substratum by mucilage.
3. **Cells:** The 'frustule' is straight, needle-shaped pointed towards both ends. The needle shape helps it to adapt to a free-floating planktonic existence. Raphe is absent for which it is non-motile. Only a pseudo-raphe is present (*See* page 235), which widens at the center of the valve to form the so-called false nodule. A pore is found at either pole of the valve through which mucilage is secreted to outside . This mucilage helps for attachment to a substratum or for joining of several individuals to form a colony.
4. **Reproduction:** Reproduction is mainly asexual through cell division or fission. Sexual reproduction takes place through formation of auxospores except in *S. affinis*.

Class Bacillariophyceae (Diatoms)

RHABDONEMA

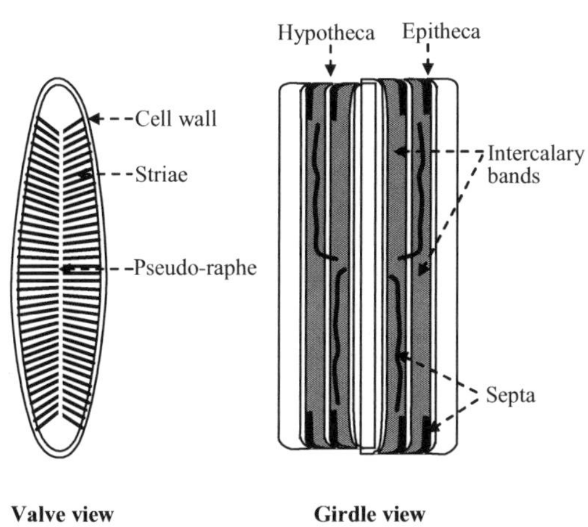

Rhabdonema arcuatum

1. **Habitat:** It is a pennate diatom (pennale) (*See* page 219) found in marine environment. Common species are *Rhabdonema arcuatum* and *R. adriaticum*.
2. **Thallus:** Unicellular, non-motile.
3. **Cells:** The 'frustule' is oblong elliptical. Raphe is absent for which it is non-motile. Only a pseudo-raphe is present (*See* page 235), which extends from one end of the valve to the other end. The striae are not parallel; rather they are arranged in a diverging manner from the center. As many as 28 intercalary bands may occur in each theca, the number being often unequal in epitheca and hypotheca. Intercalary bands are bands present between the valve and their connecting bands (girdles). They are usually well seen in the girdle-view. The intercalary bands are produced internally forming incomplete partitions running parallel to the valves. These are called septa. In *Rhabdonema*, the septa are slightly curved, are marked with transverse ribs and are perforated by 1-3 apertures.
4. **Reproduction:** Reproduction is mainly asexual through cell division or fission. Sexual reproduction takes place through formation of auxospores.

Figure 11.15: Identifying characteristics of some microscopic algae (*Synedra* and *Rhabdonema*)

Class Bacillariophyceae (Diatoms)

SURIRELLA

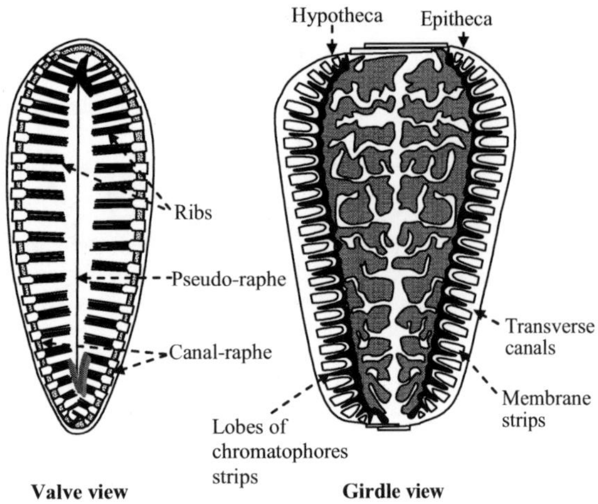

Surirella capronii

1. **Habitat:** It is a pennate diatom (pennale) (*See* page 219) found in freshwater. Important species are *Surirella capronii, S. baldjickii, S. calcarata, S. colombensis, S. gamma, S. multicostata, S. neumeyeri, S. saxonica, S. spiralis, S. splendida* and *S striatula*.
2. **Thallus:** Unicellular, motile.
3. **Cells:** The 'frustule' is elliptical or oval in valve-view and is cuneate or sub rectangular in girdle view. The valve has a prominent median pseudo-raphe (See page 235) with a system of strong ribs on both the sides, but nodule is absent. The two margins of each valve are winged. The entire length of the somewhat dilated outer edge of each wing is occupied by a narrow slit-like canal (canal-raphe), which communicates with the external medium. Each valve possesses two raphes, but these too have no nodule. The wings, as seen in the girdle view, contain a system of rather narrow transverse canals through which the protoplasm of the cell communicates with that in the raphe. These canals are separated from one another by broad intervening strips of membrane.
4. **Reproduction:** Reproduction is mainly asexual through cell division or fission. Sexual reproduction takes place through formation of auxospores.

Class Bacillariophyceae (Diatoms)

CYCLOTELLA

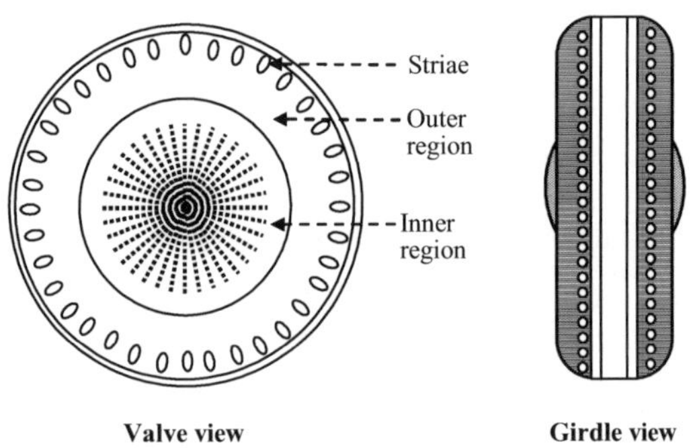

Cyclotella comta

1. **Habitat:** It is a centric diatom (centrale) (*See* page 220) found in freshwater and marine environments as free-floating plankton. Important species are *Cyclotella comta, C. plancotonica* and *C. socialis*.
2. **Thallus:** Usually unicellular, non-motile.
3. **Cells:** The 'frustule' is disc-shaped, looking like a circular pillbox. It is circular in valve view and rectangular in girdle view, with slight elevation at the center. There are no special processes. The valve is radially symmetrical, the markings being arranged radially. The valve has two concentric regions; an inner smooth region with no marking and an outer peripheral region with radially arranged striae. Raphe is absent, for which it is non-motile. This is true for all centrales.
4. **Reproduction:** Reproduction is mainly asexual through cell division or fission. Sexual reproduction takes place through formation of auxospores.

Class Bacillariophyceae (Diatoms)

BIDDULPHIA

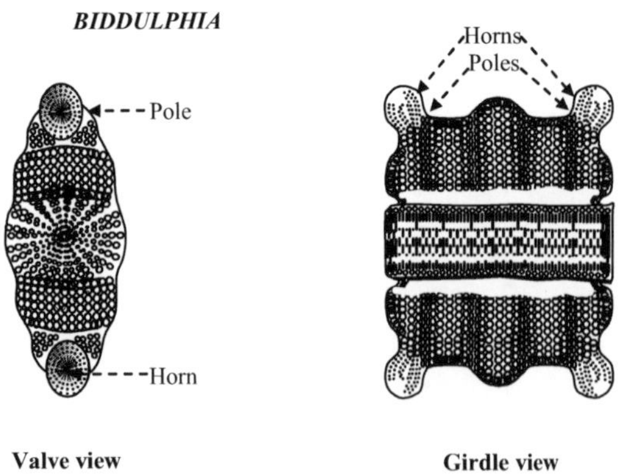

Biddulphia pulchella

1. **Habitat:** It is a centric diatom (centrale) (*See* page 220) found in marine environment as free-floating plankton. Important species are *Biddulphia pulchella, B. mobiliensis, B. pellucida* and *B. sinensis*.
2. **Thallus:** Unicellular, non-motile.
3. **Cells:** The 'frustule' is elliptical in valve view with only two planes of symmetry. Valves have two poles with horns projecting form them. Raphe is absent, for which it is non-motile.
4. **Reproduction:** Reproduction is mainly asexual through cell division or fission. Sexual reproduction takes place through formation of auxospores.

Figure 11.16: Identifying characteristics of some microscopic algae (*Surirella*, *Cyclotella* and *Biddulphia*)

Class Bacillariophyceae (Diatoms)

COSCINODISCUS

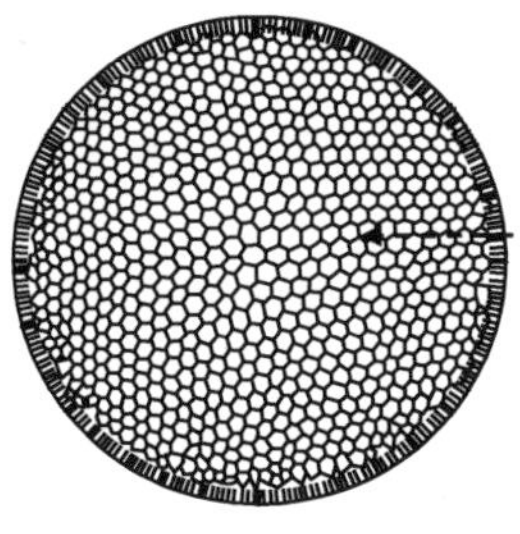

Coscinodiscus excentricus

1. **Habitat:** It is a centric diatom (centrale) (*See* page 220) found in marine environment as free-floating plankton. Important species are *Coscinodiscus excentricus, C. apiculatus, C. asteromphalus, C. biconicus* and *C. concinnus* .
2. **Thallus:** Unicellular, non-motile.
3. **Cells:** The frustule is disc-shaped. As the cell is radially symmetrical, it is a centric diatom, unlike the pinnate diatoms, which are bilaterally symmetrical. Raphe or pseudo-raphe is absent, for which it is non-motile. Valve is circular without any special process. The valve has polygonal markings called areolae arranged radially.
4. **Reproduction:** Reproduction is mainly asexual through cell division or fission. Sexual reproduction takes place through formation of auxospores.

Class Bacillariophyceae (Diatoms)

MELOSIRA

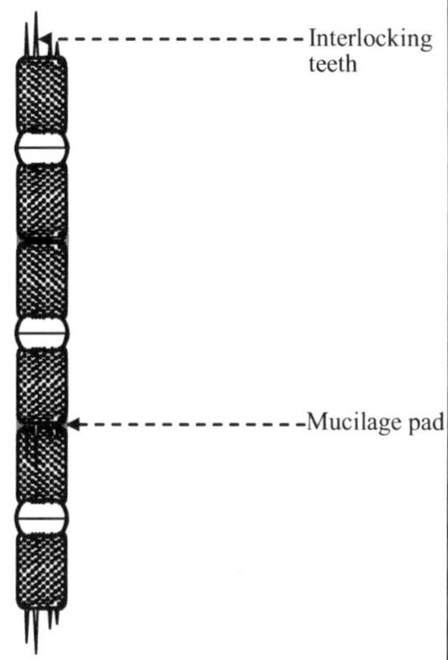

A filament

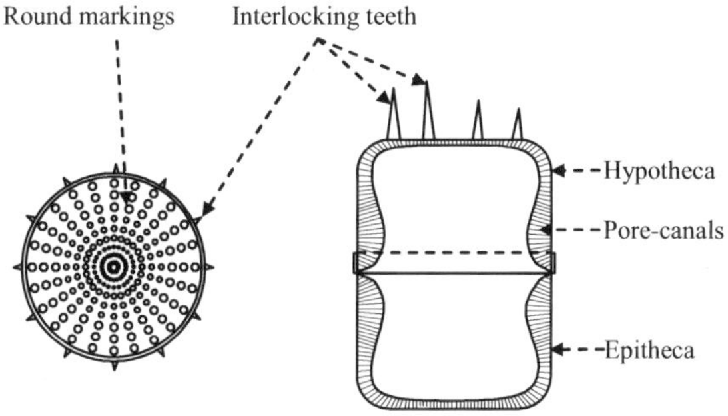

Valve view **Girdle view**

Melosira arenaria

1. **Habitat:** It is a centric diatom (centrale) (*See* page 220) found in freshwater environment as free-floating plankton. Important species are *Melosira arenaria*, *M. baicalensis*, *M. islandica*, *M. italica*, *M. jurgensii*, *M. roeseana*, *M. undulata* and *M. varians*.
2. **Thallus:** Thallus is filamentous. The cells are non-motile, which are joined end-to-end by mucilage to form the trichome. A trichome is a row of cells without any sheath. The connecting mucilage is difficult to recognise, as the frustules are joined by a larger area of their valve faces. In some species, with convex valves, the intervening pad of mucilage is faintly visible after staining. Besides mucilage, special outgrowths on the cells on alternate edges, called interlocking teeth, also help to unite the cells. They are present all round the edge of the circular valves.
3. **Cells:** The 'frustule' is cylindrical. It is circular in valve view and rectangular in girdle view. Its wall has simple structure. It is traversed by numerous fine pore-canals forming a dense network, which opens both on inner and outer sides. Valve has round markings arranged radially. Raphe is absent, for which it is non-motile.
4. **Reproduction:** Reproduction is mainly asexual through cell division or fission. Sexual reproduction takes place through formation of auxospores.

Figure 11.17: Identifying characteristics of some microscopic algae (*Coscinodiscus* and *Melosira*)

Class Bacillariophyceae (Diatoms)

SCELETONEMA

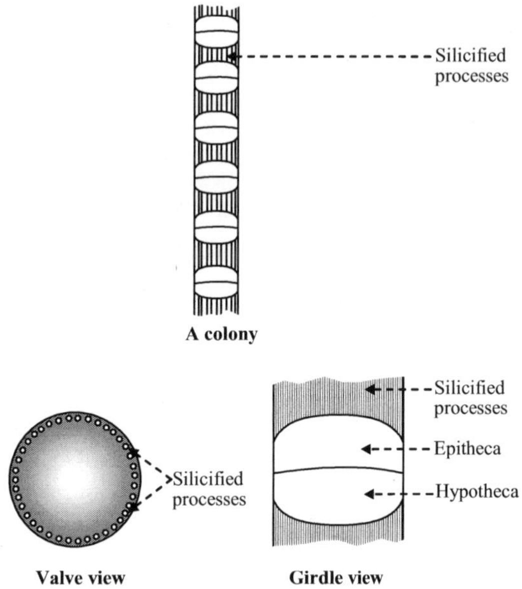

Sceletonema costatum

1. **Habitat:** It is a centric diatom (centrale) (*See* page 220) found in marine environment as free-floating plankton. Important species are *Sceletonema (Skeletonema) costatum* and *S. tropicum*.
2. **Thallus:** Thallus consists of a colony of cells joined in a line by a number of silicified processes arising near the edge of the valve-face. Each process is traversed by a fine canal, through which the cementing material that joins their tips is secreted. These connecting processes are very delicate.
3. **Cells:** The 'frustule' looks like a circular pillbox. It is circular in valve view and rectangular in girdle view. The valve surface is convex. The valve is radially symmetrical. Raphe is absent, for which it is non-motile.
4. **Reproduction:** Reproduction is mainly asexual through cell division or fission. Sexual reproduction takes place through formation of auxospores.

Class Bacillariophyceae (Diatoms)

THALASSIOSIRA

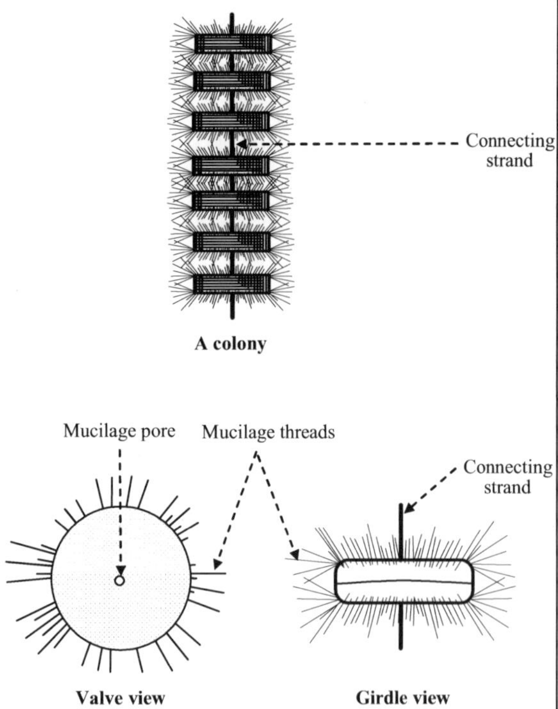

Thalassiosira gravida

1. **Habitat:** It is a centric diatom (centrale) (*See* page 220) found in freshwater and marine environments as free-floating plankton. Important species are *Thalassiosira gravida, T. subtilis* and *T. rutula.*
2. **Thallus:** Thallus consists of a colony of cells, which remain embedded in foliaceous mucilage expanses. The successive frustules are joined by a more or less delicate connecting strand made of a bundle of mucilage threads held together by a sheath of cellulose.
3. **Cells:** The 'frustule' is cylindrical. It is circular in valve view and rectangular in girdle view. The frustule has threads of mucilage arising from the valve face. A large mucilage pore is detectable in the valve face. In few species, there are a group of small mucilage pores in the center of the valve. Raphe is absent, for which it is non-motile.
4. **Reproduction:** Reproduction is mainly asexual through cell division or fission. Sexual reproduction takes place through formation of auxospores.

Figure 11.18: Identifying characteristics of some microscopic algae (*Sceletonema* and *Thalassiosira*)

Class Bacillariophyceae (Diatoms)

RHIZOSOLENIA

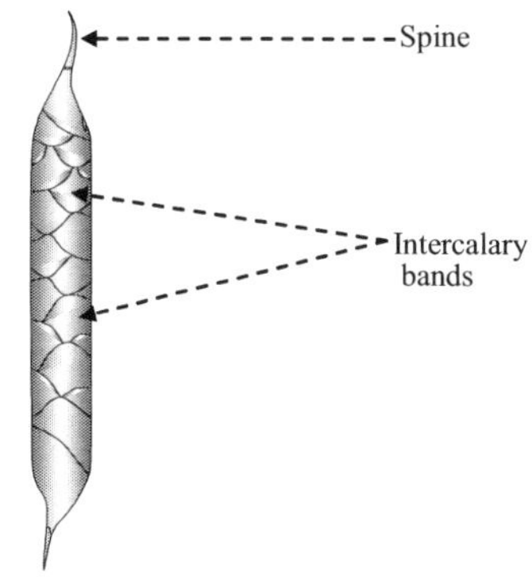

Rhizosolenia eriensis

1. **Habitat:** It is a centric diatom (centrale) (*See* page 220) found in marine environment as free-floating plankton. Important species are *Rhizosolenia eriensis*, *R. alata* and *R. rostrata.*
2. **Thallus:** Usually unicellular, non-motile.
3. **Cells:** The 'frustule' is much longer than it is broad. It is cylindrical and needle-shaped with asymmetrical calyptra-like valves terminating in an eccentric spine or long seta. The long intervening girdle is composed of numerous, usually scale-like intercalary bands, which are often more or less imbricate. Raphe is absent for which it is non-motile.
4. **Reproduction:** Reproduction is mainly asexual through cell division or fission. Sexual reproduction takes place through formation of auxospores.

Class Bacillariophyceae (Diatoms)

CHAETOCEROS

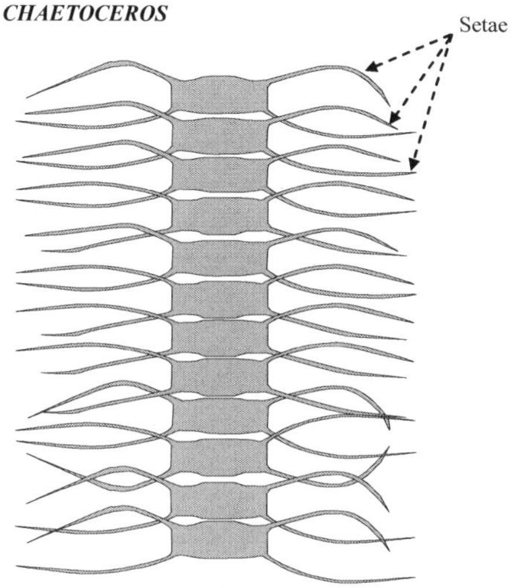

A colony

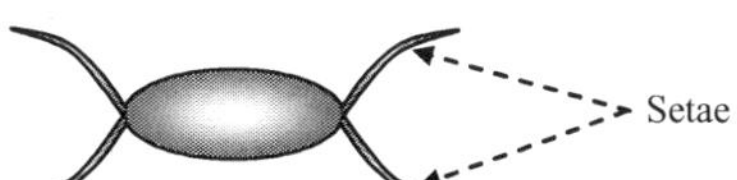

Valve view

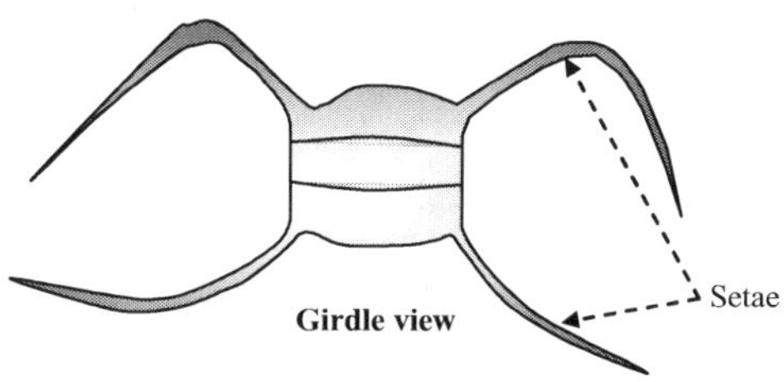

Girdle view

Chaetoceros socialis

1. **Habitat:** It is a centric diatom (centrale) (*See* page 220) found in marine environment as free-floating plankton. Important species are *Chaetoceros (Chaetoceras) socialis, C. medium, C. subtilis, C. borealis* and *C. decipiens*.
2. **Thallus:** Thallus consists of a colony of cells joined in a line with the help of the basal portions of the pairs of long setae.
3. **Cells:** The 'frustule' is elliptical in valve view and rectangular in girdle view. The valve surface is convex. Each cell has two pairs of long setae. Setae are the outgrowths of the valve, which project beyond the valve margin. Raphe is absent, for which it is non-motile.
4. **Reproduction:** Reproduction is mainly asexual through cell division or fission. Sexual reproduction takes place through formation of auxospores.

Figure 11.19: Identifying characteristics of some microscopic algae (*Rhizosolenia* and *Chaetoceros*)

Class Dinophyceae ***GYMNODINIUM*** 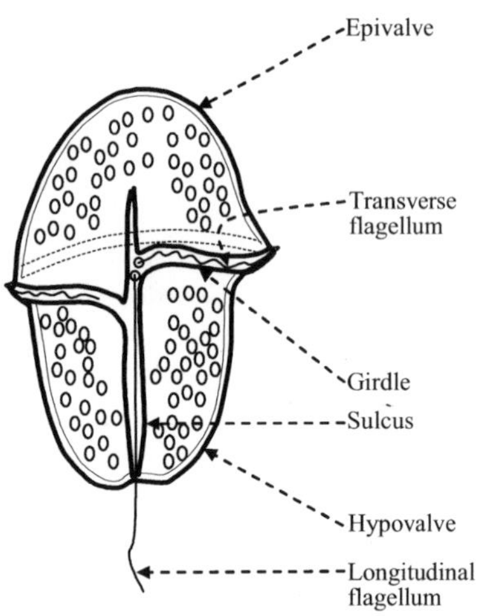 *Gymnodinium pachydermaticum*	1. **Habitat:** It is a dinoflagellate algae found in both freshwater and marine environments as free-floating plankton. Some species inhabit the shore causing green-brown discolouration of the sand at certain times when the sand is exposed. Important species are *Gymnodinium pachydermaticum, G. coerulium, G. heterostriatum, G. hiemale, G. lunula* and *G. aeruginosum*. 2. **Thallus:** Unicellular, motile. 3. **Cells:** Cell is pyramidal in outline and flattened dorso-ventrally so that the end view is sub-elliptical. It is unarmoured (has no plates). It has two furrows; the transverse furrow is called 'girdle' and the longitudinal furrow 'sulcus'. The girdle completely encircles the cell and separates it into two halves; the apical half is called 'epivalve' and the antapical half 'hypovalve'. The sulcus is confined to the hypovalve, opening into the girdle at its upper end and continuing across it for some distance into the epivalve. Two flagella arise from the cell close together, but differing in structure and orientation. The one, directed transversely, is band-shaped and exhibits an undulatory movement. The other, directed longitudinally and posteriorly, is thread-like. Both the flagella arise from the ventral surface of the cell through definite pores. 4. **Reproduction:** Reproduction is mainly asexual through cell division or fission. Cell division takes place obliquely along the longitudinal axis.
Class Dinophyceae ***GONYAULAX*** 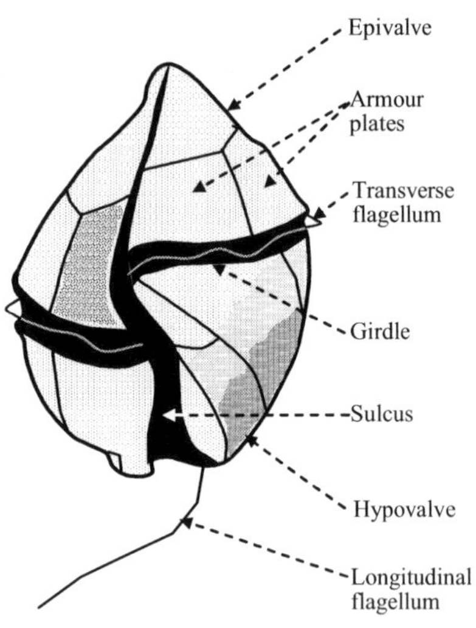 *Gonyaulax fragilis*	1. **Habitat:** It is a dinoflagellate algae found in marine environment as free-floating plankton. Important species are *Gonyaulax fragilis, G. spinifera* and *G. series*. 2. **Thallus:** Unicellular, motile. 3. **Cells:** Cell is pyramidal in outline and flattened dorso-ventrally so that the end view is sub-elliptical. It is an armoured dinoflagellate as it has firm envelope or armour. The armour is composed of a series of separate plates, grouped in a characteristic manner. The girdle is markedly spiral and separates the envelope to the apical epivalve and antapical hypovalve. The epivalve and hypovalve are made up of a series of unequal polygonal plates. Adjacent plates of the envelope overlap by their knife-like margins, which are firmly cemented together. The suture between them is clearly recognisable. The sulcus extends from the hypovalve and reaches the anterior extremity of the epivalve. Two flagella arise from the cell close together, but differing in structure and orientation. The one, directed transversely, is band-shaped and exhibits an undulatory movement. The other, directed longitudinally and posteriorly, is thread-like. Both the flagella arise from the ventral surface of the cell through definite pores. 4. **Reproduction:** Reproduction is mainly asexual through cell division or fission. Cell division takes place obliquely along the longitudinal axis.

Figure 11.20: Identifying characteristics of some microscopic algae (*Gymnodinium* and *Gonyaulax*)

Class Dinophyceae

CERATIUM

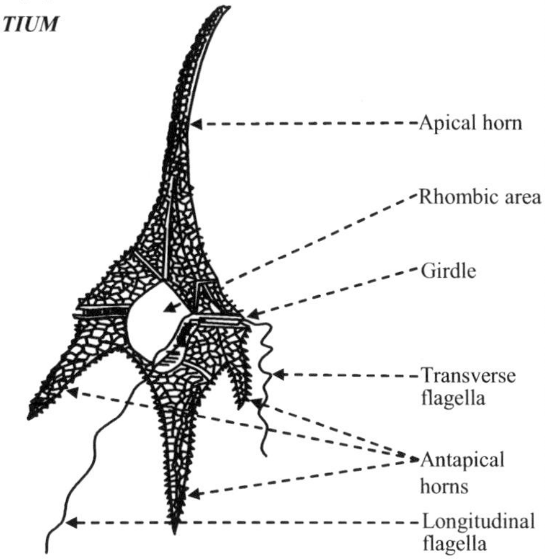

Ceratium hirundinella

1. **Habitat:** It is a dinoflagellate algae found in freshwater and marine environments as free-floating plankton. Important species are *Ceratium hirundinella, C. cornutum* and *C. tripos.*
2. **Thallus:** Unicellular, motile.
3. **Cells:** The cell is markedly asymmetric and strongly flattened dorso-ventrally. It is produced into one apical and two or three antapical hollow horns occupied by cytoplasm. The apical horn bears an apical aperture. The girdle is nearly horizontal and divides the body into two approximately equal but dissimilar halves. The plates composing the membrane are markedly areolated, being connected by narrow sutures. On the middle of the ventral surface, there is a large rhombic unsculptured hyaline area, which interrupts the transverse furrow. One transverse and one longitudinal flagella are present.
4. **Reproduction:** Reproduction is mainly asexual through cell division or fission. Cell division takes place obliquely along the longitudinal axis.

Class Dinophyceae

NOCTILUCA

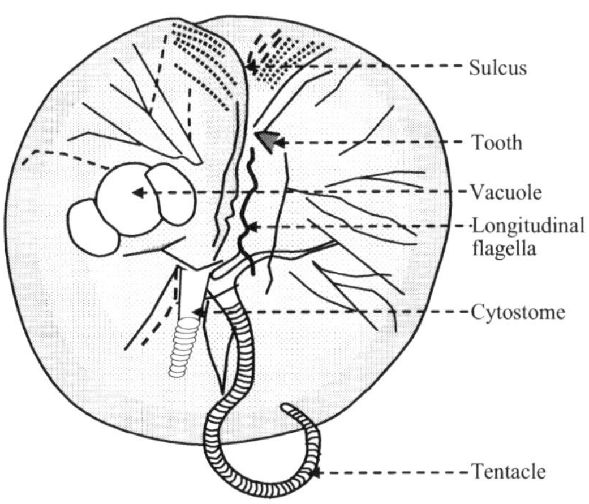

Noctiluca scintillans

1. **Habitat:** It is a cystoflagellate algae found in marine environment as free-floating plankton. An important species is *Noctiluca scintillans,* also called *N. miliaris.* It can be bioluminescent when disturbed, as are various other dinoflagellates, and large blooms can sometimes be seen as flickering lights on the ocean.
2. **Thallus:** Unicellular, motile.
3. **Cells:** The cell has sub-reniform or spheroidal protoplast, which is inflated by numerous large vacuoles. These vacuoles help it to float in the water. The longitudinal flagellum is small but recognisable, while the transverse one is represented only by a tooth. The transverse furrow is strongly reduced, while the sulcus is elaborately developed and includes a cytostome. There is a prominent tentacle.
4. **Reproduction:** Reproduction is mainly asexual through cell division or fission. At times, multiple fission leads to the formation of numerous small swarmers, each possessing a transverse furrow, a well-developed longitudinal flagellum and a small tentacle. These swarmers, however, do not possess transverse flagellum. Prior to division, the structures undergo simplification. Sexual reproduction takes place through conjugation of two equal individuals. The zygote lacks the tentacles and passes through a resting phase.

Figure 11.21: Identifying characteristics of some microscopic algae (*Ceratium* and *Noctiluca*)

Appendix I

Composition of Media Used in Microbiology (Mentioned in this Manual)

Amino acid decarboxylase broth (pH 7.2)	
Peptone	0.5 g
Yeast extract	0.5 g
Sodium chloride	0.5 g
Glucose	0.1 g
Bromocresol purple	0.0016 g
Amino acid	0.5g
Distilled water	100 ml

Bacteriophage broth (pH 7.6)	
Peptone	1.0 g
Beef extract	0.3 g
Yeast extract	0.5 g
Sodium chloride	0.25 g
KH_2PO_4	0.8 g
Distilled water	100 ml

Buffered glucose broth
(*See* MR-VP broth)

Carbohydrate broth (pH 6.8)	
Peptone	1.0 g
Sodium chloride	0.5 g
Required carbohydrate	1.0 g
Bromocresol purple	0.0016 g
Distilled water	100 ml

Cysteine broth (pH 7.5)	
Peptone	0.5 g
Beef extract	0.3 g
Sodium chloride	0.5 g
Cysteine	0.01 g
Distilled water	100 ml

DNase agar (pH 7.2)	
Tryptone	2.0 g
DNA	0.2 g
Sodium chloride	0.5 g
Agar	2.0 g
Distilled water	100 ml

Fraizer's gelatin agar (pH 7.2)	
Peptone	0.5 g
Beef extract	0.3 g
Sodium chloride	0.5 g
Gelatin	0.4 g
Agar	2.0 g
Distilled water	100 ml

Glucose phosphate broth
(*See* MR-VP broth)

Hugh-Leifson glucose broth (pH 7.4)	
Peptone	0.2 g
Yeast extract	0.5 g
Sodium chloride	0.5 g
Glucose	1.0 g
Bromocresol purple	0.0015g
Agar (added after pH adjustment)	0.3g
Distilled water	100 ml

Indole broth
(*See* Tryptone broth)

Litmus milk broth (pH 6.8)	
Skimmed milk powder	10.0 g
Litmus	0.075 g
Distilled water	100 ml

MR-VP broth (pH 6.9)	
Peptone	0.7 g
Dextrose	0.5 g
K_2HPO_4	0.5 g
Distilled water	100 ml

Nitrate broth (pH 7.2)	
Peptone	0.5 g
Beef extract	0.3 g
Potassium nitrate	0.5 g
Sodium chloride	0.5 g
Distilled water	100 ml

Nutrient agar[1] (pH 7.0)	
Peptone	0.5 g
Beef extract	0.3 g
Sodium chloride	0.5 g
Agar	1.5 g
Distilled water	100 ml

Nutrient broth (pH 7.0)	
Peptone	0.5 g
Beef extract	0.3 g
Sodium chloride	0.5 g
Distilled water	100 ml

Phenylalanine agar (pH 7.2)	
Yeast extract	0.3 g
Phenylalanine	0.2 g
Na_2HPO_4	0.1 g
Sodium chloride	0.5 g
Agar	2.0 g
Distilled water	100 ml

Sabouraud agar (pH 5.6)	
Peptone	1.0 g
Dextrose	4.0 g
Agar	1.5 g
Distilled water	100 ml

Simmons citrate agar (pH 6.9)	
Sodium citrate	0.2 g
Sodium chloride	0.5 g
K_2HPO_4	0.1 g
$NH_4H_2PO_4$	0.1 g
$MgSO_4$	0.02 g
Bromothymol blue	0.008 g
Agar	1.5 g
Distilled water	100 ml

Starch agar (pH 7.2)	
Peptone	0.5 g
Beef extract	0.3 g
Sodium chloride	0.5 g
Starch	0.2 g
Agar	2.0 g
Distilled water	100 ml

Tributyrin agar (pH 7.2)	
Peptone	0.5 g
Beef extract	0.3 g
Sodium chloride	0.5 g
Agar	2.0 g
Distilled water	100 ml
Tributyrin[2]	1.0 g

Triple sugar iron agar
(*See* TSI agar)

Tryptone broth (pH 7.5)	
Tryptone	1.0 g
Sodium chloride	0.5 g
Calcium chloride	0.011 g
Distilled water	100 ml

Tryptophan broth
(*See* Tryptone broth)

Tryptone hard agar (pH 7.5)	
Tryptone	1.0 g
Sodium chloride	0.5 g
Calcium chloride	0.011 g
Agar	1.1 g
Distilled water	100 ml

Tryptone soft agar (pH 7.5)	
Tryptone	1.0 g
Potassium chloride	0.5 g
Agar	0.9 g
Distilled water	100 ml

TSI agar (pH 7.4)	
Peptone	1.5 g
Proteose-peptone	0.5 g
Yeast extract	0.3 g
Beef extract	0.3 g
Lactose (sugar)	1.0 g
Sucrose (sugar)	1.0 g
Glucose (sugar)	0.1 g
Ferrous sulphate (iron)	0.02 g
Sodium chloride	0.5 g
Sodium thiosulphate	0.03 g
Phenol red	0.0024 g
Agar	1.2 g
Distilled water	100 ml

Urea agar (pH 6.9)	
Peptone	0.1 g
Sodium chloride	0.5 g
Glucose	0.1 g
K_2HPO_4	0.2 g
Phenol red	0.0012 g
Agar	1.5 g
Distilled water	90 ml
Urea solution[3] (20%)	10 ml

1 After dissolving the ingredients (except agar), first pH is adjusted to 7.0 using 0.1N HCl or 0.1N NaOH. Agar is added only after pH adjustment, otherwise it hydrolyses. The medium is heated on flame to dissolve the agar. Then, it is sterilised at 121°C (15 psi pressure) for 15 minutes in an autoclave.

2 Ingredients of tributyrin agar medium (excluding tributyrin, which is the lipid component) are dissolved in distilled water. After adjusting pH, the medium is heated to melt and dissolve the agar. The medium is allowed to cool to about 90°C. Then tributyrin is added and emulsified in a Waring blender. Then, it is sterilised at 121°C (15 psi pressure) for 15 min in an autoclave.

3 20% urea solution is prepared by dissolving 20 g of urea in 100 ml of distilled water. It is sterilised by membrane filter. 10ml of the filter-sterilised urea solution is added to the sterilised and cooled urea agar medium. This is done, as urea decomposes upon heating.

Appendix II

Composition of Stains and Reagents Used in Microbiology (Mentioned in this Manual)

STAINS

1. **Acid-alcohol:** Mix 97 ml ethyl alcohol (95%) with 3 ml concentrated hydrochloric acid.
2. **Carbol fuchsin:** Solution A: 0.3 g basic fuchsin in 10 ml ethyl alcohol.
   Solution B: 5.0 g phenol in 95 ml distilled water.
   Mix solutions A and B.
3. **Copper sulphate solution:** Dissolve 20 g copper sulphate ($CuSO_4.5H_2O$) in 80 ml distilled water.
4. **Crystal violet (for basic and capsule staining):** Dissolve 1 g crystal violet (85% dye content) in 100 ml distilled water.
5. **Crystal violet (for Gram staining):**
   Solution A: Dissolve 2 g crystal violet (90% dye content) in 20 ml ethyl alcohol (95%).
   Solution B: Dissolve 0.8 g ammonium oxalate in 80 ml distilled water.
   Mix Solution A and B.
6. **Eosin:** Dissolve 1 g eosin in 100 ml distilled water.
7. **Ethyl alcohol (95%)** : Mix 95 ml ethyl alcohol (100%) with 5 ml distilled water.
8. **Gram's iodine:** Dissolve 1 g iodine and 2 g potassium iodide in 300 ml distilled water.
9. **Malachite green**: Dissolve 5 g malachite green in 100 ml distilled water.
10. **Methylene blue:** Dissolve 0.3 g methylene blue in 100 ml distilled water.
11. **Nigrosin:** Dissolve 10 g nigrosin (water soluble) in 100 ml distilled water, boil in water bath for 30 min, add 0.5 ml formalin, filter twice with double filter paper.
12. **Safranin:** Dissolve 10 ml safranin O solution (2.5 g safranin O in 100 ml 95% ethyl alcohol) in 100 ml distilled water.
13. **Lactophenol cotton blue:** Mix 20 ml lactic acid, 20 g phenol, 40 ml glycerol and 20 ml distilled water. Heat gently to dissolve in hot water. Add 0.05 g aniline blue.

REAGENTS

1. **Ferric chloride solution:** Dissolve 10 g ferric chloride in 100 ml distilled water.
2. **1N HCl :** Mix 9 ml concentrated hydrochloric acid in 100 ml distilled water.
3. **Kovac's reagent:** Dissolve 5.0 g para-dimethylaminobenzaldehyde (p-DMAB) in 75 ml amyl alcohol. Add 25 ml concentrated hydrochloric acid to it.
4. **Lugol's iodine:** Dissolve 1 g iodine in 100 ml distilled water.
5. **Mercuric chloride solution:** Dissolve 15 g mercuric chloride in 100 ml distilled water. Add 20 ml concentrated hydrochloric acid to it.
6. **Methyl red solution:** Dissolve 0.1 g methyl red in 300 ml ethyl alcohol (95%). Add 200 ml distilled water to it.
7. **Nitrate reagent (Solution A):** Dissolve 0.8 g sulphanilic acid in 100 ml 5N acetic acid (1 part glacial acetic acid in 2.5 part distilled water).
8. **Nitrate reagent (Solution B):** Dissolve 0.5 g α-naphthylamine in 100 ml 5N acetic acid (1 part glacial acetic acid in 2.5 part distilled water).
9. **ONPG solution:** Dissolve 0.6 g O-nitrophenyl-β-D-galactoside in 100 ml 0.01M Na_2HPO_4. Sterilise by membrane filter and store in refrigerator in dark bottle.
10. **Oxidase reagent:** Dissolve 1.0 g N-tetramethyl-para-phenylenediamine dihydrochloride in 100 ml distilled water. Prepare immediately before use. Darkened solution should be discarded.
11. **Toluidine blue solution** : Dissolve 0.1 g toluidine blue in 100 ml distilled water.
12. **VP solution I (Barritt's reagent Solution A):** Dissolve 5 g α-naphthol (*i.e.* 1-naphthol) in 95 ml ethanol (absolute) with constant stirring.
13. **VP solution II (Barritt's reagent Solution B):** Dissolve 40 g potassium hydroxide in 100 ml distilled water. The solution becomes warm. Allow it to cool to room temperature. Then add 0.3 g creatine to it.

Appendix III

Systematic Position of Important Bacteria (Upto Genus Level) as per Bergey's Manual of Determinative Bacteriology

KINGDOM I: ARCHAEOTA

SECTION 1 Thermoprotei, sulfolobi and barophiles

Phylum I: *Crenarchaeota*
Class I: *Thermoprotei*
Order I: *Thermoproteales*
Family I: *Thermoproteaceae*
Thermoproteus
Order II: *Pyrodictiales*
Family I: *Desulfurococcaceae*
Staphylothermus
Family II: *Pyrodictiaceae*
Pyrolobus
Class II: *Sulfolobi*
Order I: *Sulfolobales*
Family I: *Sulfolobaceae*
Acidianus
Sulfolobus
Sulfurococcus

SECTION 2 The Methanogens

Phylum II: *Euryarchaeota*
Class I: *Methanobacteria*
Order I: *Methanobacteriales*
Family I: *Methanobacteriaceae*
Methanobacterium
Class II: *Methanococci*
Order I: *Methanococcales*
Family I: *Methanococcaceae*
Methanococcus
Order II: *Methanomicrobiales*
Family I: *Methanomicrobiaceae*
Methanocalculus
Methanospirillum
Family II: *Methanosarcinaceae*
Methanolobus

SECTION 3 The Halobacteria

Class I: *Halobacteria*
Order I: *Halobacteriales*
Family I: *Halobacteriaceae*
Halobacterium
Halococcus

SECTION 4 The Thermoplasms

Class I: *Thermoplasma*
Order I: *Thermoplasmatales*
Family I: *Thermoplasmataceae*
Thermoplasma

SECTION 5 The Thermococci

Class I: *Thermococci*
Order I: *Archaeoglobales*
Family I: *Archaeoglobaceae*
Archaeoglobus
Order II: *Thermococcales*
Family I: *Thermococcaceae*
Thermococcus

KINGDOM II: BACTERIA

SECTION 6 Aquifex and relatives

Phylum I: *Aquificae*
Class I: *Aquificae*
Order I: *Aquificales*
Family I: *Aquificaceae*
Aquifex

SECTION 7 Thermotogas and Geotogas

Class I: *Thermotogae*
Order I: *Thermotogales*
Family I: *Thermotogaceae*
Thermotoga
Class .11: *Thermodesulfobacteria*
Order I: *Thermodesulfobacteriales*
Family I: *Thermodesulfobacteriaceae*
Thermodesulfobacterium

SECTION 8 The Deinococci

Phylum II: *Xenobacteria*
Class I: *Deinococci*
Order I: *Deinococcales*
Family I: *Deinococcaceae*
Deinococcus

SECTION 9 Thermi and genera of uncertain affiliation

Class I: *Thermi*
Order I: *Thermales*
Family I: *Thermaceae*
Thermus
Family II: 'The paraphyletic assemblage
Nitrospira
Leptospirillum
Magnetobacterium

SECTION 10 Chrysiogenes

Phylum III: *Chrysiogenetes*
Class I: *Chrysiogenetes*
Order I: *Chrysiogenales*
Family I: *Chrysiogenaceae*
Chrysiogerres

SECTION 11 The Chloroflexi and Herpetosiphons

Phylum IV: *Thermomicrobia*
Class I: *Chloroflexi*
Order I: *Chloroflexales*
Family I: *Chloroflexaceae*
Chloroflexus

SECTION 12 Thermomicrobia

Class I: *Thermomicrobia*
Order I: *Thermomicrobiales*
Family I: *Thermomicrobiaceae*
Thermomicrobium

SECTION 13 The Cyanobacteria
Phylum V: *Cyanobacteria*
Class I: *Prochlorophyta*
Order I: *Chroococcales*
Family I:Chroococcaceae
Chroococcus
Cyanobacterium
Gloeobacter
Gloeocapsa
Microcytis
Order II: *Pleurocapsales*
Family I: *Pleurocapsaceae*
Pleurocapsa
Order III: *Oscillatoriales*
Family I: *Oscillatoriaceae*
Arthrospira
Lyngbya
Oscillatoria
Spirulina
Trichodesmium
Order IV: *Nostocales*
Family I: *Nostocaceae*
Anabaena
Nostoc
Family II: *Scytonemataceae*
Scytonema
Family Ill: *Rivulariaceae*
Rivularia
Order V: *Stigonematales*
Family IV: *Stigonemataceae*
Chlorogloeopsis
Stigonema

SECTION 14 Chlorobia
Phylum VI: *Chlorobia*
Class I: *Chlorobia*
Order I: *Chlorobiales*
Family I: *Chlorobiaceae*
Chlorobium
Phylum VII: *Proteobacteria*

SECTION 15 The α-Proteobacteria
Class I: *Rhodospirilli*
Order I: *Rhodospirillales*
Family I: *Rhodospirillacea'*
Azospirillum
Rhodospirillum
Family II: *Acetobacteraceae*
Acetobacter
Order II: Rickettsiales
Family I: *Rickettsiaceae*
Rickettsia
Family II: *Ehrlichiaceae*
Anaplasma
Family III: *Holosporaceae*
Holospora
Order III: *Rhodobacterales*
Family I: *Rhodobacteraceae*
Rhodobacter
Order IV: *Sphingomonadales*
Family I: *Sphingomonadaceae*
Erythrobacter
Sphingomonas
Order V: *Caulobacterales*
Family I: *Caulobacteraceae*
Caulobacter
Order VI: *Rhizobiales*
Family I: *Rhizobiaceae*
Rhizobium
Family II: *Phyllobacteriaceae*
Phyllobacterium
Family III: *Bartonellaceae*
Bartonella
Family IV: *Brucellaceae*
Brucella
Family VI: *Rhodobiaceae*
Rhodobium
Family V: *Methylobacteriacea*
Methylorhabdus
Family VI: *Methylocystaceae*
Methylocystis
Family VII: *Beijerinckiaceae*
Beijerinckia
Family VIII: *Hyphomicrobiaceae*
Aquabacter
Azorhizobium
Hyphomicrobium
Family IX: *Bradyrhizobiaceae*
Bradyrhizobium
Nitrobacter

SECTION 16 The β -Proteobacteria
Class I: *Neisseriae*
Order I: *Neisseriales*
Family I: *Neisseriaceae*
Aquaspirillum
Chromobacterium
Neisseria
Order II: *Burkholderiales*
Family I: *Burkholderiaceae*
Burkholderia
Family II: *Oxalobacteraceae*
Oxalobacter
Family III: *Alcaligenaceae*
Achromobacter
Alcaligenes
Family VI: *Comamonadaceae*
Polaromonas
Order III: *Rhodocyclales*
Family I: *Rhodocyclaceae*
Rhodocyclus
Order IV: *Nitrosomonadales*
Family I: *Nitrosomonadaceae*
Nitrosomonas
Family II: *Spirillaceae*
Spirillum
Thiobacillus
Family III: *Gallionellacea*
Gallionella
Order V: Methylophilales
Family I: *Methylophilaceae*
Methylobacillus

SECTION 17 The γ-Proteobacteria

Class I: *Zymobacteria*
- Order I: *Chromatiales*
  - Family I: *Chromatiaceae*
    - *Thiocapsa*
  - Family II: *Ectothiorhodospiraceae*
    - *Ectothiorhodospira*
- Order II: *Xanthomonadales*
  - Family I: *Xanthomonadaceae*
    - *Xanthomonas*
- Order III: *Cardiobacteriales*
  - Family I: *Cardiobacteriaceae*
    - *Cardiobacterium*
- Order IV: *Thiotrichales*
  - Family I: *Thiotrichaceae*
    - *Thiobacterium*
  - Family II: *Piscirickettsiaceae*
    - *Piscirickettsia*
  - Family III: *Francisellaceae*
    - *Francisella*
- Order V: *Legionellales*
  - Family I: *Legionellaceae*
    - *Legionella*
  - Family II: *Coxiellaceae*
    - *Coxiella*
    - *Rickettsiella*
- Order VI: *Methylococcales*
  - Family I: *Methylococcaceae*
    - *Methylobacter*
    - *Methylococcus*
- Order VII: *Oceanospirillales*
  - Family I: *Oceanospirillaceae*
    - *Oceanospirillum*
  - Family II: *Halomonadaceae*
    - *Halomonas*
- Order VIII: *Pseudomonadales*
  - Family I: *Pseudomonadaceae*
    - *Azotobacter*
    - *Pseudomonas*
    - *Rhizobacter*
  - Family II: *Moraxellaceae*
    - *Acinetobacter*
    - *Moraxella*
    - *Moraxella (Branhamella)*
    - *Moraxella (Moraxella)*
    - *Psychrobacter*
- Order IX: *Alteromonadales*
  - Family I: *Alteromonadaceae*
    - *Alteromonas*
    - *Marinobacter*
    - *Marinobacterium*
    - *Pseudoalteromonas*
    - *Shewanella*
- Order X: *Vibrionales*
  - Family I: *Vibrionaceae*
    - *Photobacterium*
    - *Vibrio*
- Order XI: *Aeromonadales*
  - Family I: *Aeromonadaceae*
    - *Aeromonas*
- Order XII: *Enterobacteriales*
  - Family I: *Enterobacteriaceae*
    - *Citrobacter*
    - *Edwardsiella*
    - *Enterobacter*
    - *Escherichia*
    - *Hafnia*
    - *Klebsiella*
    - *Morganella*
    - *Plesiomonas*
    - *Proteus*
    - *Salmonella*
    - *Serratia*
    - *Shigella*
    - *Yersinia*
- Order XIII: *Pasteurellales*
  - Family I: *Pasteurellaceae*
    - *Pasteurella*

SECTION 18 The δ-Proteobacteria

Class I: *Predibacteria*
- Order I: *Desulfovibrionales*
  - Family I: *Desulfovibrionaceae*
    - *Desulfovibrio*
  - Family II: *Desulfurellaceae*
    - *Desulfurella*
  - Family III: *Desulfobacteraceae*
    - *Desulfobacter*
  - Family IV: *Desulfobulbaceae*
    - *Desulfobulus*
  - Family V: *Geobacteraceae*
    - *Geobacter*
  - Family VI: *Bdellovibrionaceae*
    - *Bdellovibrio*
- Order II: *Myxococcales*
  - Family I: *Myxococcaceae*
    - *Myxococcus*
  - Family II: *Archangiaceae*
    - *Archangium*
  - Family III: *Cystobacteraceae*
    - *Cystobacter*
  - Family IV: *Polyangiaceae*
    - *Polyangium*

SECTION 19 The ε-Proteobacteria

Class I: *Campylobacteres*
- Order I: *Campylobacterales*
  - Family I: *Campylobacteraceae*
    - *Campylobacter*
  - Family II: *Helicobacteraceae*
    - *Helicobacter*

Phylum VIII: *Firmicutes*

SECTION 20 The *Clostridia* and relatives

Class I: *Clostridia*
- Order I: *Clostridiales*
  - Family I: *Clostridiaceae*
    - *Clostridium*
    - *Oxobacter*
    - *Sarcina*
  - Family II: *Peptostreptococcace*
    - *Peptostreptococcus*
  - Family III: *Eubacteriaceae*
    - *Eubacterium*

Family IV: *Lachnospiraceae*
Lachnospira
Family V: *Peptococcaceae*
Desulfotomaculum
Peptococcus
Family VI: *Syntrophomonadaceae*
Syntrophomonas
Order II: *Haloanaerobiales*
Family I: *Haloanaerobiaceae*
Haloanaerobium
Family II: *Halobacteroidaceae*
Halobacteroides

SECTION 21 The Mollicutes
Class I: *Mollicutes*
Order I: *Mycoplasmatales*
Family I: *Mycoplasmataceae*
Mycoplasma
Family II: Spiroplasma group
Spiroplasma
Family III: *Acholeplasmataceae*
Acholeplasma
Family IV: *Asteroleplasmataceae*
Asteroleplasma
Family V: *Erysipelothrichaeceae*
Erysipelothrix

SECTION 22 The Bacilli and Lactobacilli
Class I: *Bacilli*
Order I: *Bacillales*
Family I: *Bacillaceae*
Bacillus
Halobacillus
Family II: *Planococcaceae*
Planococcus
Sporosarcina
Family III: *Caryophanaceae*
Caryophanon
Family IV: *Sporolactobacillaceae*
Sporolactobacillus
Family V: *Paenibacillaceae*
Paenibacillus
Family VI: *Alicyclobacillaceae*
Alicyclobacillus
Family VII: *Thermoactinomycetaceae*
Thermoactinomyces
Order II: *Lactobacillales*
Family I: *Lactobacillaceae*
Lactobacillus
Family II: *Leuconostocaceae*
Leuconostoc
Family III: *Streptococcaceae*
Pediococcus
Streptococcus
Family IV: *Enterococcaceae*
Enterococcus
Family V: *Carnobacteriaceae*
Carnobacterium
Lactosphaera
Family VI: *Aerococcaceae*
Aerococcus
Family VII: *Listeriaceae*
Listeria
Family VIII: *Staphylococcaceae*
Macrococcus
Salinicoccus
Staphylococcus
Family IX:'Genera incertae sedis
Acetobacterium
Amphibacillus
Oscillospira
Pasteuria
Trichococcus

SECTION 23 The Actinobacteria
Class I: *Actinobacteria*
Subclass I: *Acidimicrobidae*
Order I: *Acidimicrobiales*
Suborder I: *Acidimicrobidae*
Family I: *Acidimicrobiaceae*
Acidimicrobium
Subclass II: *Rubrobacteridae*
Order II: *Rubrobacterales*
Suborder I: *Rubrobacteridae*
Family I: *Rubrobacteraceae*
Rubrobacter
Subclass III: *Coriobacteridae*
Order III: *Coriobacteriales*
Suborder I: *Coriobacteridae*
Family I: *Coriobacteriaceae*
Coriobacterium
Subclass IV: *Sphaerobacteridae*
Order IV: *Sphaerobacterale'*
Suborder I: *Sphaerobacteridae*
Family I: *Sphaerobacteraceae*
Sphaerobacter
Subclass V: *Actinobacteridae*
Order V: *Actinomycetales*
Suborder I: *Actinomycineae*
Family I: *Actinomycetaceae*
Actinomyces
Suborder II: *Micrococcineae*
Family II: *Micrococcaceae*
Arthrobacter
Leucobacter
Micrococcus
Family III: *Brevibacteraceae*
Brevibacterium
Family IV: *Cellulomonadaceae*
Cellulomonas
Family V: *Dermabacteraceae*
Dermabacter
Family VI: *Dermatophilaceae*
Dermatophilus
Family VII: *Intrasporangiaceae*
Intrasporangium
Family VIII: *Jonesiaceae*
Jonesia
Family IX: *Microbacteriaceae*
Microbacterium
Family X: *Promicromonosporaceae*
Promicromonospora

Suborder III: *Corynebacterineae*
Family I: *Corynebacteriaceae*
Corynebacterium
Family II :*Dietziaceae*
Dietzia
Family III. *Gordoniaceae*
Gordonia
Family IV: *Mycobacteriaceae*
Mycobacterium
Family V: *Nocardiaceae*
Nocardia
Family VI: *Tsukamurellaceae*
Tsukamurella
Suborder IV: *Micromonosporaceae*
Family I: *Micromonosporaceae*
Micromonospora
Suborder VI: *Propionibacterineae*
Family I: *Propionibacteriaceae*
Propionibacterium
Family II: *Nocardioidaceae*
Nocardioides
Suborder VII: *Pseudonocardineae*
Family I: *Pseudonocardiaceae*
Pseudonocardia
Suborder VIII: *Streptomycineae*
Family I: *Streptomycetaceae*
Streptomyces
Suborder IX: *Streptosporangineae*
Family I: *Streptosporangiaceae*
Streptosporangium
Family II: *Nocardiopsaceae*
Nocardiopsis
Family III: *Thermomonosporaceae*
Thermomonospora
Suborder X: *Frankineae*
Family I: *Frankiaceae*
Frankia
Family II: *Geodermatophilaceae*
Geodermatophilus
Family III: *Microsphaeraceae*
Microsphaera
Family IV: *Sporichthyaceae*
Sporichthya
Family V: *Acidothermaceae*
Acidothermus
Family VI: Incertae sedis
Cryptosporangium
Suborder XI: *Glycomycineae*
Family I: *Glycomycetaceae*
Glycomyces
Order VI: *Bifidobacteriales*
Family I: *Bifidobacteriaceae*
Bifidobacterium
Family II: 'Unknown Affiliation
Actinobispora
Actinokineospora
Excellospora

Phylum IX: Wall-less forms
SECTION 24 The Planctomycetes and Chlamydia
Class I: *Planctomycetacia*
Order I: *Planctomycetales*
Family I: *Planctomycetaceae*
Planctomyces
Order II: *Chlamydiales*
Family I: *Chlamydiaceae*
Chlamydia
SECTION 25 The Spirochetes
Phylum X: *Spirochetes*
Class I: *Spirochaetes*
Order I: *Spirochaetales*
Family I: *Spirochaetaceae*
Spirochaeta
Treponema.
Family II: *Serpulinaceae*
Serpulina
Family III: *Leptospiraceae*
Leptospira
SECTION 26 The Fibrobacters
Phylum XI: *Fibrobacter*
Class I: *Fibrobacteres*
Order I: *Fibrobacterales*
Family I: *Fibrobacteraceae*
Fibrobacter
Family II: *Acidobacteriaceae*
Acidobacterium
SECTION 27 The Bacteroides
Phylum XII: *Bacteroids*
Class I: *Bacteroides*
Order I: *Bacteroidales*
Family I: *Bacteroidaceae*
Bacteroides
Family II: *Rikenellaceae*
Rikenella
Family III: *Porphyromonadaceae*
Porphyromonas
Family IV: *Prevotellaceae*
Prevotella
SECTION 28 The Flavobacteria
Phylum XIII: *Flavobacteria*
Class I: *Flavobacteria*
Order I: *Flavobacteriales*
Family I: *Flavobacteriaceae*
Bergeyella
Flavobacterium
Polaribacter
Family II: *Myroideaceae*
Myroides
Psychromonas
Family III: *Blattabacteriaceae*
Blattabacterium

SECTION 29 The Sphingobacteria

Phylum XIV: *Sphingobacteria*
Class I: *Sphingobacteria*
Order I: *Sphingobacteriales*
Family I: *Sphingobacteriaceae*
Sphingobacterium
Family II: *Saprospiraceae*
Saprospira
Family III: *Flexibacteraceae*
Cyclobacterium
Cytophaga
Flexibacter
Family IV: *Flammeovirgaceae*
Flammeovirga
Family V: *Crenothrichaceae*
Crenothrix

SECTION 30 The Fusiforms

Phylum XV: *Fusobacteria*
Class I: *Fusobacteria*
Order I: *Fusobacteriales*
Family I: *Fusobacteriaceae*
Fusobacterium
Leptotrichia
Streptobacillus
Family II: Genera incertae sedis
Cetobacterium

SECTION 31 Verrucomicrobium and relatives

Phylum XVI: *Verrucomicrobia*
Class I: *Verrucomicrobiae*
Order I: *Verrucomicrobiales*
Family I: *Verrucomicrobiaceae*
Prosthecobacter
Verrucomicrobium

Bibliography

Almas, K. A., 1981. **Chemistry and Microbiology of Fish and Fish Processing**, Department of Biochemistry, Norwegian Institute of Technology, University of Trondheim, Trondheim, Norway, 123 pp.

Banwart, G. J., 1974. **Basic Food Microbiology**, CBS Publishers and Distributors, New Delhi, 781 pp.

Cappuccino, J. G. and Sherman, N., 1987. **Microbiology- A Laboratory Manual**, The Benjamin/ Cummings Publishing Company, Inc., California, 458 pp.

Frazier, W. C., 1958. **Food Microbiology**, McGraw-Hill Book Company, Inc., New York, 472 pp.

Giese, A. C., 1979. **Cell Physiology**, W.B. Saunders Company, Philadelphia, 609 pp.

James, M. J., 1987, **Modern Food Microbiology**, CBS Publishers and Distributors, New Delhi, 642 pp.

Mac Faddin, J. F., 1980. **Biochemical Test for Identification of Medical Bacteria**, Williams and Wilkins Co., Baltimore, 527 pp.

Madigan, M. T., Martinko, J. M. and Parker, J., 2000. **Brock Biology of Microorganism,** Prentice-Hall, Inc., New Jersey, 991 pp.

McKane, L. and Kandel, J., 1986. **Microbiology: Essentials and Applications**, McGraw Hill Book Co. 777pp

Pelczar, M. J. (Jr.), Chan, E. C. S. and Krieg, N. R., 1997. **Microbiology**, Tata McGraw-Hill Publishing Company Ltd., New Delhi, 918 pp.

Prescott, L. M., Harley, J. P. and Klein, D. A., 2005. **Microbiology**, 6th Edition, McGraw-Hill, New York, 992 pp.

Salle, A. J., 1988. **Fundamental Principles of Bacteriology,** Tata McGraw-Hill Publishing Company Ltd., New Delhi, 1094 pp.

Schlegel, H. G., 1995. **General Microbiology**, 7th Edition, Cambridge University Press, 655 pp.

Sen, D. P., 2005. **Advances in Fish Processing Technology**, Allied Publishers Pvt. Ltd., New Delhi, 818 pp.

Glossary

ABC transportation (*A*TP-*b*inding *c*assette): A process of transportation of substances across the cell membrane of bacteria in which a periplasmic-binding protein in the periplasm specifically binds to the substance, a membrane-spanning protein, which spans across the membrane, transports it across the membrane and a cytoplasmic ATP–hydrolysing protein present in the cytoplasm supplies the energy for the transport event.

Accelerated freeze-drying: Freeze-drying at a very fast rate.

Acid curd: Curd formed by growth of certain bacteria in milk with production of acids, which in presence of calcium ions precipitate the milk protein casein as calcium caseinate.

Acid-fast bacteria: Bacteria, which are extremely difficult to be stained, but once stained, it is equally, difficult to remove the stain out of their cells, even with vigorous use of acid-alcohol as decolourising agent.

Acid-fast staining: A method of differential staining of bacteria cells to differentiate between acid-fast and non-acid-fast bacteria.

Acidic staining: A method of staining bacteria cells using only one acidic stain like eosin or nigrosin, which stains the cells negatively by making the surrounding coloured, leaving the bacteria cells colourless.

Acidophiles: (= Acidophilic bacteria).

Acidophilic bacteria (*Acido*: acid; *philic*: loving): Bacteria that grow best at pH lower than 6.0 (*i.e.* in acidic conditions)

Aerobes: (=Aerobic bacteria).

Aerobic bacteria: Bacteria requiring the presence of free oxygen (or air) for their growth.

Agar: A powder extracted from certain seaweeds, which is used as a solidifying agent in microbiological culture media.

Agar agar: (=Agar)

Agar deep tube: Test tube containing sterilised culture medium for cultivation of bacteria, which has been allowed to solidify in upright position.

Agar plate: Petri dish containing a thick layer of sterilised solidified culture medium used for cultivation of bacteria.

Agar slant: Test tube containing sterilised culture medium for cultivation of bacteria, which has been allowed to solidify in slanting position.

Akinetes: Thick-walled spores of filamentous algae.

Algal bloom: A thick layer of algae floating on the surface of stagnant water bodies.

Algicidal chemicals: Chemicals, which kill algae.

Algicides: (=Algicidal chemicals)

Algology: Study of algae.

Alkaliphiles: (= Alkaliphilic bacteria).

Alkaliphilic bacteria (*Alkali*: alkaline; *philic*: loving): Bacteria that grow best at pH higher than 8.0 (*i.e.* in alkaline conditions).

Amino acid decarboxylase test: A biochemical test performed to find out the ability of a species of bacteria to decarboxylate different amino acids such as lysine, ornithine and arginine, by producing respective amino acid decarboxylase enzymes.

Aminoglycoside antibiotics: Antibiotics, which contain amino sugars bonded by glycosidic bonds to other amino sugars.

Amphitrichous flagellation (*Amphi*: both; *trichous*: hair): Flagella are present at both ends of the bacteria cell either singly or in tuft.

Anaerobes: (=Anaerobic bacteria).

Anaerobic bacteria: Bacteria, which can grow only in the absence of free oxygen. They are killed by oxygen, for which they are also called obligate anaerobes (*obligate*: strict).

Antibiotics: Antimicrobial chemicals produced by certain microorganisms that inhibit or kill other microorganisms.

Antimicrobial chemicals: Chemicals that kill or inhibit the growth of microorganisms.

Antiporters: Membrane-transporting systems present in the cell membrane of bacteria, which transport one type of molecule and always transport another type of molecule in the opposite direction.

Antiseptics: Antimicrobial chemicals used to kill the microbes present only on the body surface of living organism, which are exposed to external infection. They are sufficiently non-toxic to be applied to living tissues.

Appendaged bacteria: Bacteria, which possess extension of their cells, as long tubes in the form of stalk or hypha, or as buds.

Arcula: (=Box-shaped bacteria)

Aseptic techniques: Techniques in microbiological studies in which contamination with external microbes, other than those of interest, is completely inhibited.

Autoclave: A closable container, which can be sealed airtight, that generates and maintains steam under pressure inside it for sterilisation of materials to be used in microbiological studies.

Autoclaving: A process of heat sterilisation, in which the materials to be sterilised is heated at 121°C (15 psi pressure) for 15 minutes by super-saturated steam (steam with temperature above 100°C) in an autoclave.

Autoradiography: A cytochemical technique, in which the location of a particular chemical constituent in an object is determined by observing the site, at which a radioactive material becomes positioned.

Autospore: Non-motile spore, which resembles the parent cell producing it in shape and structure.

Autotrophic organisms (*Auto*: self; *trophein*: to nourish): Organisms capable of nourishing themselves by preparing the required food substances within their bodies from inorganic materials of the environment.

Auxochrome: Component of a dye that imparts the electrolytic dissociation property (salt forming property) to it.

Auxospore: A type of spore formed in diatoms, which grows to original size similar to the parent cell.

Bacilli: (Plural of bacillus)

Bacillus: Bacteria, which are cylindrical or rod-shaped.

Bacteria: Prokaryotic, unicellular microorganisms, which lack chlorophyll pigments.

Bacteriochlorophyll: Photosynthetic pigments present in photosynthetic bacteria, which are different from true chlorophyll pigments present in algae and higher plants in their chemical structure.

Bacteriocidal chemicals: Chemicals, which kill bacteria.

Bacteriocides: (= Bacteriocidal chemicals)

Bacteriocins: Antimicrobial chemicals produced by some bacteria that kill closely related species or even different strains of the same species.

Bacteriology: Study of bacteria.

Bacteriophages: Viruses, which infect bacteria.

Bacteriostatic agents (*Bacterio*: of bacteria; *static*: unchanged): Agents, which inhibit the growth of bacteria.

Bacteriostatic chemicals: Chemicals, which inhibit the growth of bacteria.

Basal body: Lower part of a bacterial flagellum that forms its base and is anchored in the cytoplasmic membrane and cell wall. It provides anchorage to the flagellum as well as functions as a motor, thereby imparting the rotary motion to the flagellum.

Basic staining: A method of staining bacteria cells using only one basic stain like methylene blue, crystal violet or carbol fuchsin, which binds tightly to the bacteria cells and imparts a deep colour of the stain to the cells, whereas the surrounding medium gets a light colour of the stain.

BGA: (=Blue green algae).

Binary fission (*Bi*: two; *fission*: division): Process of reproduction in bacteria and many other unicellular organisms, in which a single cell divides to two daughter cells.

Biochemical tests: Tests performed for the identification of bacteria species based on the differences in the biochemical activities of different bacteria.

Blue green algae: Algae belonging to the class Cyanophyceae, which include photosynthetic gram-negative prokaryotes.

Boiling: A process of heating materials in boiling water at 100°C for about 30 minutes to destroy microbes present in it.

Box-shaped bacteria: Flat, box-shaped bacteria, with perfectly straight edges and sharp 90° angles at the corners.

Bright-field microscope: Microscope, in which the microscopic field (the circular area visible under microscope) is brightly illuminated and the microbes (or biological specimen) appear darker, as they absorb some of the light passing through them.

Broad-spectrum antibiotics: Antibiotics that act on both gram-positive and gram-negative bacteria.

Broth: Clear liquid medium containing water and nutrients in simpler forms for growth of bacteria, which has been sterilised in autoclave.

Brown algae: Algae belonging to the class Phaeophyceae, whose characteristic brown colour is due to the presence of the golden brown xanthophyll pigment, 'fucoxanthine'.

Buds: Cellular appendages of bacteria or yeast, which directly develop as daughter cells from the mother cells, without the intervening formation of hyphae.

Buffers: Chemicals, which resist the change in pH of solutions following addition of strong acid or base.

Bulk pasteurisation: A process of heat treatment of milk at 63-66°C for 30 minutes, which kills certain pathogenic microbes as well as some spoilage microbes present in it, thereby making it safe to drink as well as increasing its storage life considerably.

Calyptra: Thickened membrane on the tip of the apical cell of few filamentous algae.

Capsid: The protein coat of virus particle, which protects its nucleic acid from destruction by DNase.

Capsule staining: A method of differential staining of bacteria cells to stain the capsule, which surrounds capsulated bacteria.

Capsule: A polymer coat consisting of a dense, well-defined viscous layer closely surrounding the bacteria cells in many species.

Carbohydrate fermentation test: A biochemical test, performed to find out the ability of a species of bacteria to ferment carbohydrates (sugars) with the production of an acid or acid and gas.

Catalase test: A biochemical test, performed to find out the ability of a species of bacteria to degrade hydrogen peroxide by producing the enzyme catalase.

Cell membrane: Thin membrane that completely encloses the protoplasm of cells.

Cell wall: Rigid structure that immediately surrounds the cell membrane of bacterial cells as well as that of plant cells.

Cellular growth of bacteria: Increase in the size of an individual bacteria cell when environmental conditions are favourable.

Centrales: (= Centric diatoms).

Centric diatoms: Diatoms, which are radially symmetrical.

Chemotaxis: Tendency of an organism to move towards or away from a chemical.

Chemotherapeutic agents: Antimicrobial chemicals, which can be used internally to control infectious diseases in man and animals and are not toxic to them. These are commonly used as medicines.

Chilling: The process of lowering the temperature of a material to about 0°C, but not below it.

Chloroplast: A type of cytoplasmic organelle called 'plastid' present in photosynthetic eukaryotic organisms, which contains chlorophyll pigments; both chlorophyll a and chlorophyll b.

Chromatophores of algae: A type of cytoplasmic organelle called 'plastid' present in eukaryotic algae, which contains chlorophyll a and other pigments except chlorophyll b.

Chromatophore of bacteria: Special organelles present in phototrophic bacteria and cyanobacteria (blue green algae), in which photosynthesis is carried out. They are formed by the invagination of the cell membrane and contain enzymes and pigments for photosynthesis.

Chromogen: Compound formed by combination of chromophore and benzene in a dye molecule.

Chromophore: Colouring component of a dye molecule.

Citrate utilisation test: A biochemical test, performed to find out the ability of a species of bacteria to utilise citrate as the sole source of carbon.

Cleaning: Acts such as sweeping, wiping, washing and brushing of a material, which removes most of the microbes present on it.

Coagulase test: A biochemical test, performed to find out the ability of a species of bacteria belonging to the genus *Staphylococcus*, to coagulate blood by producing the enzyme coagulase.

Cocci: (Plural of coccus)

Coccobacillus: Rod-shaped bacteria (bacillus), which are so short and stumpy that they appear ovoid. They look like coccus and bacillus.

Coccus: Bacteria, which are spherical or ovoid in shape.

Coenobium: A colony of algal cells in a specific arrangement and number that does not increase once mature.

Coliphage: Virus (phage) that infects the bacteria, *Escherichia coli.*

Colonies: Individual, macroscopically visible masses of bacteria cells grown on the surface of a solid medium, each representing the multiplication of a single bacteria cell.

Compound microscope: Most commonly used microscope for general purposes, which magnifies the image of minute objects by a series of two lenses; the objective lens and the ocular lens.

Conidia: Chains of cells produced from the sterigma by budding in filamentous fungi.

Conidiophores: A number of hyphae, which stand erect from the vegetative mycelium of filamentous fungi.

Conjugales: One group of green algae having no flagella in any stage of life, which reproduces by conjugation.

Conjugation: A mode of reproduction in green algae in which the gamet of one cell moves to another cell by amoeboid action and fuses with its gamet to produce the zygote.

Connecting band: Circular projection at the margin of the valve of diatom frustule.

Contractile vacuoles: Large, clear circular membrane-bound organelles present in the cytoplasm of amoeba that regulates internal water pressure.

Core polysaccharide: Inner polysaccharide (chain of sugars) attached to the lipid A molecule in the cell wall of gram-negative of bacteria.

Core: Innermost content of bacterial endospore, which contains the usual structures of a bacteria cell, such as cell wall (core wall), enclosing the spore protoplast. The spore protoplast consists of the cell membrane, cytoplasm, nucleoid, ribosomes, inclusions and so on.

Cortex: Third covering layer from outside of bacterial endospore, which is made of loosely cross-linked peptidoglycan.

Counter-stain: A stain used in staining of bacteria to stain decolourised bacteria cells.

Cultivation of bacteria: Growing of bacteria in sterilised nutritionally rich liquid or solid media, so as to make them perceptible to naked eye as suspension or colony respectively.

Culture media: Substances containing adequate quantity of nutrients in simpler forms for rapid growth and multiplication of bacteria.

Curing: Process by which plasmids can be eliminated from the host bacteria cell.

Cyanobacteria: Blue green algae, which belong to the Class Cyanophyceae. As they are prokaryotic similar to bacteria, many consider them to be bacteria and group them as Cyanobacteria.

Cyst: A desiccation-resistant form of certain bacteria, produced under adverse conditions, in which the whole cell is surrounded by a thick protective layer called 'coat'. Upon return of favourable conditions, the coat ruptures and the cell becomes active again. Thus, cyst is completely different from spore, which are released from the bacteria cell.

Cytoplasm: Viscous fluid-like substance, which fills the compartment within the cell membrane.

Cytoplasmic membrane: (=Cell membrane).

Dark-field microscope: Microscope, in which the object is brilliantly illuminated against a dark background.

Deaminate: To remove the amino group, usually from an amino acid.

Death phase: (=Decline phase)

Decarboxylate: To remove the carboxyl group, usually from an amino acid.

Decline phase: A phase in the growth curve of bacteria, during which the number of bacteria cells in the culture decreases exponentially (logarithmically).

Decolourisation: Making bacteria cells colourless by removal of the colour incorporated into them during staining.

Decolourising agent: A solvent used in staining of bacteria to remove the stain (decolourise) from stained bacterial cells.

Decontamination: A method that reduces, to varying extents, the initial number of bacteria in a given material by their removal from it.

Deoxyribonuclease test: A biochemical test, performed to find out the ability of a species of bacteria to hydrolyse deoxyribonucleic acid (DNA) by producing the enzyme deoxyribonuclease (DNase).

Desmids: Unicellular conjugales.

Destruction: A method by which bacteria present in a given material are destroyed to varying extents, thereby reducing the initial number.

Diatoms: Algae belonging to the class Bacillariophyceae in which the cell wall of the individuals are highly sculptured and symmetrically ornamented.

Differential staining: A method of staining bacteria cells using more than one stains.

Dipicolinic acid: A chemical not found in vegetative bacteria cells, but found in bacterial endospores, which is associated with the resistance of the endospores to adverse conditions.

Diplobacillus: Rod-shaped bacteria (bacillus), in which the bacilli are arranged in pairs.

Diplococcus: Spherical bacteria (coccus), in which the cocci are arranged in pairs.

Diploptene: One of the most important hopanoids present in the unit membrane of several bacteria as a strengthening agent, similar to the sterols present in the unit membrane of eukaryotes. It has 30 carbon atoms.

Discolouration: Change in original desirable colour to some undesirable colour.

Disinfectants: Antimicrobial chemicals used to kill the microbes present only on inanimate objects.

DNase test: (= Deoxyribonuclease test).

Doubling time: (=Generation time)

DPA: (=Dipicolinic acid).

Dyes: Chemicals used for general purposes colouring such as, for colouring textile materials and for colouring walls.

Ectoplasm: Outer layer of cytoplasm of amoeba with clear appearance.

Electromagnetic radiation: Radiations such as microwaves, ultraviolet (UV) radiation, light rays, gamma rays, X-rays and electron beams.

Electron microscope: Microscope, in which electron beams are used to produce highly maginified images of very small objects and in which magnification is obtained by a system of electromagnetic fields.

Electron microscopic techniques: Techniques used in processing and observation of minute specimen under elecron microscope for specific purposes.

Endoenzymes: (= Intracellular enzymes).

Endoplasm: Inner cytoplasmic region of amoeba with granular appearance.

Endospore: A differentiated cell formed within the cell of certain gram-positive rod-shaped bacteria, which can withstand severe adverse conditions like heat, cold, radiation, ageing, toxic chemicals and lack of nutrients. It is formed within the bacterial cell and released to outside as 'spore' to survive the adverse conditions. These are the most commonly found spores. Therefore, very often spore and endospore are used synonymously.

Endotoxins: Substances present in the bacteria cell as its internal component, which can cause disease in a host. It is the lipid A fraction of the lipopolysaccharide of gram-negative cell wall.

Enumeration of bacteria: Estimating the number of bacteria present in a given sample.

Episomes: Plasmids, which can integrate into the host chromosomal DNA.

Epitheca: Older and outer half of diatom frustule, which, like the top half of the petri dish, fits closely over the younger and inner half, hypotheca.

Eukaryotes: Organisms, in which the chromosomes are confined within a membrane-bound nucleus. They include all higher plants and animals.

Eukaryotic cells (*Eu*: modern; *karyotic*: about nucleus): Cells, in which there is a membrane-bound nucleus as found in most of the higher plants and animals.

Exoenzymes: (= Extracellular enzymes).

Exospore: A differentiated cell formed external to the vegetative cell by budding at one end of the bacteria cell and released to outside as 'spore' to survive the adverse conditions.

Exosporium: Outermost layer of bacterial endospore, which is a thin, delicate covering, made of protein.

Exotoxins: Substances synthesised inside the bacteria cells and released to outside, which can cause disease, if present in or enters into the host's body.

Exponential growth: A very rapid type of growth occurring in bacteria, in which the number of cells doubles during each unit time (generation time). Though apparently it follows geometric growth, after few generations it grows as 1, 10,100,1000,10000.......(10^0,10^1,10^2,10^3,10^4....) whose logarithmic values are 0,1,2,3,4 ... respectively.

Exponential phase: (=Log phase).

Extracellular enzymes: Enzymes secreted by cells to the surrounding to hydrolyse high molecular weight or complex substances such as proteins, polysaccharides and fats, which cannot permeate the cell membrane, because of their large size or complex nature.

Extreme halophiles (*Halo*: salt; *philic*: loving): Salt-loving bacteria, which require NaCl at high concentrations of 15-30% for their growth.

Eyespot: Light sensitive pigmented spot present in some unicellular organisms.

Facultatively anaerobic bacteria: Bacteria growing in the presence or absence of free oxygen.

Facultatives: (=Facultatively anaerobic bacteria).

Filament: An individual trichome of filamentous algae surrounded by a sheath.

Filament: Long hair-like filamentous portion of a bacterial flagellum, which emerges from the hook. It is several times longer than the bacteria cell. It is made of a single type of protein, 'flagellin', whose molecular weight is about 40,000.

Filamentous bacteria: Very long thin filament-shaped bacteria.

Filter sterilisation: A process of passing a liquid or gas through a filter having very small pores, which do not allow microbes to pass through, but allow the liquid or gas. The liquid or gas that comes out from the filter is free of microbes and is therefore sterile.

Fimbriae: Thin filamentous hair-like appendages present in few bacteria, which are structurally similar to flagella, but are not involved in the motility of bacteria.

Flagella staining: A method of differential staining of bacteria cells to visualise flagella of flagellated bacteria.

Flagella: Thin filamentous hair-like helical appendages present in few bacteria that protrude through the cell wall and are responsible for the motility of bacteria.

Flagellation: The arrangement of flagella on a bacteria cell.

Flaming: A process of sterilisation of materials like scalpel, scissor and glass spreader, which are first dipped in spirit and then just run over the flame allowing the spirit to catch fire and burn off. They are not allowed to become red hot.

Flash pasteurisation: A process of heat treatment of milk at 71°C for 15 seconds, which kills certain pathogenic microbes as well as some spoilage microbes present in it, thereby making it safe to drink as well as increasing its storage life considerably.

Fluid-mosaic model: Model representing cell membrane and many other biological membranes. It consists of a phospholipid bilayer with protein molecules embedded in it. The phospholipid bilayer is always in the state of motion like a 'fluid' and the embedded proteins provide the membrane with a 'mosaic' appearance.

Fluorescence microscope: Microscope used to view fluorescent microbes and microbes stained with fluorescent dyes for specific purposes.

Fluorescent substance: Substance, which after absorbing light of a particular wavelength and energy, emit light of a longer wavelength and lesser energy.

Food vacuoles: Membrane-bound organelles present in the cytoplasm of amoeba containing engulfed food undergoing digestion.

Freeze-drying: Drying under low temperature.

Freeze-etching: An electron microscopic technique, by which ultra-thin sections of an object is obtained by freezing it inside a block and then sectioning it, while still contained inside the block in frozen condition.

Freezing: The process of lowering the temperature of a material below its freezing point.

Frustule: Diatom cell with a wall of usually two equal halves.

Fungicidal chemicals: Chemicals, which kill fungi.

Fungicides: (=Fungicidal chemicals)

Fungistatic chemicals: Chemicals, which inhibit the growth of fungi.

Gas vacuoles: Spindle-shaped gas-filled structures found in the cytoplasm of some bacteria cells.

Gelatinase test: A biochemical test, performed to find out the ability of a species of bacteria to hydrolyse gelatin by producing the enzyme gelatinase.

Gene: Any segment of a DNA, which is responsible for a particular character of the host organism.

Generation time: Time required for a given population of bacteria to double.

Genome: Sum total of all the genes present in a cell.

Germicides: (=Disinfectants).

Germination: Process of conversion of endospores (spores) of spore-forming bacteria to vegetative cells under favourable condition.

Girdle: Overlapping region of the connecting bands of epitheca and hypotheca of diatom frustule, which remain united by some cementing organic substance.

Glycocalyx (*Glyco*: carbohydrates; *calyx*: part of flower below the petals extending outward from the stalk): Polysaccharide-containing material lying outside the bacteria cell in many species as a loose network of polymer fibers extending outward from the cell.

Glycogen granules: Starch–like polymers made of glucose subunits, which act as storage depots of carbon and energy in bacterial cytoplasm.

Golden-brown algae: Algae belonging to the class Crysophyceae, in which the plastids (chromatophores) are brown or orange coloured.

Gram-negative bacteria: Bacteria, which after staining with crystal violet, undergo decolourisation by washing with a decolourising agent (ethanol or acetone).

Gram-negative cell wall: Cell wall of gram-negative bacteria. It is very complex and more fragile than gram-positive cell wall. It is made of a thin layer of peptidoglycan, which constitutes about 10% of the wall. It is surrounded by a protective coating called lipopolysaccharide (LPS) layer, which resists penetration of some potentially toxic chemicals into the bacteria cell.

Gram-positive bacteria: Bacteria, which after staining with crystal violet, resist decolourisation by washing with a decolourising agent (ethanol or acetone).

Gram-positive cell wall: Cell wall of gram-positive bacteria. It is very simple and is made of a thick layer of peptidoglycan, which constitutes about 90% of the wall.

Gram staining: A method of differential staining of bacteria cells to differentiate between gram-positive and gram-negative bacteria.

Green algae: Algae belonging to the class Chlorophyceae, which include photosynthetic eukaryotic algae, whose colour is green due to abundance of the green pigments 'chlorophyll a' and 'chlorophyll b' over other pigments in the plastids called chloroplasts.

Group translocation: A process of transportation of substances across the cell membrane of bacteria, in which the transported substance is chemically altered during passage across the membrane.

Growth curve: The curve obtained by plotting the log of bacteria number versus time.

Growth of bacteria: An increase in the number of bacteria cells.

Growth rate of bacteria: Increase in the number of bacteria cells per unit time.

GvpA (*G*as *v*acuole *p*rotein A): Major gas vacuole protein, which is small and highly hydrophobic. It is the shell protein and makes up 97% of the total protein of the gas vacuoles. GvpA molecules are aligned as parallel 'ribs' forming a watertight surface. They fold as a β-sheet and thus, give considerable rigidity to the overall vacuole structure.

GvpC (*G*as *v*acuole *p*rotein C): Minor gas vacuole protein, which is a large protein. It strengthens the shell of the gas vacuoles by acting as cross-linker, binding several GvpA ribs together like a clamp.

H_2S test: (= Hydrogen sulphide test).

Half aperture angle: The angle subtended by the optical axis (the line joining the centers of all the lenses) and the outermost ray still covered by the objective of a microscope.

Halophiles: (= Halophilic bacteria).

Halophilic bacteria (*Halo*: salt; *philic*: loving): Salt-loving bacteria, which require at least some salt (NaCl) for their growth.

Halophobic bacteria (*Halo*: salt; *phobic*: hating): Salt-hating bacteria, which die at salt concentrations above 1%.

Halotolerant bacteria: Bacteria, which can tolerate and grow at some concentrations of salt, but growth is best in absence of salt.

Halotolerants: (= Halotolerant bacteria).

Hanging drop preparation: A light microscopic technique for observing the motility of bacteria. A very small drop of bacteria suspension is hung from the center of a cover slip into the cavity of a cavity slide. The hanging drop is observed under a compound microscope using oil-immersion objective.

Heat-fixation: Fixing a smear of bacteria on a glass slide to prevent its washing away during staining. This is done by quickly passing the slide containing the smear of bacteria, high above a flame, 2-3 times, with the smear surface facing upward, so that the smear does not get heated up.

HEPA filters: A filter used to deliver clean air into an enclosure such as a cubicle or room, so as to keep it dust-free and sterile.

Heterocysts: Specialised enlarged vegetative cells with thick wall found in some blue green algae, which are the sites of nitrogen fixation.

Heterotrophic organisms: Organisms incapable of preparing food by themselves and depend upon food substances prepared by other organisms.

Holdfast: A structure at the end of the stalk of appendaged bacteria, by which the stalk is attached to the substratum.

Hook: Bent middle part of a bacterial flagellum that connects the basal body to the filament of the flagellum.

Hopanoids: Strengthening agents present in the unit membrane of several bacteria, which are similar to the sterols present in the unit membrane of eukaryotes.

Hormogonia: Short sections of trichome of filamentous algae separated from each other by dead cells called necridium.

House-keeping genes: Genes, which are needed for basic survival of bacteria. It is distributed between the two daughter cells during cell division.

Hydrogen sulphide test: A biochemical test, performed to find out the ability of a species of bacteria to produce hydrogen sulphide by reduction of sulphur compounds.

Hyperthermophiles: (=Hyperthermophilic bacteria).

Hyperthermophilic bacteria (*Hyperthermo*: very high temperature; *philic*: loving): Very-high-temperature-loving bacteria, which have very high optimum temperatures for growth, of 80°C or above.

Hyphae of fungi: Branching filaments, which constitute the thallus of some fungi.

Hyphae of bacteria: Cellular appendages formed by direct cellular extension of the mother bacteria cell containing cell wall, cell membrane, ribosomes and occasionally DNA.

Hypotheca: Younger and inner half of diatom frustule, which, like the bottom half of the petri dish, fits closely inside the older and outer half, epitheca.

Incineration: A process of sterilisation by burning a material to ashes.

Inclusions: Non-living reserve materials, suspended in the cytoplasm, bounded by a thin non-unit membrane consisting of lipids, separating them from the surrounding cytoplasm. Their function is the storage of energy or structural building blocks.

Inclusion staining: A method of differential staining of bacterial cells to stain the cell inclusions like volutin granules, glycogen granules and PBH granules.

Indicators: Chemicals, which change colour with the change in pH.

Indole test: A biochemical test, performed to find out the ability of a species of bacteria to hydrolyse the amino acid tryptophan to indole.

Inhibition: A method, by which the growth of bacteria in a given material is inhibited. As a result, they cannot grow and their number remains almost unchanged.

Integral proteins: Proteins, which are tenaciously held in the phospholipid bilayer structure of cell membrane.

Intercalary growth: Growth of bacteria taking place throughout the surface of each cell.

Intracellular enzymes: Enzymes functioning inside the cells, which are mainly responsible for synthesis of new protoplasmic substances and production of cellular energy from simple substances permeating into the cells through the cell membrane.

Ionising radiations: Electromagnetic radiations, which have energy sufficiently high (more than 10eV) to ionise cell components so that the cells can no longer perform critical functions and consequently, damage the cells.

Isogamous conjugation: A mode of sexual reproduction in algae involving fusion of morphologically and physiologically similar gametes.

Isolation of bacteria: Segregation of different species of bacteria from their mixed population.

β-Lactam antibiotics: Antibiotics, which possess β-lactam ring. All of them are potent inhibitors of cell wall synthesis.

Lag phase: A phase in the growth curve of bacteria between the inoculation and beginning of the normal logarithmic growth.

L-forms: (= protoplast). L stands for Lister Institute in London.

Light microscope: Microscope, in which light waves are used to produce enlarged images of very small objects and in which magnification is obtained by a system of optical lenses.

Light microscopic techniques: Techniques used for observation of microscopic objects under light microscopes.

Limit of resolution of objective: The distance between any two closest points on the microscopic object, which can be resolved into two separate and distinct points on the enlarged image produced by the objective of a microscope.

Lipid A: Lipid component of the lipopolysaccharide molecule present in the cell wall of gram-negative bacteria. When gram-negative pathogenic bacteria is killed inside the host's body, the lipid A is released, which elicits toxic reactions and disease symptoms. That is why, lipid A is also called 'endotoxin' (*endo*: internal). It is made of fatty acids bonded to a disaccharide composed of two NAGA phosphates.

Lipid hydrolysis test: A biochemical test, performed to find out the ability of a species of bacteria to hydrolyse lipids (fats).

Litmus milk test: A biochemical test, performed to find out the abilityof a species of bacteria to transform different milk components into varied end products.

Log phase: A phase in the growth curve of bacteria, during which bacteria grows at the fastest rate in a logarithmic (exponential) manner.

Logarithmic growth: (=Exponential growth).

Lophotrichous flagellation (*Lopho*: tuft; *trichous*: hair): A tuft or cluster of flagella is present at one end of bacteria cell.

LPS layer: Thick lipopolysaccharide layer that surrounds the thin peptidoglycan layer in the cell wall of gram-negative bacteria. It resists penetration of some potentially toxic chemicals into the bacteria cell. The LPS layer consists of a lipoprotein layer and an outer membrane. The outer membrane has LPS molecules embedded in its outer leaf.

LPS molecule: Lipopolysaccharide molecule embedded in the outer leaf of the outer membrane of the LPS layer of the cell wall of gram-negative bacteria. Each LPS molecule is made of a lipid A molecule and a polysaccharide molecule.

Lyophilisation: (=Freeze-drying).

Magnetic bacteria: (=Magnetotactic bacteria).

Magnetosomes: Granules of the iron mineral, magnetite (Fe_3O_4), which impart a permanent magnetic dipole to the cells of some bacteria allowing them to respond to magnetic fields.

Magnetotactic bacteria: Bacteria, which show magnetotaxis.

Magnetotaxis: Tendency of some bacteria to orient and migrate along geomagnetic field.

Maintenance of pure culture: Growing of isolated microbes in the laboratory by repeated transfer to fresh slants at regular intervals for their subsequent identification by various staining, biochemical, serological and molecular techniques as well as for their future use.

Membrane-transporting systems: Specific proteins, present on and in the cell membrane of bacteria, which allow and facilitate transport of specific substances across it by active and passive transport. This enables a bacteria cell to concentrate specific substances inside the cell and remove specific substances from the cell to the outside. Structurally, the membrane transporting systems are proteins made of 12 alpha helices that wind back and forth through the membrane to form a channel, through which the substances to be transported are carried into or out of the cell. These proteins can bind to specific substances to be transported and move them into or out of the cell across the membrane as required.

Mesophiles: (=Mesophilic bacteria).

Mesophilic bacteria (*Meso*: moderate temperature; *philic*: loving): Moderate-temperature-loving bacteria, which have moderate optimum temperatures for growth, of 20-45°C.

Mesosomes: Membranous invaginations of the cell membrane of bacteria cell into the cytoplasm, which increase the surface area for efficient absorption.

Metachromasy: Phenomenon of colour change of the basic dye, toluidine blue to reddish violet, when it combines with the polyphosphate granules (volutin granules) present in few bacteria.

Metachromatic granules: (= Volutin granules).

Methyl red test: A biochemical test, performed to find out the ability of a species of bacteria to utilise glucose with the production of a stable acid as the end product.

MIC: (=Minimum inhibitory concentration).

Microaerophiles: (=Microaerophilic bacteria).

Microaerophilic bacteria: Bacteria, which can grow better in the presence of very little free oxygen.

Microcapsule: A viscous layer surrounding the bacteria cell in many species, which is so thin that it cannot be visualised by light microscopy.

Microlid antibiotics: Antibiotics, which contain large lactone rings connected to sugar moieties.

Micrometer: A micro-scale used in the measurement of the dimensions of microscopic objects under microscope.

Micrometry (*Micro*: microscopic, *metry*: measurement): Measurement of the dimensions of microscopic objects in terms of length, breadth, diameter and thickness.

Microorganisms (*Gk*: *Micros*: small, *organismos*: organism): Living forms, whose size is so small that they are usually not visible to naked human eye.

Microscope: Instrument, which can produce enlarged images of very small objects, making it possible to view them, which, otherwise, cannot be seen distinctly by naked human eye.

Microscopic algae: Eukaryotic, autotrophic microorganisms that fail to show any cellular differentiation into true tissues like root, stem or leaf and in which vascular system is absent.

Microscopic fungi: Eukaryotic, heterotrophic microorganisms that fail to show any cellular differentiation into true tissues like root, stem or leaf and in which vascular system is absent.

Microscopic techniques: Techniques used in processing and observation of minute specimen under microscopes for specific purposes.

Microwave radiation: A type of electromagnetic radiation, whose antimicrobial effect is due, at least, to its thermal (heating) effects.

Mild halophiles (*Halo*: salt; *philic*: loving): Salt-loving bacteria, which require NaCl at low concentrations of 1-6% for their growth.

Minimum inhibitory concentration: Minimum amount of an antimicrobial chemical needed to inhibit the growth of a test microorganism.

Moderate halophiles (*Halo*: salt; *philic*: loving): Salt-loving bacteria, which require NaCl at moderate concentrations of 6-15% for their growth.

Modified atmosphere packaging: A bacteriostatic process used to extend the shelf life of fresh fish, meat, fruits and vegetables during chilled storage by packing them in airtight containers, within which the atmosphere is modified desirably by flushing-in of required gases in required proportion.

Monotrichous flagellation (*Mono*: single; *trichous*: hair): A single flagellum is present at one end of the bacteria cell.

Mordant: A chemical used in staining of bacteria that binds to the primary stain, which has entered into the bacteria cells, so as to form a dye-mordant complex; thus making the escape of the stain from the bacteria cells difficult.

Motility test: (=Hanging drop preparation)

MR test: (=Methyl red test).

Mucopeptide: (=Peptidoglycan).

Murein: (=Peptidoglycan).

Mycelium: Network of the branching filaments of filamentous bacteria or of loosely or compactly interwoven fungal hyphae.

Mycology: Study of fungi.

NAGA: A sugar, N-acetylglucosamine, present in the cell wall of bacteria.

NAMA: A sugar, N-acetylmuramic acid, present in the cell wall of bacteria, to which are attached short side chains of four or five amino acids bonded to each other through peptide bonds.

Narrow-spectrum antibiotics: Antibiotics, which act only on a single group of bacteria.

Necridium: Dead cells in the trichome of filamentous algae.

Negative staining: An electron microscopic technique used to observe minute details of very small objects such as viruses and bacterial flagella. An electron-opaque material like phosphotungstic acid or its salt is allowed to form a coat of thick deposit on the surface of the object, without entering into it. When electrons from the electron gun of the electron microscope cannot pass through these coated surfaces, these structures become clearly visible.

Neutrophiles: (= Neutrophilic bacteria).

Neutrophilic bacteria: Bacteria that have optimum pH for growth between 6.0 and 8.0 (*i.e.* in neutral conditions, which are neither acidic nor alkaline).

Nitrate reduction test: A biochemical test, performed to find out the ability of a species of bacteria to reduce nitrates.

Nodules: Thickened cell wall of diatom frustule at the ends (polar nodules) or at the center (central nodule).

Non-acid-fast bacteria: Bacteria, which are easily stained and are also easily decolourised by acid-alcohol as decolourising agent.

Non-spore-formers: Bacteria, which always remain as metabolically active vegetative cells and die under adverse conditions, as they cannot change to metabolically inactive highly resistant spore to survive severe adverse environmental conditions.

Non-spore-forming bacteria: (=Non-spore-formers)

Nucleoid: A relatively transparent region of chromosomal material present in the cytoplasm of bacteria cells containing the aggregated mass of DNA that makes up the chromosome of bacteria.

Numerical aperture: The light gathering capacity of a lens system (condenser or objective).

O/F Test: (= Oxidation-fermentation test).

Obligate acidophiles: (= Obligate acidophilic bacteria).

Obligate acidophilic bacteria: Bacteria that can grow only at low pH and cannot grow at high pH or even at neutral pH.

Octet: (= Sarcinae)

Ocular micrometer: A circular glass disc with micro-scale etched on it, that fits into the ocular of the microscope and is used in the measurement of the dimensions of microscopic objects under microscope.

ONPG Test: (= Ortho-nitrophenyl galactoside test).

O-polysaccharide: Outer polysaccharide (chain of sugars) attached to the core polysaccharide away from the lipid A molecule in cell wall of gram-negative bacteria.

Optical microscope: (=Light microscope)

Ortho-nitrophenyl galactoside test (ONPG Test): A biochemical test, performed to find out the ability of a lactose-non-fermenting bacteria to hydrolyse ortho-nitrophenyl-β-D-galactoside, by producing the enzyme β-galactosidase.

Osmophiles: (=Osmophilic bacteria).

Osmophilic bacteria: Bacteria, which can grow in high osmotic environments containing high concentration of solutes (salt or sugar).

Oxidase test: A biochemical test, performed to find out the ability of a species of bacteria to oxidise reduced cytochrome C by producing the enzme cytochrome oxidase.

Oxidation-fermentation test: A biochemical test, performed to find out the ability of a species of bacteria to utilise glucose aerobically (oxidatively) or anaerobically (fermentatively).

Palisades: Rod-shaped bacteria (bacillus), in which the bacilli bend at the points of division following the cell division resulting in a palisade arrangement resembling a picket fence and angular patterns that look like Chinese letters.

Parenchyma cells: Simple thin-walled plant cells, which are isodiametric in that, they expand equally in all sides.

Pasteurisation: A process of heat treatment upto 100°C using moist heat, which kills certain types of microbes in a given material, but does not kill all the microbes present in it.

Pellicle: Elastic layer present outside the cell membrane of some unicellular organisms.

Pennales: (=Pennate diatoms).

Pennate diatoms: Diatoms, which are bilaterally symmetrical.

Peptidoglycan (*Peptido*: chain of amino acids; *glycan*: sugar) (=murein or mucopeptide): It is the constituent of cell wall of bacteria, which consists mainly of amino acids and sugars. Two sugars namely N-acetylglucosamine (NAGA) and N-acetylmuramic acid (NAMA) are bonded to each other alternately through glycosidic bonds (β 1-4 linkage) to form long parallel chains. Attached to the NAMA molecules are short side chains of four or five amino acids bonded to each other through peptide bonds, which form cross-linkages between adjacent chains to form a network or layer.

Peptonisation: (= Proteolysis)

Peripheral proteins: Proteins, which are loosely anchored on the surface of the phospholipid bilayer structure of cell membrane.

Periplasm: Fluid or plasma that fills the periplasmic space between the cell wall and the cell membrane of bacteria cell.

Periplasmic space: Thin space between the cell wall and the cell membrane of bacteria cell.

Peritrichous flagellation (*Peri*: around; *trichous*: hair): Flagella are present throughout the surface of the bacteria cell.

Phages: (=bacteriophages).

Phase-contrast microscope: Microscope, in which a microscopic object can be seen in unstained condition, due to the difference in the refractive index of the object and its surrounding medium.

Phenylalanine deaminase test: A biochemical test, performed to find out the ability of a species of bacteria to deaminate the amino acid phenylalanine by producing the enzyme phenylalanine deaminase.

Phycology: Study of algae.

Pili: Thin filamentous hair-like appendages present in few bacteria, which are structurally similar to flagella, but are not involved in motility of bacteria. They are also structurally similar to fimbriae, but are generally longer and only one or a few pili are present on the surface of a bacteria cell.

Placoderm desmids: Desmids in which the cell wall has more than one piece and has pores on it.

Plaques: Clear zones in a confluent lawn of bacteria formed by the lysis of the host bacteria cells by bacteriophages (viruses, which infect bacteria).

Plasma membrane: (=Cell membrane).

Plasmids: Few non-chromosomal DNA found in the cytoplasm of some bacteria, each consisting usually of a small circular piece of double stranded DNA, which can replicate independently of the chromosome.

Plastids: Membrane-bound cytoplasmic organelle found in eukaryotic plant cells, which contain pigments. They are of different types such as, (1) Chloroplasts present in green leaves, which help in photosynthesis, as they contain the green photosynthetic pigments chlorophyll; both chlorophyll a and chlorophyll b, (2) Chromoplast present in coloured flowers and fruits, which impart different shades of colours, as they contain the coloured non-photosynthetic pigments, (3) Leucoplasts present in white parts of plants, which contain no pigment, but help in the storage of synthesised foods such as starch (in amyloplasts), lipids (elaioplasts) or proteins (proteinoplasts) and (4) Chromatophores present in few algae, which help in photosynthesis, as they contain the green photosynthetic pigments, chlorophyll a and other pigments except chlorophyll b.

Plates: (=Agar plates)

Pleomorphic bacteria: Bacteria, which do not have any characteristic shape. They can change their shape.

Polar growth: Growth of a bacteria cell at a single point (pole) as a small outgrowth of the cell.

Poly-β-hydroxyalkanoate (PHA) granules: All classes of carbon/energy storage polymers found in bacterial cytoplasm. The most common PHA granules are the PHB granules. The length of the monomers in the polymer can vary, from as short as C_4 (in PHB granules) to as long as C_{18} (in other PHA granules) in certain bacteria.

Poly-β-hydroxybutyric acid (PHB) granules: Granules present in the cytoplasm of certain bacteria, consisting of poly-β-hydroxybutyric acid (PHB), which is a lipid-like substance. Monomers of β-hydroxybutyric acid are bonded to each other in a chain by ester linkages to form the polymer of poly-β-hydroxybutyric acid. The polymers aggregate into granules.

Pond scum: Extensive masses of the free-floating algae, *Spirogyra* in freshwater ponds.

Pond silk: (=Pond scum)

Porins: Proteins present in the outer membrane of the lipopolysaccharide layer (LPS layer) of gram-negative bacterial cell wall, which make the outer membrane relatively permeable. Each porin contains three identical subunits. Each subunit is cylindrical with a central pore, through which materials can pass.

Pour plate technique: A technique of cultivation of bacteria, in which 1 ml of the bacteria suspension is dropped aseptically in a sterilised empty petri dish and then liquefied nutrient agar medium is poured over it. The petri dish is swirled gently, so as to allow the suspension to mix with the medium uniformly. It is allowed to cool and solidify. Then it is incubated to get isolated colonies of bacteria on the agar plate.

Preservatives: Antimicrobial chemicals used in processing of foods including fish, meat and vegetable products to retard or prevent microbial spoilage.

Prokaryotes: Organisms, in which the chromosome is not confined within a membrane-bound nucleus. They include blue green algae (BGA) and bacteria.

Prokaryotic cells (*Pro*: primitive; *karyotic*: about nucleus)**:** Primitive cells, like the cells of bacteria and blue green algae, in which the chromosome is not confined within a membrane-bound nucleus.

Prosthecae: Cytoplasmic extensions from bacteria cells, which form appendages like hypha, stalk or bud.

Proteolysis: Hydrolysis of milk proteins, primarily casein, to their basic building blocks, namely amino acids by bacterial enzymes.

Protoplast: Cell wall-deficient bacteria cells consisting of only protoplasm enclosed by cell membrane. They are produced by exposure of gram-positive bacteria cells to chemicals like lysozyme, which hydrolyses the cell wall.

Protozoa: Eukaryotic, unicellular microorganisms, which lack cell wall.

Protozoology: Study of protozoa.

Pseudopodia: : Protoplasmic projections in amoeba that function for its locomotion.

Pseudovacuoles: Vacuole-like structures present in the protoplasm of few algae, which are not actually vacuoles, rather they are cylindrical gas vesicles observable in both longitudinal and cross-section.

Psychrophiles: (=Psychrophilic bacteria).

Psychrophilic bacteria (*Psychro*: low temperature; *philic*: loving): Low-temperature-loving bacteria, which have low optimum temperatures for growth, of 0-20°C.

Psychrotolerant bacteria: (= Psychrotrophic bacteria).

Psychrotolerants: (= Psychrotrophic bacteria).

Psychrotrophic bacteria: Bacteria, which can grow at 0-20°C, but have moderate optimum temperatures for growth, of 20-40°C. Unlike psychrophilic bacteria, which are cold-loving, psychrotrophic bacteria are not cold-loving, rather they can tolerate cold.

Psychrotrophs: (= Psychrotrophic bacteria).

Pure cultures: Isolated species of bacteria, grown separately on agar slants.

Pyrenoids: Proteinaceous bodies present in the chloroplasts of green algae, which are associated with the formation of storage products.

Pyrogens: Broken cell wall debris of heat-killed gram-negative pathogenic bacteria, which can induce disease symptoms similar to those produced by the living bacteria itself.

Radiation: Energy transmitted through space in a variety of forms.

Raphe: A longitudinal slot in pennate diatoms extending from one end of the valve to the other along the middle of the axial strip, which helps diatom for their movement.

Real image: Image, which can be captured on a screen.

Red algae: Algae belonging to the class Rhodophyceae, whose characteristic red colour is due to the presence of two red phycobilins pigments, phycoerythrin and phycocyanin.

Rennet curd: Curd formed by growth of certain rennin-producing bacteria in milk. The rennin acts on the milk protein casein to form paracasein, which, in presence of calcium ions, is precipitated as calcium paracaseinate and forms an insoluble clot.

Resolving power of objective: Ability of the objective of a microscope to resolve each point on the minute object into widely spaced points so that the points, in the image can be seen as distinct and separate from one another, so as to get a clear unblurred image.

Rhizoids: Root-like structures in algae and fungi.

Ribosomes: Granular bodies present in the cytoplasm, in which protein synthesis takes place.

Rosettes: A type of arrangement of cells in some bacteria, in which the stalks of several individuals remain attached together.

Sacoderm desmids: Desmids, in which the cell wall is a single piece and has no pore.

Sarcinae: Spherical bacteria (coccus), in which the cocci are arranged in a cuboidal manner, as the cells are formed by regular cell division in three planes.

SASPs: Small acid-soluble spore proteins, which are synthesised during sporulation in spore-forming bacteria.

Scanning and transmission electron microscope: Electron microscope having both transmission and scanning electron microscope functions.

Scanning electron microscope: Electron microscope, in which an electron beam scans the surface of the microscopic object, thereby inducing it to release a shower of electrons to be collected by a detector to generate the image.

SEM: (=Scanning electron microscope).

Serial dilution-agar plating method: A method of enumeration of bacteria in a given sample by diluting it serially using nine volumes of a diluent in each dilution, followed by inoculation by pour plate or spread plate technique and incubation at a suitable temperature.

Shadow-casting: An electron microscopic technique, in which the microscopic object is dried in a special grid placed inside a vacuum jar and an extremely thin layer of metal (*e.g.* platinum) is deposited on it from a highly heated filament at an oblique angle, so that the object produces a shadow on the uncoated side. Examination of the shadowed image provides information as to the shape of the object (topographic features of the surface of the object), which can be observed by scanning electron microscope.

Sheaths: Long hollow tubular structures, which enclose chains of bacteria cells forming 'trichomes'.

Simple microscope: Microscope used to obtain small magnifications, with the help of a single biconvex lens.

Simple staining: A method of staining bacterial cells using only one stain.

Simple transportation: A process of transportation of substances across the cell membrane of bacteria, in which the energy from the proton motive force is used.

S-Layer: A layer found on the surface of most of the pathogenic bacteria, which is composed of two-dimensional array of proteins with crystalline appearance in various symmetries such as hexagonal, tetragonal or trimeric.

Slime: A diffuse mass of polymer fibers surrounding the bacteria cells in many species, which is seemingly unattached to any single cell. The viscous layer is so thick that many cells are embedded in the slime matrix.

Smear: A thin film of bacterial suspension formed on a glass slide by spreading a drop of the bacterial suspension on it and then air-drying it.

Spheroplast: Cells of bacteria, from which the cell wall has been removed incompletely. Therefore, the protoplasts retain pieces of cell wall, due to which the cells take amoeboid shape, protruding out where there is no cell wall.

Spiral bacteria: Rod-shaped bacteria, which have more than one twist in the cell, unlike the vibrios, which have less than one complete turn or twist in the cell.

Spirillum: Spiral bacteria, which have rigid spiral structure. Spirillum with many turns can superficially resemble spirochetes. They do not have outer sheath and endoflagella; but have typical bacterial flagella.

Spirochetes: Spiral bacteria, which are flexible and can twist or contort their shape. They have outer sheath and endoflagella, but lack typical bacterial flagella.

Spore coat: Second covering layer from outside of bacterial endospore, which is made of layers of spore-specific proteins.

Spore cycle: Cyclic process of conversion of vegetative cells of spore-forming bacteria to endospores (spores) under adverse conditions through the process of sporulation (sporogenesis) and back from spores to vegetative cells under favourable conditions through the process of germination.

Spore staining: A method of differential staining of bacteria cells to stain endospore of spore-forming bacteria.

Spore: (=Endospore)

Spore-formers: Bacteria, in which the metabolically active vegetative cells can change to metabolically inactive highly resistant spore to survive severe adverse environmental conditions.

Spore-forming bacteria: (=Spore-formers).

Sporogenesis: (=Sporulation)

Sporulation: Process of conversion of vegetative cells of spore-forming bacteria to endospores (spores) under adverse conditions.

Spread plate technique: A technique of cultivation of bacteria, in which 0.1 ml of the bacteria suspension is dropped aseptically on a prepared sterilised agar plate. Then, the drop of suspension is spread uniformly on the agar plate by a sterilised glass spreader and incubated to get isolated colonies of bacteria on the agar plate.

Square-shaped bacteria: (=Box-shaped bacteria)

Stage micrometer: A special glass slide with micro-scale etched on it, which is clipped to the stage of a compound microscope and is used to calibrate the graduations of the ocular micrometer.

Staining: A method of imparting colour to the otherwise colourless transparent microorganisms with the help of various biological dyes called stains for their microscopic observation.

Stains: Chemicals used for colouring biological or microbiological specimen. Chemically, these are organic compounds containing a benzene ring, a chromophore group and an auxochrome group.

Stalks: Cellular appendages used by certain aquatic bacteria for attachment to solid substratum.

Staphylococcus: Spherical bacteria (coccus) in which the cocci are arranged in a grape-like cluster formed by irregular cell division in three plains.

Starch hydrolysis test: A biochemical test, performed to find out the ability of a species of bacteria to hydrolyse starch.

Stationary phase: A phase in the growth curve of bacteria, during which the number of bacteria cells in the culture of bacteria remains almost constant.

STEM: (=Scanning and transmission electron microscope).

Sterigma: The ultimate branches of conidiophores of filamentous fungi.

Sterilants: Antimicrobial chemicals, which, under appropriate circumstances, can kill all microbial life and can actually be used to sterilise inanimate objects and surfaces.

Sterilisation: A method by which a given material is rendered completely free of microbes either by killing them (bacteriocidal) or removing them from the material (decontamination).

Stigma: (= Eyespot).

Stock cultures: Standard pure cultures of microorganisms maintained in internationally recognised microbiology laboratories whose identification has been established to genus, species, sub-species, type, or sub-type level.

Streak plate technique: A technique of cultivation of bacteria in which the bacteria-containing sample (swab) is touched on the surface of an agar plate and streaked on it aseptically using a flame-sterilised loop for growing the bacteria as isolated colonies on the plate.

Streptobacillus: Rod-shaped bacteria (bacillus), in which the bacilli are arranged in chains, as the cells divide in one plane.

Streptococcus: Spherical bacteria (coccus), in which the cocci are arranged in chains, as the cells divide in one plane.

Striae: Two rows of ridges arranged on both the side of an axial strip on the valve surface of pennate diatoms to produce beautiful ornamentation.

Sulphur granules: Granules of elemental sulphur produced by its accumulation in the bacterial cytoplasm.

Swarmer: A flagellated daughter cell formed from a mother bacteria cell by polar growth.

Symporters: Membrane-transporting systems present in the cell membrane of bacteria, which transport one type of molecule and always transport another type of molecule along with it in the same direction.

TEM: (=Transmission electron microscope).

Tetracyclines: Antibiotics, which contain a naphthacene ring structure.

Tetrads: Spherical bacteria (coccus), in which the cocci are arranged in packets of four cells, as the cells divide in two plains.

Thallus: A plant body, which is not differentiated into true tissues like root, stem or leaf.

Thermophiles: (=Thermophilic bacteria).

Thermophilic bacteria (*Thermo*: high temperature; *philic*: loving): High-temperature-loving bacteria, which have high optimum temperatures for growth, of 45-80°C.

Total magnification: Product of objective magnification and ocular magnification in a microscope.

Total plate count: Total number of bacteria present in unit amount of a given sample as can be enumerated following serial dilution-agar plating method.

TPC: (= Total plate count)

Transmission electron microscope: Electron microscope in which an electron beam is transmitted through an ultra-thin section of the microscopic object and the image is magnified by the electromagnetic fields.

Trichome of algae: A row of cells of filamentous algae without any sheath.

Trichome of bacteria: A row of cells of rod-shaped bacteria (bacillus), in which the bacilli are arranged with larger area of end-to-end contact between the cells.

Triple sugar iron test: A biochemical test, performed to find out the ability of a species of bacteria to utilise any one or more of the three sugars such as glucose, sucrose and lactose as well as its ability to produce hydrogen sulphide (H_2S), which reduces iron.

TSI test: (=Triple sugar iron test).

Tyndalisation: A process of fractional heat sterilisation using moist heat, performed over three days so as to sterilise a material completely.

Ultra-thin sectioning: An electron microscopic technique used to observe minute details of the intracellular fine structures. The cell is embedded in a block of plastic material and cut into ultra thin sections (as thin as 60 nm).

Uniporters: Membrane-transporting systems present in the cell membrane of bacteria, which transport one type of molecule only in one direction across the membrane.

Unit membrane: Protein-embedded phospholipid bilayer structure (fluid-mosaic model) that constitutes the cell membrane and most of the other biological membranes. The phospholipid bilayer consists of two opposite facing layers, each consisting of a layer of phospholipid molecules. Each phospholipid molecule has a head and a pair of tails emerging from it. The head is charged and hydrophilic (water-loving) for which it remains towards the aqueous environment. The tails are uncharged and hydrophobic (water-hating) for which they remain hidden inside the membrane away from the aqueous environment. The protein molecules are either tenaciously held in the bilayer (integral proteins) or loosely anchored on the surface (peripheral proteins).

Urease test: A biochemical test, performed to find out the ability of a species of bacteria to hydrolyse urea by producing the enzyme urease.

Useful magnification: Magnification that makes visible the smallest resolvable particle.

UV radiation: Electromagnetic radiation (UV= ultraviolet) with wavelength between 220 and 300 nm.

Valve: The main surface of the epitheca and hypotheca of diatom frustule.

Vegetative cell: Metabolically active form of bacteria found when the environmental conditions are favourable for their normal metabolic activities. In this form, they take up nutrients, grow and reproduce. On the other hand, when the environmental conditions become severely adverse beyond their tolerance, they die. Some bacteria, survive under such adverse conditions by changing themselves to highly resistant metabolically inactive forms called 'spores'.

Vibrios: Comma-shaped bacteria with less than one complete turn or twist in the cell.

Viricidal chemicals: Chemicals, which kill viruses.

Viricides: (=Viricidal chemicals)

Viristatic chemicals: Chemicals, which do not kill viruses, but inhibit their growth.

Virology: Study of viruses.

Virtual image: Image, which cannot be captured on a screen.

Viruses: Ultra-microscopic, non-cellular living particles, composed solely of a nucleic acid (DNA or RNA) core, surrounded by a protein envelope called capsid.

Voges-Proskauer test: A biochemical test, performed to find out the ability of a species of bacteria to utilise glucose with the production of acetylmethylcarbinol (acetoin) as the neutral end product.

Volutin granules: Granules, composed of polyphosphates, found in the cytoplasm of some bacteria. The basic dye, toluidine blue becomes reddish violet when it combines with the polyphosphate granules.

VP test: (=Voges-Proskauer test).

Water net: Colony of the freshwater algae *Hydrodictyon* found in ponds and pools, which has beautiful net-like appearance.

Wet mount: A light microscopic technique for observing the natural shape, size and arrangement of bacteria cells in living condition. A drop of bacteria suspension is placed on a slide, covered with a cover slip and observed under a compound microscope using oil-immersion objective.

Xerophiles: (=Xerophilic bacteria).

Xerophilic bacteria: Bacteria, which can grow in very dry environments.

Yellow green algae: Algae belonging to the class Xanthophyceae, whose characteristic yellow green colour is due to the presence of chlorophyll a, chlorophyll e, β-carotene and several xanthophylls.

Index